Pediatric Nursing Skills & Procedures

Pediatric Nursing Skills & Procedures

BARBARA L. MANDLECO, RN, PhD

Associate Professor and Undergraduate Coordinator
College of Nursing
Brigham Young University
Provo, Utah

THOMSON

DELMAR LEARNING™   Australia   Canada   Mexico   Singapore   Spain   United Kingdom   United States

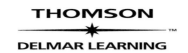

THOMSON
™
DELMAR LEARNING

Pediatric Nursing Skills & Procedures

by Barbara L. Mandleco, RN, PhD

Vice President,
Health Care Business Unit:
William Brottmiller

Editorial Director:
Cathy L. Esperti

Executive Editor:
Matthew Kane

Senior Developmental Editor:
Elisabeth F. Williams

Marketing Director:
Jennifer McAvey

Marketing Channel Manager:
Tamara Caruso

Marketing Coordinator:
Michele Gleason

Production Editor:
John Mickelbank

Library of Congress Cataloging-in-Publication Data

Mandleco, Barbara L.
  Pediatric nursing skills & procedures / Barbara Mandleco.
      p. ; cm.
  Includes bibliographical references and index.
  ISBN 1-4018-2580-X
  1. Pediatric nursing.   I. Title: Pediatric nursing skills and procedures.   II. Title.
  [DNLM: 1. Pediatric Nursing—methods. WY 159 M273p 2005
  RJ245.M29 2005
  618.92'000231—dc22   2004061890

NOTICE TO THE READER

CONTENTS

PREFACE

Caring for children requires special consideration. This statement was the genesis for *Pediatric Nursing Skills & Procedures*, which is an exciting new product designed to prepare nurses to perform both basic and advanced procedures on their younger clients. Understanding that the family is an integral part of a child's world, this book stresses communicating and caring for children within the context of their families.

Each unit or topic area opens with a brief overview discussion that takes into account the special needs of pediatric clients. Important information that may influence the successful completion of a procedure, such as the child's developmental level or body weight, is provided as appropriate. Specific skills include a listing of equipment needed, general guidelines, the step-by-step procedure to execute the skill, documentation notes, and an estimated time needed to complete the procedure. This practical format enhances readability and fosters competence and confidence in completing the skills.

Organization

Pediatric Nursing Skills & Procedures is organized into 18 units, subdivided into topics and procedures. Unit I opens with fundamental information that lays the groundwork for helping children and their families manage health issues and concerns. Communication of the nurse-child-family triad is discussed in detail, as are basic concepts of health care such as informed consent, adherence, and protective precautions.

General pediatric procedures are covered in Unit II. These include guidelines on preparing children for procedures, transporting a child, and restraining a child to ensure safety.

Health assessment is the focus of Unit III. Beginning with obtaining a health history and conducting a physical examination, the nurse is then guided through standard procedures in health assessment such as obtaining growth measurements, measuring vital signs, and performing nutritional, developmental, and other standard assessments.

Specimen collection is covered in detail in Unit IV, with attention to promoting client comfort, avoiding infection, and obtaining accurate results. A similar approach is seen in Unit V, which focuses on diagnostic tests.

Two units (VI and VII) are devoted to procedures relating to medication administration and intravenous access. Thorough discussion is included of the unique needs and developmental considerations of children based on their body size, weight, fluid balance, and potential for serious risks and complications related to medication administration.

Units VIII through XIII take a body systems approach to the care of the child who is ill. Procedures such as oxygen administration, suctioning, catheter care, cast care, and applying a dressing are covered in detail.

Unit XIV addresses the child who is having surgery, including pain management and preoperative and postoperative care.

Emergency care is the focus of Unit XV, starting with fever management and moving through respiratory and cardiac emergencies. This content is followed by a Unit XVI on community and camp procedures.

The final two Units focus on health promotion topics such as hygiene, bathing, umbilical cord care, and circumcision care for the newborn.

Features

The EQUIPMENT list informs the reader of the standard tools or equipment necessary to perform a given procedure.

Many units and sections include GENERAL GUIDELINES which apply across several procedures and are designed to ensure safe, competent care.

STEP-BY-STEP PROCEDURES walk the nurse through the sequential activities involved in performing each skill.

The DOCUMENTATION section provides a summary of essential information to record about a procedure and a specific client.

ESTIMATED TIME TO COMPLETE PROCEDURE supplies an appraisal to the nurse regarding the approximate amount of time it should take to conduct the procedure from beginning to end.

ILLUSTRATIONS and PHOTOGRAPHS offer visual reinforcement of the detailed procedures.

RATIONALE for procedures helps nurses understand why certain procedures are necessary. Rationales are italicized.

CONTRIBUTORS

Debra Ann Mills, RN, MS
Associate Teaching Professor
College of Nursing
Brigham Young University
Provo, Utah

Nicki L. Potts, RN, PhD
Former Associate Professor
School of Nursing, Austin Community College
Austin, Texas
Former Assistant Professor
School of Nursing, University of Texas at Austin
Austin, Texas

Mary Tiedeman, RN, PhD
Associate Professor
College of Nursing
Brigham Young University
Provo, Utah

REVIEWERS

Principles and Concepts
of Pediatric Care

Nurse, Child, and Family Communication
Informed Consent
Adherence
Protective Precautions

Nurse, Child, and Family Communication

OVERVIEW

Effective communication requires sensitivity to the child and family's needs and a well-developed and carefully thought-out plan. In fact, the nurse's ability to establish a therapeutic relationship with children and their caregivers is strongly tied to communication abilities and must be a high priority for all nurses as they interact with clients and families. Nurses always need to be aware of family and client needs for education and use communication interactions as an entrée into providing new or reinforcing old information. Increasing knowledge and providing information regarding a child's illness, symptoms, care needed, or developmental level can empower families and ultimately increase well-being.

Elements of Communication

Before communication can be effective, several key elements must be addressed, including establishing rapport, building trust, showing respect, conveying empathy, listening actively, providing appropriate feedback, and establishing professional boundaries.

Rapport and Trust

Nurses must develop trust and rapport with clients, and clients must be willing to talk, listen, and provide honest answers. Nurses may also need to be available and open to questions parents and children may have. To build rapport with a child and caregivers, the nurse must be accepted by the child and family and be willing to discus nonhealth-related issues to convey warmth and friendliness. To establish trust, a nurse must follow through on promises, keep appointments, respect client confidentiality, and carefully explain procedures in a way that is acceptable for the family.

Respect

To establish respect, the nurse should address the child by name (use formal name unless given permission to use a nickname) and the caregivers by Mr., Ms, or Mrs. Before addressing a caregiver by first name, it is imperative that the caregiver's approval is given. Respect is also conveyed by considering the family's feelings, cultural views, and values. Nurses need to convey that they have time to spend with the child and family. This will allow the family to share their thoughts and concerns, as they will not be worried or hesitant to ask questions. If nurses communicate that they do not have time by standing near the doorway, frequently looking at the clock while talking, or confiding to the child and family how busy they are, parents and children will soon learn that the nurse is too busy or doesn't really care. These messages interfere with establishing trust and respect and should be avoided. Interference also occurs when a child is in isolation and nurses are required to wear gloves and masks. Indeed, children in these situations may feel isolated since they are not visited frequently and verbal communication is muffled or difficult to understand. Therefore, the nurse should make a concerted effort to speak more clearly without appearing to yell. Smiling is also important; although the child cannot see it through the nurse's mouth, the child will see it in the nurse's eyes.

Empathy

Empathy forms the basis of a helping relationship and is an important element in communication. Empathetic nurses are able to appreciate and understand children and parents as unique individuals, and this allows them to feel cared about and accepted. For this to happen, the nurse's empathy needs to be combined with verbal and nonverbal behavior. Empathy, however, is not to be confused with sympathy. The empathetic nurse maintains a sense of objectivity and is supportive, understanding, and able to plan and implement helpful behaviors by teaching and giving examples that facilitate the child and parent's ability to function in difficult and sad situations. The sympathetic nurse who offers condolence and pity may not be able to establish a therapeutic relationship with families. Such behaviors may also hinder the family's ability to function in difficult situations. The nurse empathizer is able to establish an accurate understanding of the child and parents from their perspective, build rapport, and relate with parents and children in such a way as to allow them to express feelings and concerns.

Listening

Listening consists of providing verbal and nonverbal clues that communicate interest and is an activity requiring attention and effort as one not only listens to the words of the child and parents but also to how words are used and whether what is said is what is meant. Accurate listening does not happen without effort. It takes actively attending to what is verbalized, observed, and created by the entire communication context. It is important not to allow one's mind to wander, daydream, or prejudge what is being said or think about what will be said as a response; to listen attentively; and wait for others to finish what they are saying. Attentive listening goes beyond hearing and includes what is not said or what is conveyed through gestures as well. Active listening also includes maintaining eye contact, assuming an open and relaxed posture, and facing the child/family; see Box I-1 for some helpful tips.

BOX I-1:   Four Bs of Effective Listening

Be attentive; eliminate distractions.
Be clear about the message; clarify if necessary.
Be empathetic; convey concern and caring.
Be open-minded; avoid prejudices.

When working with children and parents, the nurse should encourage and allow each to give input, discuss concerns, express feelings, and acknowledge problems. Respecting other's feelings and views and appreciating other's understandings and fears even though they are different than one's own are also important. While listening to children, nurses need to consider their developmental level, cognition, and emotional behavior. Children who are social and verbal may seem to be more in control and better able to understand and think more logically and rationally than children who engage in shy, clinging, and dependent behaviors. Nurses should use developmentally appropriate language and behavior with children and listen to behavioral cues for concerns and fears. For example, a child may keep talking and asking questions to avoid beginning a treatment.

Providing Feedback

Providing feedback can include a nod of the head, reflecting back to the client what was said, asking questions to clarify, seeking validation from the client to ensure one is talking about the same thing, and focusing on a single idea and exploring it further. Focusing means to direct the conversation based on a statement made by the client. For instance,

during a conversation with a child regarding her broken leg, the child mentions that another child on the playground has been pushing her around. The nurse may want to direct the conversation to delve more deeply into the potential problem of interacting again with that child from the playground, fear that the child-client may be experiencing due to the playground incident, and interactions the child-client may have had in the past with the other child.

Professional Boundaries

The nurse should create and maintain professional boundaries in relationships. Therapeutic relationships should be caring and empathetic but should avoid emotional involvement and overprotectiveness. It is always helpful to explain to children and families the care provided, time frame when care will be provided, and how both parents and children can assist in the care if needed. Identifying needs and establishing expectations will enhance and facilitate interactions. The nurse should never interfere with the parent-child relationship. Rather, the nurse can best serve the child by assisting parents in caring for and nurturing the child and by recognizing the parent's need to feel accepted by the professional and be an important contributor to their child's well-being. Finally, nurses should avoid personal behaviors that signal overinvolvement such as socializing with the child or their family, sharing personal information such as home addresses or telephone numbers, and giving or accepting gifts. See Box I-2 for more information about how to avoid becoming overinvolved.

BOX I-2:   Avoiding Overinvolvement

Do not have contact with children and families after discharge.
Do not purchase gifts for children/families.
Do not share personal information with children and families.

Additional Skills Useful in Communicating with the Family

Several additional skills have been found especially useful when communicating with children and their families. These include observing; using silence; being aware of the environment; using humor, play, writing, or drawing; using third parties; and storytelling.

Observing

Observational skills enable the nurse to validate and interpret what children and parents do not say. Nonverbal behavior provides meaningful information about what the child and parent are communicating to each other and to the nurse. How words are delivered is as important as the words used. Consistency between the meaning of the verbalizations and all other behaviors validates messages. Observing the eyes (position, movement, gaze, and expression), mouth, furrowing of the brow and nasolabial area, general emotional mood, bodily movements, and posture is important. Cues also need to be interpreted from within the child's cultural perspective to avoid erroneous interpretations. For example, in some cultures, eye contact and directness are signs of paying attention. However, in other cultures, looking someone directly in the eye is considered rude. The nurse should also observe the ways parents and children respond to each other's request for attention and how they behave and interact in disciplinary and nurturing situations. These observations can help assess the effectiveness of child-parent communication patterns and develop health-related strategies respectful of their relationship.

Silence

Silence may be another method used to communicate. Silence should be interpreted in relation to the environment where communication occurs and the normal behavior of those interacting. A child who is shy and hesitant with strangers may be silent when the nurse approaches for care. A parent who is silent after being told of a child's terminal diagnosis is likely to be experiencing shock and disbelief and trying to come to grips with the reality of what was just heard. Children may be silent out of separation anxiety and fear, as with the four-year-old who is hospitalized and must spend time in a strange environment without parents nearby. Silence also may demonstrate comfort, respect, and concern, such as when a nurse sits with parents after upsetting news is heard or when the child is falling asleep after an upsetting procedure.

Environment

The environment can also affect communication events between the nurse and the child or parents even more than the spoken words. The way we exist in the environment and use space to make people more or less comfortable as they seek care is important. Nurses who are effective in nurse-client communication have developed and demonstrate a respect for a client's sense of physical and personal space. For example, when sensitive issues or feelings of anxiety need to be discussed and the environment is in a four-bed unit where roommates can overhear the conversation, sharing fears and anxieties and asking questions may be difficult. A quiet, private environment should be provided before discussion begins. Nursing behaviors such as knocking before entering a child's room, calling the child and parents by name, addressing each directly, and asking permission to examine demonstrate respect and engender a sense of ownership of

physical and personal space. Clients in caregiving settings such as hospitals and clinics will experience less stress, irritability, and fatigue when they remain in relative control of their physical and personal space. Therapeutic communication environments reduce psychological distress experiences so that children can attend to their health care situation. When children are relaxed or not experiencing fear, they are able to cope with people and their environment and are more willing to converse. However, children may vary in communication based on personality, temperament, experiences, and developmental levels. The nurse should use her concern, care, and knowledge of child development and remain flexible in using various communication approaches with the same child during different interactions and with different children in similar interactions.

Humor

Humor is healing and can bridge communicative gaps even when the direct communication is feared and/or offensive, and it is an effective method of helping children and adolescents cope with illness, pain, and hospitalization. For example, a person who is able to laugh at himself may be forgiven, and a person who can make someone laugh is not all bad or scary. The nurse should use tasteful humor in dealing with pediatric clients and their families and promoting therapeutic interactions.

Play

Play, a natural childhood behavior, should be encouraged in health care environments and employed as a method of communicating. The nurse can engage the child by using puppets, dolls, or stuffed animals; drawing pictures with crayons and paints; or using a storytelling approach to give information. Because play is familiar and a daily form of natural behavior, children do not associate it with stress, anxiety, or fear. Play helps the child to relax and shed inhibitions, however temporary, brought about by health care environments.

Writing and Drawing

Writing is an especially effective method of communicating with older school-age children and adolescents, and writing can include keeping a journal or diary or writing a letter that is not delivered. Other examples include encouraging the child or adolescent to write down thoughts or feelings that are not easy to express verbally, keeping track in written form of experiences related to a health care situation, or writing a story or essay about an experience. Sometimes just being able to articulate thoughts and feelings in writing can serve as a springboard for later discussions or concerns.

Drawing can be helpful for younger children since it provides clues to a child's emotional state and feelings. Evaluating the drawings or having a child tell a story about the drawing allows a window into their inner self. One needs to be cautious, however, since evaluating drawings needs to occur in conjunction with other information such as observation of behavior and direct communication with the child. Examination of drawings needs to include the gender of the figures, order in which the figures are drawn and position in relation to other figures in the drawing, exclusion of certain individuals, accentuation or absence of particular body parts, placement and size of the drawing on the page, whether the drawing is made with bold or light strokes, and the colors used.

Third-Party Communication

The nurse can also promote dialogue with children by using indirect methods such as a third party. Here, the nurse directs her attention to the child through a trusted friend (stuffed toy). By doing this, the nurse is taking an interest in the child's normal activity, employing a stress-reducing communication method to create a therapeutic environment, and assisting the child to focus on the content of the message rather than anxieties and fears.

Another third-party approach used with older children and adolescents is to attribute feelings or thoughts to other children. This method can be a safe form of interaction that uses thoughts and feeling of the group rather than of the child/adolescent directly. Using group feelings helps a child/adolescent feel comfortable talking to an adult because someone else is talking, as the adult is told what the third-party person thinks without the child being responsible for the statement.

Storytelling

Storytelling is another effective communication strategy nurses may use to promote therapeutic environments with children. Storytelling techniques can be used to establish rapport, assess and help resolve children's anxieties and fears, explain treatments and procedures, teach health, and prepare for painful or emotional events. The nurse can devise or use stories so that the child can participate in either of the two storytelling roles: teller or listener. For example, a child can be read or told a story about the boy who had surgery or asked to tell a story about a boy who has had surgery. The former might be used to explain what will happen when going to surgery. The latter is a way of eliciting information about the child's experience where the nurse devises a story and takes turns with the child in filling in the content. Called mutual storytelling, the nurse might say, "I'll start the story, and when I nod, you fill in the next part of the story." The nurse begins with "Once upon a time a boy broke his leg and had to have surgery. He—." The nurse nods to the child to finish the sentence. The nurse then uses the child's response to connect with another statement, followed by nodding to the child again for a response. The nurse then analyzes the themes presented by the child that may reveal important feelings. See

Boxes I-3 and I-4 for principles of communicating with children and parents.

BOX I-3:   Principles of Effective Communication in Pediatric Settings

1. Talk to parents initially if child is shy or appears hesitant.
2. Use objects (toys, dolls, stuffed animals) instead of questioning child directly.
3. Provide opportunities for older children and adolescents to talk privately with care provider.
4. Use clear, specific, simple phrases in confident, quiet, unhurried speech.
5. Position self so communication is at eye level.
6. Allow expression of thoughts and feelings.
7. Provide honest answers.
8. Offer choices only if they exist.
9. Use a variety of age-appropriate methods and techniques.

BOX I-4:   Communicating with Parents

1. Explain equipment and procedures thoroughly.
2. Answer parents' questions and concerns honestly.
3. Teach parents what to expect their child to feel and look like during treatment.
4. Help parents understand the bigger picture—that is, the long range as well as the short-range effect of treatment.
5. Teach and allow the parents to carry out as many aspects of their child's care as feasible.
6. Make reassurance a part of family interactions; ask parents how they are doing as time passes.

Developmental Factors Affecting Communication

Effective communication will enhance preparation of a child and family for their experiences related to health and illness. However, the nurse must incorporate knowledge of human growth and development when communicating with children. Children should be encouraged to become active contributors to their health as soon as they are developmentally able to understand and carry out health-promoting behaviors. Until then, the nurse works directly with parents and reinforces their self-confidence in caring for and teaching their child. See Table I-1 for communication principles based on developmental level.

Table I-1 Communication principles based on developmental level

Developmental Level	Communication Principles
Infants	Allow time to warm up to strangers. Respond to cries in a timely manner. Use motherese* and a soothing and calm voice. Talk to infant directly.
Toddlers	Approach carefully; child may be fearful. Integrate toddler's words for familiar objects/activities into care. Prepare for procedures right before they are to be carried out. Integrate dolls, storytelling, and picture books into conversations.
Preschoolers	Allow choices as appropriate. Use play, storytelling, puppets, and third parties. Speak honestly, use simple language, and be concise. Prepare for procedures one to three hours before they are to be experienced.
School-age children	Use books, diagrams, and videos in preparing for procedures. Prepare for procedures several days in advance. Allow for honest expression of feelings and adequate time for questions to be answered.
Adolescents	Prepare up to one week prior to experiences. Respect need for privacy. Use appropriate medical terminology. Used creative methods to explain experiences and procedures.

*Motherese is child-directed speech that adults use when talking to young children. It uses simple, short sentences spoken slowly in a high-pitched voice. There is also repetition and exaggerated emphasis on key words, which are usually words for activities and objects.

Infants

Infancy is a time when communication is achieved through nonverbal means. Even though the adult may use language to relate to an infant, the tone, pitch, speed, touch, and bodily movements accompanying the words generate meaning to the infant more so than the words used. However, loud, sudden noises may cause startle reactions and crying, while soft, songlike tones delivered in an upbeat tempo may soothe and comfort. Gentle rubbing or patting while securely holding an infant is also a method of communicating pleasure and security. Infant responses include vocal cues such as crying, cooing, and whining and body language such as stiffness or relaxation, arm or leg movement, pushing away with hands and feet against the adult, opening or closing the mouth, and gripping or pushing objects (e.g., rattles and blankets). Infant expressions of comfort and discomfort become more direct and overtly explicit with age. That is, a two-week-old infant will cry and flail arms and legs when hungry, while a six-month-old infant may kick the legs and arm-wave or suck on toys, fingers, or blankets when hungry.

Toddlers

The toddler continues to experience the world through hearing, seeing, smelling, tasting, and touching and remains dependent on parents. Independence emerges and satisfaction is derived from repetition and routines while exploring the environment. Language in the form of two-word combinations emerges, as does the ability to participate in turn-taking rules of social communication (e.g., an answer follows a question, and someone listens when someone speaks). Gestures and simple language are used to convey wants and needs. One-word sentences that are part babble with "bye-bye" may be used to express whole ideas, aided by accompanying gestures that provide clues to the meaning. "Bye-bye" with hat in hand may mean "I want to go out and play," while "bye-bye" after being kissed by Dad prior to walking out the door may mean "I want to go bye-bye with Dad." Two-word utterances become common at about two years of age. The two-word sentence consists of a noun and verb, such as "me do." By the age of three years, complete sentences are constructed using all parts of speech, and the child's vocabulary has progressed to approximately 900–1,000 words. Toddlers also engage in monologues as a way of practicing speech, and as they mature egocentric thought and monologue speech become more socialized. Increasingly they engage in more conversation with others.

Nurses interacting with toddlers need to be observant of situations surrounding one-word utterances and gestures. Learning the words toddlers use for common items or behaviors and using them in conversation is recommended. For instance, instead of saying it is "time for bed," a child may respond to an expression that for the particular child means bedtime, such as "It is time to hear the night, night angel sing." This statement that indicates bedtime or naptime and the child's ritual of falling asleep while a music box plays are comforting, familiar ways of interacting that bring safe experiences to the child's mind. Using play or books to demonstrate or describe activities or procedures immediately before they are to occur is a good way to prepare toddlers for experiences. Refraining from wordy explanations and preparing for procedures well in advance are not toddler-friendly. Being aware of the child's response and approaching the child calmly and positively are important.

Preschoolers

During the preschool years, articulation becomes clearer; there are improvements in correct grammatical usage, and an expansion of word combinations occurs. The vocabulary rapidly expands, and the child is able to use words appropriately even when the meaning is not fully appreciated. Since the preschooler is striving for independence but still needing adult encouragement and support, it is important to allow the child to initiate activities and make choices if possible. For example, let the child decide whether to have water or a mouthful of Jell-O after medicine. Nurses may need to remind children how to cooperate in an activity or wait for their turn. Asking the child's cooperation by giving something to do or hold may engage the child cooperatively and provide the attention sought for and required. Using picture books, stuffed toys, and puppets to prepare a child for a procedure will allow the child to experience the procedure in a nonthreatening way. A child may also answer the nurse's question if it is asked through a teddy bear rather than directly.

Preschoolers are egocentric, and magical thinking predominates; they see things only from their perspective. When they lack information or do not understand something, they fill in the gaps with their imagination. Since an avid imagination can be far worse than any reality, it is better to communicate with honesty in simple sentences and concrete language. The nurse should never smile or laugh when giving an injection, say something won't hurt when it will, or use words with double or literal meanings such as "a shot" or "a stick in the arm." It is also not helpful to tell the child about others or what "good boys or girls" do. Allowing preschoolers to touch and manipulate equipment they will see and experience is essential. Telling preschoolers how it will feel when they come in contact with the equipment (cold, warm, pressure, tickles, etc.) and how they can behave is also important. For example, tell them it is okay to squeeze the teddy bear, cry, or bang on the bed with their hand.

School-Age Children

A school-age child's relational experiences expand to people and environments outside the family and home. They are taught rhymes, chants, and rituals by other children, which can serve as a means of emotional-social control in frightening and confusing contexts. We all remember examples such as "cross your heart and hope to die," "star light, star bright, first star I see tonight," and "knock on wood" that we used to minimize the bad that could befall us. Humor and riddles—e.g., "Knock, knock, who's there?"—are tension releasers and assist a child with social identity. During the early school years, interaction with other children increases and close friendships are developed. Children of this age group may be verbally aggressive, bossy, opinionated, and argumentative.

School-age children learn to accept responsibility for their actions; rules are understood, and children become oriented to rules and sanctions. They are interested in learning and have increased attention spans. They learn to master classification, serialization, and spatial, temporal, and numerical concepts. Concrete thinking emerges and predominates. They learn to focus on more than one aspect of an experience and to explore and consider many alternatives to a problem. They are increasingly able to understand their body and their environment and to use language as a means of control and as a method used by others to control them. School-age children also have expanding vocabularies that enable them to describe feelings, thoughts, and concepts. They are able to carry on conversations with others and to appreciate their viewpoints. However, words with multiple meanings and words describing things they have not experienced are still not thoroughly understood.

When working with the school-age child, the nurse should spend time with the child to explain treatments and procedures well in advance of the scheduled time. Photographs, books, drawings, and videos may be used to aid understanding and assist in answering questions. Immediate and subsequent opportunities should be allowed for questions, and repetition of explanations and enhanced details of what will happen to them should be provided. Fears and concerns about body integrity should be assessed and truthfully answered. Conversation that encourages critical thinking should be promoted.

Adolescents

Adolescents are able to think logically and abstractly and are able to verbalize and comprehend most adult concepts. They are able to create hypothetical situations and generate explanations for and about situations they encounter. Privacy and independence are sought in activities and relationships. The adolescent makes personal discoveries about relationships and events and will discuss them with peers and trusted adults in an effort to construct ideals.

Adolescents' preoccupation with what "should or could be" produces conflict in relationships with people who are unwilling to listen to them express their thoughts. They need to verbalize what the world "should be like" in order to analyze their own ideas and come to their position short of the ideal. The ideal world they construct must be merged with the real world by listening to themselves and others.

Attentiveness and acceptance are necessary. Parents and adults need to be patient and actively listen to matters the adolescent considers significant, even though trivial to adults. The adolescent should be allowed the freedom to work through issues and provided the guidance necessary to develop and decide on a positive course of action. Since adolescents may be moody and argumentative, interactions between adolescents and parents or adults are more cooperative when the adolescent participates in working toward a solution and is permitted to participate in the selection of the final decision(s) and subsequent course of action.

The nurse should communicate support during interactions with adolescents by actively listening without demonstrating surprise or disapproval and without trivializing. Avoid questioning, giving personal advice, or taking sides. It may be necessary to initiate multiple interactions before an adolescent feels safe and secure enough to ask questions or discuss concerns. Short, nonthreatening contacts may serve as icebreakers to more involved conversations.

Cultural Impact on Communication

The nurse's relationship with children and their families should be caring, supportive, and respectful and, just as important, congruent with their acceptable cultural perspective. This is important so that the nurse's intentions and behavior are not perceived as culturally insensitive. This requires the nurse to know and understand how personal cultural values and beliefs affect behavior in providing nursing care and to learn about and be nonjudgmental of the cultural values and beliefs of those cared for. Nurses also need to know how to respond to gestures or questions, how to listen to concerns, how and when to be sensitive to child/family reactions, when to use an interpreter, and how to consider illness and health-related beliefs when delivering care. Refer to Table I-2 for information related to specific cultures and their communication patterns, Box I-5 for information about using

Table I-2   Communication patterns of various cultures

Chinese	Self-expression repressed Silence valued Hesitant to ask questions Nonverbal and contextual cues important May smile even if does not understand Touching limited
Japanese	Listens empathetically Stoic Values politeness, personal restraint, self-control Attitudes, actions, feelings more important than words Direct eye contact considered a lack of respect Touching limited
Vietnamese	Disrespectful to question authority figures Value harmony and modesty of speech and action Avoid direct eye contact Relaxed concept of time
	Respectful of titles and family and generational relationships
Filipino	Value personal dignity, nonverbal communication, preserving self-esteem Avoid direct eye contact and expressions of disagreement, especially with authority figures, and discussions of personal topics Small talk important before serious discussions
African Americans	Cautious, distrustful of majority group Value direct eye contact Use nonverbal expressions Sensitive to incongruence between verbal and nonverbal messages Tend to "test" majority before submitting to their suggestions and care
Hispanic Americans (Mexican)	Use direct eye contact Use gestures and voice tone changes in speech Unassertive if others appear busy or rushed May smile and nod even if do not understand Perceive touch as reassuring, comforting, sympathetic Frequently bilingual Small talk important before serious discussions
Puerto Ricans	Appreciate open-ended questions, nondirective approach Important for father to be present when speaking with a male child Discussions of personal topics easier if nurse is same gender as client
Cubans	Value personal and family privacy; questions regarding family considered presumptuous and disrespectful Relaxed concept of time May not use standard English Many bilingual Most new immigrants bilingual Small talk important before serious discussions
Native Americans	Value nonverbal communication Silence essential to understanding and respecting another Direct eye contact considered insulting Reticent in forming opinions of health care providers Pauses are common after being questioned; signify thoughtful consideration Hesitant to discuss personal affairs unless trust has developed; prefer these discussions occur with person of same gender

continues

Table I-2   (*continued*)

	Sensitive about having behaviors and words written down
	Believe it is ethically wrong to speak for another
Middle Eastern	Use silence to show respect
	Men and women do not touch each other unless they are immediate family or married
	Touching or embracing common among same gender
European Americans	Hugs/embraces tolerated among intimates and close friends
	Understanding or agreement noted by nods
	Use neutral facial expressions in public
	Separate into gender-specific groups at social events, unless activity is for couples
	Prefer personal space
	Speak warmly and pleasantly, and smile to put others at ease
	Firm handshake symbolizes goodwill; pat on shoulder/back denotes camraderie

Adapted from Estes (2002).

BOX I-5   Surmounting Language Barriers between Health Care Providers and Children/Families.

A. With an interpreter

1. Determine language(s) and dialect (if relevant) a client is familiar with and speaks at home; the language may not be identical to the one commonly used in the country of origin. Some clients may be multilingual, and a language other than their mother tongue can be used.
2. Avoid using interpreters from groups (countries, regions, religions, tribes) where there may be past or present conflicts.
3. Be sensitive to and make allowances for differences with regard to age, culture, gender, and socioeconomic status between client and interpreter.
4. Request as verbatim a translation as possible.
5. Be aware that an interpreter not related to the client may request compensation.
6. Maintain a list of potential interpreters.
7. Contact institutions (hospitals, universities, etc.), organizations, and translation services, including telephone companies, that may be able to provide interpreters, emergency translations, and other relevant information.

B. Without an interpreter

1. Always be polite, formal, patient, and attentive to the client's (or client's family's) attempts to communicate.

2. When greeting the client, smile, use the client's complete or last name, indicate your name by saying it while gesturing to oneself, and offer a handshake or nod.
3. Speak in a low and moderate tone.
4. If possible, use words from the client's language.
5. Use simple words—no idioms, jargon (medical or otherwise), or slang. Avoid the use of contractions and pronouns, which may be less clear to the client.
6. Give instructions clearly, in simple language (with a minimum of words), and in the correct order.
7. Talk about one topic at a time.
8. Use hand gestures freely, and act out actions while talking.
9. Check the client's understanding by requesting a description/illustration of the procedure; have the client pantomime the meaning or repeat the instructions.
10. Try using Latin phrases or phrases from other languages that have become universal.
11. Write simple sentences in English or another language, since some people understand the written but not spoken languages, and some accents may be confusing.
12. See if a family member or friend can act as an interpreter for the client. If not, and if the health provider cannot find one, enlist the family in networking to find one.
13. Use phrase books and flash cards.

Adapted from Munoz (2005).

BOX I-6:   When Parents Speak English as a Second Language

Enunciate clearly and speak slowly.
Avoid situations preventing the listener from seeing lip movements, facial expressions, and gestures.
Speak in the active voice.
Avoid using contractions, slang, and idioms.
Speak in a normal volume.

---

an interpreter, and Box I-6 for how to communicate with parents for whom English is a second language.

The care that is planned and implemented with a child and/or parent should be congruent with their values and consistent with their meaning for health care. During contact, the nurse needs to incorporate questions and make observations to elicit information about the family's practices that impact care. These include questions about their communication and decision-making strategies, child rearing, and health and illness practices. Once this information is obtained, it can be used to determine priorities and develop an individualized treatment plan that is culturally consistent with t values and beliefs and more likely engenders the ment and compliance. Refer to Box I-7 for que· ing pertinent information about health care beliefs.

For family members who would normally depend on their extended family for support and find themselves without them in their present environment, extra time or assistance may be necessary in making critical health care decisions. Appropriate nursing intervention includes anticipating the arrival of members who must travel to reach a child and family or providing a quiet place for the family to telephone distant extended family members.

?OX I-7:   Questions Eliciting Pertinent Information .bout Health Care Practices/Beliefs

Who do you discuss your child's health/illness problems with?

Who assists you in making decisions about your child's health/illness problems?

Who assists you or your family when you need help related to health care?

Informed Consent

OVERVIEW

Informed consent is the duty of a health care provider to discuss the risks and benefits of a treatment or procedure with a client prior to giving care. While pediatric clients are entitled to informed consent, it is usually the role of the child's parent or legal guardian to give the informed consent. After receiving informed consent, the child's parent or guardian has the right to accept or refuse any health care. If a hospital or health care provider treats a child without receiving proper informed consent from a parent or guardian, the provider may be charged with assault and held liable for any damages.

A child should be asked to give assent prior to receiving a treatment or procedure. Assent means that the pediatric client has been informed about what will happen during the treatment or procedure and is willing to permit a health care provider to perform it.

The elements of informed consent as well as the nurse's role in informed consent and pediatric considerations follow:

Elements of Informed Consent

1. **Disclosure:** Information presented to the person responsible for making the decision.
   a. Present all relevant information. This includes (i) the nature of the ailment and the child's current medical status; (ii) treatment alternatives and the risks and benefits of each; (iii) probability of success, including a statement that no outcome can be guaranteed; and (iv) professional opinion as to best alternative.
   b. Present information in simple, easy-to-understand terms.
   c. Answer all questions and concerns honestly.

2. **Comprehension:** Person responsible for making decision understands information presented. Barriers to understanding include (a) language, (b) culture, (c) terminology, and (d) anxiety and fear.

3. **Competence:** Capacity to understand and the legal right to consent. The law varies from state to state; know the law where you practice. Some general guidelines:
   a. Person giving consent must be over the age of majority (generally 18 years of age) unless an emancipated minor.
   b. Some states allow adolescents to give consent regarding some treatments, e.g., birth control and substance abuse treatment.
   c. When caregivers are divorced, health care provider must determine which has right to give consent.

4. **Voluntary:** Consent must be given freely, without coercion, manipulation, or duress. *Threatening a caregiver/guardian in a manner that creates a fear of battery is an assault.*

Nurse's Role in Informed Consent

1. Informed consent for medical or surgical treatment is the responsibility of the physician.
2. General consent for care is obtained at admission. Specific consent is needed for the following:
   a. Major surgery.
   b. Minor surgery, e.g., cut-down, I&D.
   c. Invasive diagnostic procedures, e.g., lumbar puncture, bone marrow aspiration.
   d. Treatments that involve high risk, e.g., chemotherapy, radiation, dialysis.
   e. Any procedure considered research.
   f. Photographs of clients/families.

3. Nurse's role as witness to informed consent includes:
   a. Witnessing the exchange between the physician and caregiver/guardian.
   b. Establishing that caregiver/guardian understands, i.e., is really informed.
   c. Witnessing caregiver/guardian signature.

NOTE: *If only the signature is witnessed and not the disclosure, the nurse should state "witnessed signature only."*

4. If the nurse has any reservations about the four elements of consent, the physician should be notified before the procedure is performed.
5. If the caregiver/guardian refuses to sign the consent, notify the physician so consequences of refusal can be discussed.
   a. Obtain a signed release indicating the refusal to consent and releasing the agency from responsibility for the outcome of this act.
   b. Notify child protective agencies to obtain court approval to perform the procedure, if refusal to give consent is life-threatening.

Pediatric Considerations

1. Although the caregivers/guardians make the final decision, children have the right to be consulted and their feelings and wishes (as developmentally appropriate) should influence all aspects of their treatment. *Enhances cooperation and participation.*
2. In situations where the caregiver/guardian is not present:
   a. The person in charge of the child (e.g., teacher, babysitter) may give consent for emergency treatment, if that person has signed, written permission from the caregiver/guardian to authorize care in his or her absence.
   b. If caregiver/guardian can be contacted by phone, verbal consent can be obtained with two witnesses listening simultaneously.
   c. In life-threatening situation, lifesaving treatment may be given without first obtaining consent.

⏳ **Estimated time to obtain informed consent:** *5–10 minutes.*

Adherence

OVERVIEW

Adherence is the extent to which a person's behavior (following a diet, making lifestyle changes, taking medications, using monitoring devices) corresponds with the suggested health or medical regimen. Other terms that have a similar meaning are compliance, cooperation, therapeutic alliance, and engagement.

Factors enhancing adherence are related to aspects of the care delivery system, individual and family aspects, or the actual treatment regimen. They are described as follows:

1. Care delivery system: includes how positive the interactions are with health care providers, how individualized the care is, how convenient the care setting is for the child/family, how satisfied the child/family is with the care, how long the waiting time is for the appointment, and whether there is continuity from one visit to the next.
2. Individual aspects: includes the degree of autonomy, the belief system, and the amount of self-esteem the child has as well as how well the child understands and remembers to carry out the treatment regimen and, finally, perceptions of the provider-client relationship.
3. Family aspects: includes how successful the family believes the treatment will be, how supportive the family is to the child, and how effective family communication is.
4. Treatment regimen: includes how easy or hard it is to learn the treatment, how bearable the side effects are, how disruptive the treatment is to the child/family's life, the cost of the treatment, how long the treatment will last, and how apparent the benefits of the treatment are.

Adherence can be assessed by a variety of methods:

1. Self-report of the child/family on their ability to carry out the treatment.
2. Observation by the nurse or health care provider of the child/family carrying out the treatment.
3. Examining attendance at scheduled appointments to determine if the child actually was seen by the nurse or health care provider.
4. Clinical judgment of the nurse or health care provider based on the child's condition and family reports.
5. Determining the therapeutic response to discover if the child's condition changed while receiving the prescribed treatment.
6. Counting the number of pills left in the original container and then comparing that number with the number that should be left in the container if the child received the prescribed medications.
7. Chemical assay of plasma drug levels to determine the amount of a medication recently ingested; often used

when children are prescribed anticonvulsants, antibiotics, or a cardiac glycocide.

Nursing strategies for enhancing adherence are primarily concerned with educating parents and children about the reasons and benefits for following the prescribed treatment plan as well as helping the family solve any problems or situations that seem to interfere with adherence. Answering questions, supporting families, and providing rewards and praise for adherence have also proved helpful.

Protective Precautions

OVERVIEW

In order to protect health care workers from pathogenic microorganisms, the CDC (Centers for Disease Control and Prevention) and the HICPAC (Hospital Infection Control Practices Advisory Committee) developed two levels of precautions. The first level, Standard Precautions, should be used whenever caring for any client. The second level, Transmission-based Precautions, is used in conjunction with the Standard Precautions whenever caring for a client who has a documented or suspected infection caused by a pathogen that is highly transmissible or epidemiologically important.

In 1996, the CDC revised the Guidelines for Isolation Precautions in Hospitals by combining the major features of Universal Precautions and Body Substance Isolation into a single set of Standard Precautions. The Standard Precautions are designed to reduce the risk of transmitting organisms from recognized and unrecognized sources of infection, and apply to blood, all body fluids, secretions, excretions, nonintact skin, mucous membranes, and contaminated items whether or not they contain visible blood or other body substances. The following guidelines should be followed:

1. Before and after any client contact, wear gloves. Wash hands during client contact if needed.
2. Wear gloves whenever there is a possibility of contacting blood, body fluids, excretions, mucous membranes, nonintact skin, or secretions. Gloves should be changed each time they are contaminated, and hands should be washed every time gloves are changed.
3. If there is a chance that body fluids will splash on the health care provider, additional protective equipment (gown, mask, goggles) may be needed.
4. Protective equipment should be worn to clean up any body fluid spill, and any waste should be discarded in proper body substance waste containers. The spill area should be cleaned with bleach or appropriate cleaner, and any contaminated laundry should be placed in appropriate bags.
5. Lancets, needles, and scapels should be discarded in labeled sharps containers without recapping.
6. Clients who may have airborne or droplet infections should be assigned private rooms.

The three types of transmission-based precautions, implemented until a diagnosis is confirmed, include airborne precautions, contact precautions, and droplet precautions:

1. Airborne precautions. Used for diseases (e.g., measles, chickenpox, TB) spread via the air. Health care providers need to wear special air filter respirators when in contact with the client. The clients need to wear surgical masks whenever out of the room. If the client has TB, the client's room should have a negative airflow ventilation system. All client rooms need to be labeled with a sign asking all visitors to check with the nurses' station before entering.
2. Contact precautions. Used for diseases that are spread either via direct contact with the skin or by indirect contact with a contaminated object; these include GI illness (E. coli, Hepatitis A), genital infections (chlamydia, gonorrhea, herpes simplex, syphilis), or skin infections (impetigo) or infestation (scabies). Gloves should be worn whenever caring for the client, and gowns need to be worn if the health care professional's clothing might come in contact with the client or contaminated surfaces in the room.
3. Droplet precautions. Used for diseases spread by droplet; these include Haemophilus influenzae type b, mumps, pertussis, pneumonia, and rubella. Masks should be worn by health care providers when within three feet of the client. Clients should wear a mask if out of the room. The room door does not need to be closed.

UNIT II

General Procedures

Preparing Children for Procedures

OVERVIEW

Preparing children for procedures facilitates cooperation, decreases anxiety, enhances mastery of experiencing a potentially stressful event, and supports or helps children develop new coping skills. Most strategies used in preparing children/families for painful procedures are done informally and individually. Although general principles and specific guidelines based on the child's developmental level are listed below, the nurse also needs to consider the child's previous experiences with the procedure, temperament and current methods of coping with stressful events, and attention span and interest level.

Physical preparation of the procedural site rarely involves more that just cleansing the area with an appropriate agent. Occasionally, however, a local anesthetic agent (EMLA cream, Numby Stuff, lidocaine) is used when an injection is necessary (e.g., bone marrow aspirate).

Support during the procedure is important and often is a factor in obtaining the child's cooperation. Most procedures are carried out in a treatment room instead of the child's hospital room, and if possible the nurse responsible for preparing the child should also be the nurse responsible for supporting the child during the actual procedure. Involving the child in some aspect of the procedure (opening bandages, removing old dressings) provides him/her with some sense of control and encourages cooperation. Distraction or diversion (telling a story, counting to ten, squeezing someone's finger) is also useful. Finally, children need to be allowed to express their feelings (crying, being angry or afraid) about the procedure/treatment, as long as the expression does not harm themselves or others.

Support after the procedure is also important, as the child often needs reassurance that he/she handled the experience as well as could be expected and still is accepted and loved. Encouraging constructive expression of feelings about the experience and praising the child for doing the best he/she could during the procedure, are critical.

General Principles

1. Confirm the details of the procedure to be carried out.
2. Involve parents/guardians in teaching if appropriate and if parents are comfortable with involvement.
3. If parents/guardians are involved in the procedure, explain how they can help (comfort child, stand so child can see parent/guardian).
4. Preparation should be age or developmentally appropriate. Consider all aspects of development—cognitive, psychosocial, and physical.
5. Preparation is best done by the staff member who has been working with the child and family.
6. The younger the child, the less time there should be between the preparation and the procedure.
7. The nature of the procedure influences timing, e.g., preparation for surgery should occur further in advance than preparation for a blood draw.
8. Stress the benefits of undergoing the procedure.
9. Prepare children for procedures using sensory information, i.e., tell them what they will see, hear, feel, taste, and smell.
10. Explain any words that are not familiar to the child/family.
11. Use concrete terms (developmentally appropriate) and visual aids (such as drawings or dolls) to describe procedure.
12. Allow children, especially toddlers and preschoolers, to handle equipment. Seeing and doing are more effective ways to learn. For example, the child may want to handle the stethoscope and listen to his or her own heart or that of a caregiver, nurse, or doll.
13. Provide information in sequential fashion, i.e., tell children what to expect in the order it will occur.
14. Use minimally threatening or soft language, e.g., "You may feel sore" rather than "This part will hurt." Or "make a small opening" rather than "cut."
15. Stress that no other body part will be involved other than the one undergoing the procedure.
16. Avoid potentially ambiguous words. Some examples:
    a. "Stool collection" *(why do they want to collect little chairs?);* use child's familiar term.
    b. "The doctor will give you some dye" *(to make me die?);* use "medicine that will help the doctor see your _____ more clearly."

16. Be truthful.
17. Allow choices when possible.
18. Tell children how they can help. State directions positively, e.g., "Hold your arm still" rather than "Don't move your arm."
19. Review the parents' and child's current level of understanding, and allow time for child/parent questions to be answered/discussed.

Preparation for Procedures: Infant

1. Most preparation is directed to the primary caregivers, including how they can participate and support their infant. *Reduces anxiety, which can be conveyed to the infant. Helps caregivers provide effective support to their infant.*
2. When possible, encourage caregivers to be present during procedures. Be sensitive to their needs and allow them to make the choice. *Some caregivers are uncomfortable being present for procedures, especially potentially painful procedures.*
3. Provide comfort after procedure is completed, e.g., hold, cuddle. *Pleasurable sensory stimuli provide comfort and help trust development.*
4. Allow infant to have favorite toy, blanket, etc. *Promotes a sense of security.*
5. Use sensory soothing measures during procedure (pacifier, gentle stroking). *Promotes comfort.*

Preparation for Procedures: Toddler

1. Prepare nonverbal toddler just before the procedure. The verbal toddler can be prepared in advance of the procedure. *Facilitates cooperation.*
2. Use pictures and/or a doll to demonstrate what will be done. *This is less threatening than pointing directly to the area on the child's body.*
3. Keep explanations simple and focused on what the child will experience. *Toddlers are egocentric and need to know what they will experience; cognitive abilities are not mature enough for scientific explanations and rationale.*
4. Tell child that it is acceptable to yell, cry, or express discomfort. *Gives child permission to express feelings.*
5. Give child one direction at a time. *Simple, directed instructions are more easily understood.*
6. If caregivers understand the procedure, have them explain it to the child. *Even if toddlers do not understand explanation, it will help them to know that significant adults do.*
7. When possible, encourage primary caregivers to be present during the procedure. Be sensitive to caregivers' needs, and allow them to make the choice. *Some*

caregivers may be uncomfortable being present for procedures, especially potentially painful procedures. Caregiver anxiety may be conveyed to the child and interfere with the caregiver's ability to be supportive.
8. Provide comfort after a procedure, e.g., holding. *Pleasurable sensory stimuli provide comfort and help maintain trust.*
9. Allow favorite toy, blanket, and so forth. *Promotes a sense of security.*

Preparation for Procedures: Preschooler

1. Prepare in advance and use simple terms. *Facilitates cooperation.*
2. Use body outline, doll, or other visual aid. *This is less threatening.*
3. Use play and the child's imagination. Allow child to manipulate dolls, doll-size equipment, or actual equipment if appropriate. *Preschoolers have an active imagination; provides a sense of control.*
4. Be explicit about what body parts will not be involved and what will be done to the body parts that are involved. *Preschoolers have anxiety related to castration and mutilation.*
5. If caregivers understand the procedure, have them explain it to the child. *Even if children do not understand the explanation, it will help them to know that significant adults do.*
6. When possible, encourage primary caregivers to be present during the procedure. Be sensitive to their needs, and allow them to make the choice. *Some caregivers are uncomfortable being present during procedures, especially potentially painful procedures.*
7. Reassure child that the procedure is not punishment. *Preschoolers may think cause of illness is magical or a consequence of breaking a rule, thus they may see procedures as punishment.*

Preparation for Procedures: School-age Child

1. Prepare for procedures in advance. Use developmentally appropriate concrete terms, and allow time for questions and answers. *Children are in Piaget's concrete operations stage and can understand information presented ahead of time.*
2. Use body outlines especially for explanation of anatomy and physiology and for visualization of postprocedure appearance. *Helps child to know what to expect.*
3. Use of a doll may be appropriate for some younger school-age children; allow child time to manipulate prop or equipment. *Reduces fear and enhances understanding of procedure.*

4. Use medical and scientific terminology. Teach scientific terminology for body parts and medical procedures after learning the child's word for them. *School-age children are curious and want explanations regarding how things work and why.*

5. Suggest ways for child to manage feelings (counting, deep breathing). *Gives child some resources for controlling reactions.*

6. Be straightforward about body parts involved. *Allays unnecessary fears.*

7. Allow child to choose if caregivers will be present during the procedure, if possible. *School-age children are developing increased independence from caregivers and may be very modest.*

Preparation for Procedures: Adolescent

1. Prepare for procedures in advance as with adults. *Adolescents are in Piaget's formal operations stage.*

2. Teach adolescent separately from the caregivers. *Adolescents are striving for increased independence and should be recognized as individuals capable of understanding and participating in their own care.*

3. Encourage questions. *Fosters sense of involvement in treatment plan.*

4. Use body outlines and diagrams to give scientific explanation. *Formal operations allow for more scientific explanations.*

5. Provide rationale for procedures. *Formal operations allow adolescents to understand reason for procedures.*

6. Provide privacy. *Respects adolescent's independence.*

7. Suggest ways for adolescent to manage feelings (deep breathing, relaxation techniques). *Gives resources for controlling reactions.*

Estimated time to prepare a child for a procedure: *10–15 minutes, depending on the procedure and age of child.*

PROCEDURE 1

TRANSPORTING A CHILD

OVERVIEW

It is not uncommon for hospitalized infants, children, and adolescents to be transported either within the pediatric unit or outside the pediatric unit to another department of the hospital (x-ray, cardiac catheter lab). Usually, it is appropriate to carry infants and toddlers or small children if the distance is not very far. However, for longer distances, the child/adolescent needs to be transported safely and appropriately. When determining the best method of transporting a child, the destination and the child's condition and developmental level need to be considered. For example, a stroller, wagon, or wheelchair might be appropriate for a trip to the playroom, whereas a crib or gurney may be more appropriate for transporting a child to surgery. Whenever transporting a child, he/she should always be visible to the adult responsible for the transport. In addition, whenever using a wheelchair or gurney, the child should always be belted in for safety. If a child is transported via a crib or hospital bed, the side rails should always be in the "up" and "locked" position.

EQUIPMENT

Appropriate transporting vehicle (wheelchair, wagon, gurney, stroller, crib, hospital bed)
Blankets (if needed)
Wheeled poles (if child has an IV)

GENERAL GUIDELINES

1. Check physician's order and agency policy regarding use of transport vehicles. *For legal purposes, is important to follow agency policy and procedures.*
2. Gather equipment. *Promotes organization and efficiency.*
3. Explain purpose of transport to child and parents. *Promotes cooperation and reduces anxiety and fear.*

PROCEDURE

1. Steps 1–3 of General Guidelines.
2. Assist child to gurney, wagon, wheel chair or stroller (if appropriate), place child on gurney if crib/bed is not being used (Figure II-1). *So the child does not fall or is*

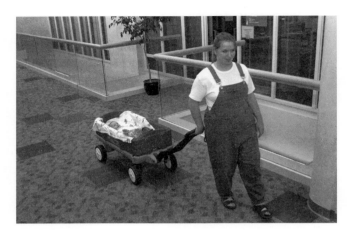

FIGURE II-1   Transporting infant.

   not injured while being moved to gurney, wagon, wheel chair or stroller.
3. Cover child with blanket (if needed). *So the child does not get cold.*
4. Secure safety belt if wheelchair, stroller, or gurney is used, raise side rails if gurney is used. If wagon is used, attach sides of wagon. If crib or bed is used, be sure side rails are raised. *So child does not fall during transport.*
5. Move IV to wheeled pole (if appropriate) and unplug any IV monitoring equipment from the wall electrical socket. *So is easier to manage transporting IV; battery will sustain IV monitoring equipment while it is unplugged.*
6. Ask for assistance to move IV on wheeled pole (if appropriate). *Is difficult for one person to manage a wheeled pole and a gurney when transporting a child to a procedure.*
7. Encourage parents to accompany child on transport if appropriate. *So child will have parental support available if needed.*

DOCUMENTATION

1. Time and reason for transport.
2. Method of transport.
3. How well child tolerated the transport.

⧗ **Estimated time to complete procedure:** *less than 5 minutes.*

Restraints

OVERVIEW

The Joint Commission on Accreditation of Healthcare Organizations (JCAHO) has established standards regarding the use of restraints. Restraints must be ordered by a physician, with the type of restraint identified and how often the child can be removed from the restraint noted. In addition, staff need to be trained and competent in the use of restraints so they are safe. The JCAHO guidelines go on to state that any client in restraint needs to be assessed and assisted as needed, and restraints need to be discontinued as soon as they are no longer needed.

There are two kinds of restraints: human and mechanical. Human restraint involves using a trained person to hold the child in a particular position for a procedure (lumbar puncture, insertion of intravenous catheter, otoscopic examination) rather than using a mechanical device. It is important when using human restraint that the person holding and positioning the child understands what body part is to be held and how to hold that particular body part firmly and safely. Two positions most commonly used in human restraint are sitting and supine.

Sitting Position: General

1. Position the child on the adult's (parent, nurse, assistant) lap with the child's legs firmly held between the adult's legs and the child's arms around the adult's waist. *Prevents child from moving during procedure.*
2. Ask the adult to use his/her arms to hold the child firmly against the adult's chest by wrapping his/her arms around the child's upper body. *The hugging position will hold the child firmly yet comfortably while the procedure is being completed.*

Sitting Position: Otoscopic Examination

1. Position the child on the adult's (parent, nurse, assistant) lap with the child's legs firmly held between the adult's legs and the child's arms around the adult's waist. *Prevents child from moving during procedure.*
2. Ask the adult to hold the child's head firmly against the adult's chest with one arm as the other arm holds the child's arms and upper chest. *Holding the child's head against the adult's chest prevents the child's head from turning while undergoing the otoscopic examination.*

Supine Position: General

1. Position the child on his/her back (supine) on the bed or stretcher. *So child is positioned correctly for the procedure.*
2. Ask the adult to extend the child's extremity that will be used for the procedure as he/she restrains the child by leaning over the child. *This position will hold the child firmly yet comfortably while the procedure is being completed.*

Supine Position: Otoscopic Examination

1. Position the child on his/her back (supine) on the bed or stretcher. *So the child is positioned correctly for the procedure.*
2. Ask the adult to restrain the child's arms and body by leaning over the child as he/she helps stabilize the child's head. *Stabilizing the child's head against the bed or stretcher prevents the child's head from turning while undergoing the otoscopic examination.*

Mechanical restraint is often used temporarily to reduce a child's head or extremity movement so that the health care provider is able to complete a procedure (insertion of intravenous line, painful dressing change) or to immobilize an extremity after surgery or a treatment. Frequently used mechanical restraints include the papoose board, the mummy restraint, the elbow restraint, the wrist and ankle (clove hitch) restraint, and the jacket restraint.

General Guidelines

1. Check physician's order and agency policy regarding use of restraints. *For legal purposes, it is important to follow agency policy and procedures.*
2. Gather equipment. *Promotes organization and efficiency.*
3. Wash hands. *Reduces transmission of microorganisms.*
4. Explain purpose of restraints to child and parents. Reassure child that restraint is not a punishment. *Promotes cooperation and reduces anxiety and fear.*

PROCEDURE 2

APPLYING A PAPOOSE BOARD

EQUIPMENT

A papoose board (a board and cloth wrapping with Velcro fasteners) of appropriate size (infant-toddler, larger children) for child.

PROCEDURE

1. Steps 1–4 of General Guidelines.
2. Place blanket, sheet, or towel on board. *So child is not placed directly on the hard board.*
3. Lie child supine on board, with child's head at top of board. *So child is positioned correctly on board.*
4. Position fabric wrappings around child and secure Velcro fasteners; be sure child is not able to move knees, elbows, and hips. *Securely wrapped fasteners will prevent child from loosening wrappings.*

5. Remain with child while he/she is on the papoose board until the procedure is complete. *So child is positioned correctly and fear is reduced.*

DOCUMENTATION

1. Type and location of restraint.
2. Time and reason for application.
3. Condition of the skin under the restraint, distal circulation, and removal of restraints for range of motion and skin care as appropriate.
4. Assessment of need for continued use.
5. When device removed.

⧗ **Estimated time to complete procedure:** *2–5 minutes.*

PROCEDURE 3

APPLYING A MUMMY RESTRAINT

EQUIPMENT

Blanket or sheet large enough to fit the child (2–3 times larger than child).

PROCEDURE

1. Steps 1–4 of General Guidelines.
2. Place blanket on secure surface.
3. Fold down one corner of the blanket until the tip reaches the middle of blanket/sheet (Figure II-2A).
4. Place the child in a diagonal position with his or her neck at the folded edge of the blanket.
5. Bring one side of the blanket over the child's arm and trunk and tuck it under the other arm and around the back (Figure II-2B). *So arm does not move.*
6. Repeat for the other arm (Figure II-2C). *So arm does not move.*
7. Excess blanket may be tucked under the child or brought up over the abdomen with the sides tucked under his or her back (Figure II-2D).
8. Remain with the child in a mummy restraint until the procedure is complete. *So child is positioned correctly and feels secure.*

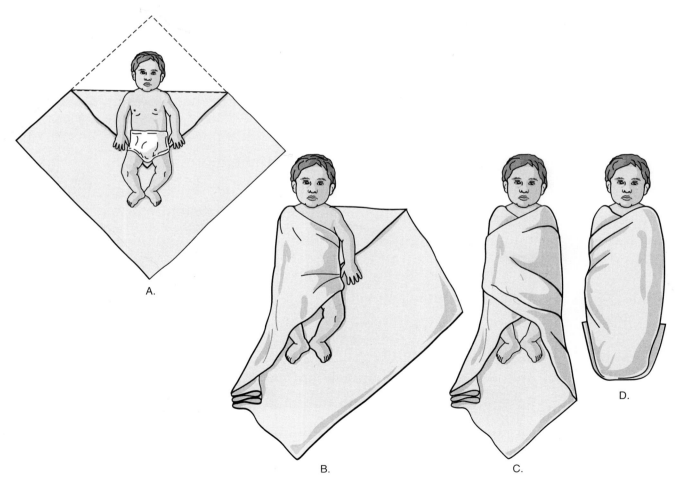

FIGURE II-2 Mummy restraint. A. Fold corner of blanket, placing infant with folded edge at shoulder/neck. B. Place infant's right arm in a comfortable position, then fold blanket over arm, then across abdomen, tucking edge snugly behind the back. C. Repeat procedure for left arm. D. Bring excess blanket over abdomen and tuck sides under back.

DOCUMENTATION

1. Type and location of restraint.
2. Time and reason for application.
3. Condition of the skin under the restraint, distal circulation, and removal of restraints for range of motion and skin care as appropriate.
4. Need for continued use.
5. When device was removed.

⊠ **Estimated time to complete procedure:** *less than 5 minutes.*

PROCEDURE 4

APPLYING A MODIFIED MUMMY RESTRAINT

EQUIPMENT

Blanket or sheet large enough to fit the child (2–3 times larger than child).

PROCEDURE

1. Steps 1–4 of General Guidelines.
2. Place blanket on secure surface.
3. Fold blanket in half. Place the child with his or her neck at the folded edge of the blanket.
4. Position arm comfortably at side, fold blanket over one arm, and tuck it snugly under the child's back (Figure II-3A). *To immobilize arm.*
5. Repeat for other arm (Figure II-3B). *To immobilize arm.*
6. Bring excess blanket over abdomen, leave chest exposed, and secure sides of blanket behind child's back (Figure II-3C).

7. Remain with the child in a mummy restraint until the procedure is complete. *So child is positioned correctly and feels secure.*

DOCUMENTATION

1. Type and location of restraint.
2. Time and reason for application.
3. Condition of the skin under the restraint, distal circulation, and removal of restraints for range of motion and skin care as appropriate.
4. Need for continued use.
5. When device was removed.

⌛ **Estimated time to complete procedure:** *less than 5 minutes.*

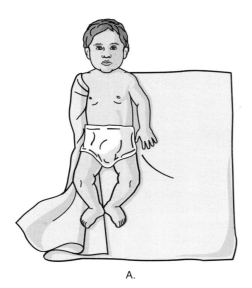 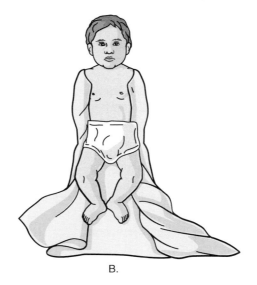 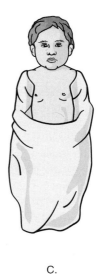

A. B. C.

FIGURE II-3 Modified mummy restraint. A. Position arm comfortably at side, fold blanket over one arm, and tuck snugly under the child's back. B. Repeat for other arm. C. Bring excess blanket over abdomen, leave chest exposed, and secure sides of blanket behind child's back.

PROCEDURE 5

APPLYING AN ELBOW RESTRAINT

EQUIPMENT

Elbow restraint
Soft padding (as needed)
Tongue blades (for certain types of restraints)

PROCEDURE

1. Steps 1–4 of General Guidelines.
2. If appropriate, insert tongue blades. Be sure tongue blades are covered by padded material. *Prevents tongue blades from irritating the skin.*
3. Pad child's arm with shirtsleeve or other soft material. *Prevents the restraint from chafing the skin.*
4. Place restraints over each elbow. Wrap snugly but not too tightly. *Ensures restraints stay in place while allowing for adequate neurovascular function (Figure II-4).*
5. Be sure the restraints do not rub the child's axilla or wrist. *Prevents restraints from chafing the skin.*
6. Secure restraints using safety pins, ties, or tape. (Exact method depends on type used.) *So restraints don't come off.*
7. For small infants and children, tie or pin restraints to shirt. *Prevents restraints from sliding down arm.*
8. Care of child while in restraints.
   a. Assess position of restraints, circulation, sensation, and skin condition every hour. *Ensures effectiveness of restraints and minimizes occurrence of potential problems.*
   b. Release restraints every 2 hours. *Allows range of motion (ROM).*
   c. Encourage diversional activity. *Diverts attention from restraints, encourages normal childhood activity, and fosters growth and development.*
   d. Encourage caregivers/hospital personnel to hold child. *Promotes feeling of security.*
9. Discontinue the use of restraints as soon as the child's condition allows. *Not needed unless specifically indicated.*

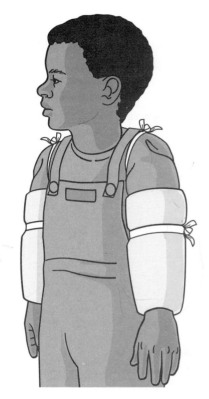

FIGURE II-4   Soft elbow restraints should not restrict circulation.

DOCUMENTATION

1. Type and location of restraint.
2. Time and reason for application.
3. Condition of the skin under the restraint, distal circulation, and removal of restraints for range of motion and skin care as appropriate.
4. Need for continued use.
5. When device was removed.

Estimated time to complete procedure: *less than 5 minutes.*

PROCEDURE 6

APPLYING A WRIST AND ANKLE RESTRAINT

EQUIPMENT

Soft padding (as needed)
Cloth restraints (several types available)
or
Kerlix gauze
or
Two 3 x 3 gauze sponges unfolded to form 6-inch rectangle
1-inch tape
4 large safety pins
Cloth diaper

PROCEDURE

1. Steps 1–4 of General Guidelines.
2. Apply restraint.
   a. Cloth restraint.
      1. Place padding around child's ankle or wrist. *Prevents restraint from chafing skin.*
      2. Wrap restraint around wrist/ankle, pulling tie through loop in the restraint. *Secures restraint and prevents it from overtightening at the wrist/ankle.*
      3. Slip two fingers under restraint to check for tightness. *Too loose a restraint can be slipped off; too tight a restraint may impair neurovascular status.*
   b. Clove-hitch restraint.
      1. Pad wrist or ankle with gauze or cloth. *Prevents restraint from chafing skin.*
      2. Using a 2–3-foot strip of gauze, make a figure 8 (Figures II-5A and II-5B).
      3. Bring loops together.
      4. Put wrist or ankle through loops and secure (Figures II-5C and II-5D).
      5. Tighten knot by pulling ends alternately and firmly. Slip little finger between wrist/ankle and knot to check for tightness. *Too loose a restraint can be slipped off; too tight a restraint may impair neurovascular status.*

NOTE: *A clove-hitch knot will not tighten when pulled.*

      6. Fasten restraints to bed frame (not side rail) or pin to diaper, allowing for some movement of extremity. *Prevents accidental injury due to moving side rails. Decreases child's ability to untie restraints* (Figure II-6).
   c. Gauze restraint.
      1. Fold gauze or softnet into an approximate 1/2- to 3/4-inch band and wrap it around the infant's wrist so that both ends are even in length when they meet.
      2. Tape the bands together at the infant's wrist snugly so the infant's hand does not slide out, but not so tight that you cannot insert your little finger under the band. *Ensures restraint stays in place. Allows for adequate circulation in the extremity.*
      3. Pin a cloth diaper on the infant over his or her disposable diaper. *So restraint can be pinned to diaper.*

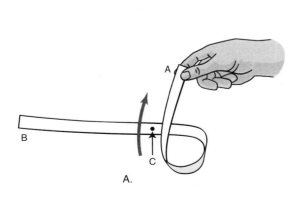

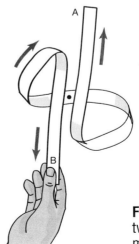

FIGURE II-5 A and B. Using a two- to three-foot strip of gauze, make a figure 8. (continues)

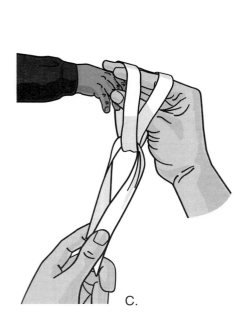

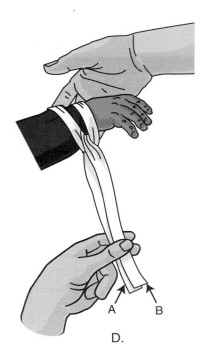

FIGURE II-5 (continued) C. Bring loops together and place clove hitch over child's hand. D. Knot is tightened by pulling ends (A and B) firmly and alternately. Knot should be loose enough to prevent impaired circulation.

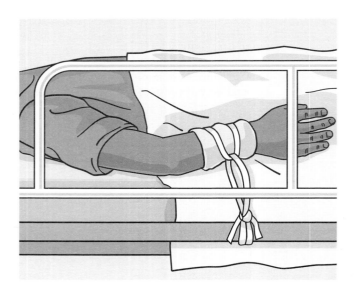

FIGURE II-6 Method for securing a soft wrist restraint to the bed frame.

4. Bring the infant's wrist(s) down and pin both ends of the band to the diaper or fasten restraints to bed frame. *Immobilize child's arms.*

DOCUMENTATION

1. Type and location of restraint.
2. Time and reason for application.
3. Condition of the skin under the restraint, distal circulation, and removal of restraints for range of motion and skin care as appropriate.
4. Need for continued use.
5. When device was removed.

Estimated time to complete procedure: *less than 5 minutes.*

PROCEDURE 7

APPLYING A JACKET RESTRAINT

EQUIPMENT

Jacket restraint

PROCEDURE

1. Steps 1–4 of General Guidelines.
2. Be sure restraint is appropriate size.
3. Place restraint over child's hospital gown or clothing with opening at front or back according to manufacturer's instructions. *Prevents restraint from rubbing child's skin, provides for privacy/modesty; improper application may lead to serious injury including suffocation.*
4. Pull tie on end of jacket flap across body and place in through the slit on the opposite side. Repeat for the other tie (Figure II-7).
5. Secure ties.
   a. In bed, secure ties to bed frame. *Allows restraint to move freely with bed if head of bed raised or lowered.*

NOTE: *Do not tie to head of bed. Prevents compression of brachial plexus in axilla.*

   b. In chair, cross ties behind seat of chair and secure to lower legs.
   c. In wheelchair, secure in a manner that ties will not get caught in wheels.

NOTE: *Use a half-bow knot to secure ties. Does not tighten or slip when attached end pulled, but unties easily when loose end pulled.*

DOCUMENTATION

1. Type and location of restraint.
2. Time and reason for application.

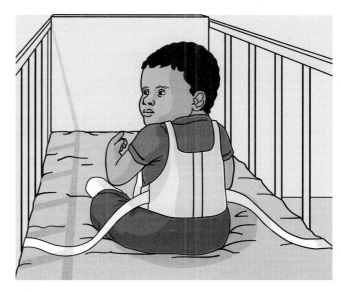

FIGURE II-7   The jacket restraint is secured in the back to prevent child from removing it. Long ties are tied to each side of bed frame.

3. Condition of the skin under the restraint, distal circulation, and removal of restraints for range of motion and skin care as appropriate.
4. Need for continued use.
5. When device was removed.

Estimated time to complete procedure: *5 minutes.*

UNIT III

Health Assessment

Health Assessment

OVERVIEW

The pediatric health assessment includes not only obtaining a health history but also completing a physical examination. Assessing and taking a history of the child begins in the waiting room or when obtaining vital signs, observing parent-child interactions, and rating the child's mood and developmental level.

PROCEDURE 8

OBTAINING A HEALTH HISTORY

OVERVIEW

The health history usually precedes the physical examination.

EQUIPMENT

Paper and pencil/pen
A general health history outline or the standard format used at the health care agency

GENERAL GUIDELINES

1. Gather equipment. *Promotes organization and efficiency.*
2. Wash hands. *Reduces transmission of microorganisms.*
3. Explain purpose of health assessment to parent/child. *Promotes cooperation and reduces anxiety and fear.*

PROCEDURE

All children, regardless of their age, should be recognized by their first name, even though most of the information obtained in the history will be given by the parent. The headings and questions listed below are traditionally used in the pediatric setting but may be modified or shortened according to the situation.

CHIEF COMPLAINT

Why is the child being seen today? (The caregiver answer usually is simple: "He has a runny nose.")

PRESENT ILLNESS

Describe the child's signs and symptoms. (Signs and symptoms should be listed in the order mentioned. Specific questions may include: Is the child coughing? What kind? How much? When? How long? How is the child acting otherwise? Has the child been exposed to an illness? What kind of treatment has been used?)

Past History

Birth. *Prenatal:* How was the mother's health during the pregnancy? Where did she receive prenatal care and for how long? If she had any illnesses or infections, when during the pregnancy did she have them? How were they treated? If she took any medications during her pregnancy, what did she take and when did she start taking them? What is her blood type, the father of the child's blood type, and the child's blood type? Did she receive any x-rays during the pregnancy? Was she on any special diet during the pregnancy? If she was hospitalized during the pregnancy, what was the reason? When was she in the hospital and for how long? How many living children does she have? Was she or her doctor worried about this pregnancy? If so, why? How long was this pregnancy?

Natal: How long was labor? Were there any problems? What type of delivery? If anesthesia was used, what kind was it and were there any problems with it? Where was the baby born? What was the weight? What was the baby's condition at birth? Did the baby cry spontaneously? Was the baby blue? Did the baby need oxygen? Who was with the mother during the delivery?

Postnatal: How long did the baby stay in the nursery? Did the baby have any problems in the nursery? If so, what were they? Did the mother and baby come home from the hospital at the same time? Was the baby ever jaundiced or cyanotic? Did the baby have any feeding problems? Did the baby develop any rashes? How much weight did the baby lose?

Allergies. Is the child allergic to any foods? Medications? Insects? Animals? Does the child seem to have any allergies during any particular time of the year? Describe what happens when the child has an allergic reaction. Does the child ever break out into a rash? If so, why?

Accidents. Has the child ever had an accident? If so, where was it (home, school, in car, on bicycle or other sporting equipment)? Describe what happened. How was it treated? Where was the child treated? How did the child react? Have there been any residual problems?

Illnesses. Has the child had any infections? When? Where? How was it treated? How was it followed up? Has the child had any childhood diseases? If so, what diseases did the child have (measles, mumps, roseola, chickenpox, whooping cough)? Has the child ever had any x-rays?

Surgeries. Has the child ever had any surgery? If so, when? For what condition? What was the outcome?

Hospitalizations. If the child has ever spent any time in the hospital, what was the reason? Where was the hospital? Has the condition resolved? Are there any residual problems?

Immunizations. Has the child had any immunizations? Which ones has the child had? Did the child have any reactions to the immunizations? If so, what was the reaction? Has the child received any boosters? If so, which ones? Has the child ever been tested for tuberculosis? If so, how? When? What was the result?

Family History

Family Members. What is the mother's age and health status? What is the father's age and health status? What are the ages and genders of this child's siblings? What is the health status of each?

Family Diseases. Within the immediate family (grandparent, first aunts/uncles, parents, siblings) are any of the following conditions present?

Eyes, ears, nose, throat: Nosebleeds, sinus problems, glaucoma, cataracts, myopia, or strabismus? Any other problems not listed?

Cardiorespiratory: Is there any asthma? Hay fever? Tuberculosis? Hypertension? Heart murmurs? Heart attacks? Strokes? Anemia? Rheumatic fever? Leukemia? Pneumonia? Emphysema? Any other problem not listed?

Gastrointestinal/Genitourinary: Does anyone have any ulcers? Colitis? Kidney infections? Bladder infections? Any other problem with the gastrointestinal or genitourinary system not listed?

Musculoskeletal: Does anyone in the family have any of the following: dislocated hips, club foot, muscular dystrophy, arthritis? Any other problems with bones, joints, or muscles not listed?

Neurological: Does anyone have seizures? Mental retardation? Mental problems? Epilepsy? Any other problems not listed?

Special senses: Is anyone blind or deaf?

Chronic: Does anyone have diabetes? Cancer/tumors? Thyroid problems? Congenital anomalies?

General: Are there any medical problems in the family that are important to know about?

Social History

Where does the family live? In a house? Apartment? Room? How large is the place where they live? Is there a yard? Is it fenced? Does anyone live with the family (grandparents, aunts, etc.)? Does the father and/or mother work? Full- or part-time? What are their occupations? If no one works, how are they supported? Is there any outside help? Does the child go to child care? Preschool? School? What are the relationships of the family like (happy, sad, chaotic, depressed, violent)?

Review of Systems

Skin. Does the child have any rashes? Birth marks? Discolorations?

Eyes, Ears, Nose, Throat. Does this child have any persistent nosebleeds? Frequent sore throats or colds (more than four a year)? Pneumonia? Trouble breathing? Epistaxis? Nasal discharge? Frequent earaches? Difficulty hearing? Pain? Ear discharge? Myringotomy? Do the child's eyes ever cross? Do they tear excessively? Have there been any eye injuries? Discharges? Puffiness? Redness? Has the child ever worn glasses? Any difficulty swallowing? Dental defects? Swollen glands? Masses? Stiffness in the neck? Neck asymmetry?

Cardiorespiratory. Does the child have any trouble breathing? Running? Finishing a three- to four-ounce bottle without tiring (if an infant)? Cough? Hoarseness? Wheezing? Does the child turn blue? Have there been any heart defects? Heart murmurs? "Heart trouble"? Pain over the heart or in the chest?

Gastrointestinal. Does the child have any problems with diarrhea? Constipation? Bleeding around the rectum? Bloody stools? Pain? Vomiting? What has the appetite been like? Abdominal pain or distension? Jaundice?

Genitourinary. Does the child have a straight, strong urinary stream, or does the urine just dribble out? How often does the child urinate? Is there any pain? Is there any discharge? How much does the child void during the day? Does she (an older girl) menstruate? If so, what was the age of onset? How often does she menstruate? Are there any problems?

Neurological. Has the child ever had a seizure? A fainting spell? Tremors? Twitches? Blackouts? Dizzy spells? Frequent headaches? Any incoordination? Numbness?

Musculoskeletal. Has the child ever broken any bones? Had any sprains? Complained of pain in the joints or swelling or redness around the joints? Difficulty moving extremities or in walking?

Special Senses. Does the child see well? Hear well? Does the child seem clumsy? Can the child see the blackboard from where he or she sits in the classroom? Does the child fall or walk into doors?

Chronic Conditions. Does the child have any long-term disease? If so, describe the child's disease.

General. Does the child have any other problems you would like to talk about? If yes, please describe.

Habits

Nutrition. How would you describe the child's appetite (good, fair, varied)? Is the child breast fed or bottle fed? If the child is receiving formula, what kind is it? How much and how often does the child eat in a 24-hour period? How is the formula prepared? What kinds of food (meat, fruits, vegetables, cereals, milk, eggs, juices, sweets, snacks) and how often does the child eat? What are the portion sizes? Does the child take vitamins? If so, what kind? How often? How much? Does the child feed himself or herself? Does the child use a cup? Utensils? Would you describe the child as messy? Does the child eat with the family? What is the emotional climate (relaxed, rushed, tense) of the family meals? What are the child's favorite foods? What foods does the child dislike?

Elimination. Describe the child's bowel and bladder patterns (frequency, consistency, color, discomfort). Is the child toilet trained? If not, is it planned in the future? When? If the child is toilet trained, describe any problems. If the child is toilet trained, does the child have any accidents? If so, when do they occur? How frequently do they occur?

Rest and Sleep. Where does the child sleep? What time does the child go to bed at night? What time does the child wake up in the morning? Does the child wake up during the night? If so, how often? Describe what the child does. Describe how the parent responds. Does the child have any nightmares? Night terrors? Does the child nap during the day? If so, when? How long does the child nap? How many hours does the child sleep in a 24-hour period? Does the child seem to need more sleep than he or she is getting?

Play and Activity. What types of play or games is the child involved in during the day? How often? If an older child: Does the child participate in sports, team activities, and/or regular exercise? Ask child and parent to describe the child's friendships.

Safety and Accident Prevention. Questions to use related to childproofing the home are found in Box III-1.

Development. How does the child's development compare with siblings and peers? When did the child first roll over? Sit? Stand? Walk? Talk? What grade is the child in at school? Does the child like school? What does the child like to do in school? Tell me about the child's playmates.

Personality. How would you describe the child's personality (quiet, outgoing, independent, dependent)? How does the child cope with stress (withdraw, aggressive, etc.)? Describe the child's temper. Describe how the child handles anger, fear, jealousy. How does the child relax? How does the child separate from parents? How does the child react to new situations? How does the child react to discipline? How does the child relate to baby sitters or others?

BOX III-1   Questions about childproofing the environment

1. Tell me how you have childproofed your home.
2. Do you have gates on the top and bottom of the stairs?
3. Are the slats on the crib less than 2 3/8 inches apart?
4. Have you taken the crib mobile down and taken out the bumper pads (applies to infants who are trying to pull up)?
5. Is all sleepwear flame retardant?
6. Is the hot water thermostat turned down to 120° Fahrenheit?
7. Have you installed potty locks to keep the toilet lid down?
8. Do you keep curtain and blind strings out of reach?
9. Have you placed all sharp items such as razors and knives out of reach of the child?
10. Do you monitor your child in the bathtub?
11. Do you always drain the water in the tub after getting out?
12. Have you placed cushioned covering on the tub's water faucet and drain lever?
13. Do you use a nonskid bath mat in the tub?
14. Are there outlet covers on every outlet in the house?
15. When you are cooking, do you keep the pot or pan handles turned in?
16. Have you taken tablecloths off all tables?
17. Do you keep the phone cord out of reach?
18. Is the slack taken up on all electrical appliances and lamp cords?
19. If you have a raised hearth, have you covered it with bumpers, pads, or towels?
20. Are all of your plants out of reach?
21. Are slip protectors under all rugs?
22. If you have a pool in the yard, is it fenced in, or is there a protective cover on top?
23. Do you empty pails that contain liquid after using them?
24. Are medications, cosmetics, pesticides, gasoline, cleaning solutions, paint thinner, and all other poisonous materials out of the child's reach?
25. Do you have your local poison control telephone number next to each phone?
26. Do you have syrup of ipecac in the house? Do you know why it is used and its expiration date?
27. Do you have smoke detectors close to or in the child's bedroom, and on each floor of the house?
28. Do you have a fire extinguisher on each floor?
29. Have you devised and practiced an escape route plan in case of fire?
30. Are you CPR trained?
31. What would you do in case of an emergency?
32. Where do you place your child's car seat—in the front or back seat, facing front or rear? Do you place your child in the car where an air bag is supplied?
33. Does your child use protective gear such as a helmet or knee and elbow pads if participating in an activity in which injuries may occur?
34. Do you keep plastic dry cleaner overwraps, latex balloons (unattended by a caregiver), plastic trash bags, and grocery bags out of the child's reach?

Family Relations. How do members of the family get along? How are disagreements handled within the family? What activities do the family participate in together? How often? What methods are used in the family for discipline? Are there any siblings? How does child get along with siblings (if present)?

DOCUMENTATION

1. Time and date history was obtained.
2. Client/family responses to the health history questions.

⏳ **Estimated time to obtain health history:** *20–30 minutes or longer, depending on how complicated child's health history is.*

PROCEDURE 9

CONDUCTING A PHYSICAL EXAMINATION

OVERVIEW

The physical examination of a pediatric client should begin immediately after entering the room and initially needs to include an observation of the client's skin color, position, and gait (if the child is observed walking), as well as the parent or caregiver's response and interaction with the child. Rapport can be established with the parent/caregiver and child by first talking with the parent/caregiver and then with the child.

The nurse can use therapeutic play as necessary to accomplish the examination. Listening to the caregiver's or a stuffed toy's heart and lungs can show children, especially toddlers, that it does not hurt. The nurse can then attempt to obtain the resting heart rate, heart sounds, respirations, and breath sounds. If possible, allowing the child to assist with the assessment and letting the child listen to his or her own heart rate will not only teach the child about the body, but also elicit his/her cooperation.

Invasive procedures and painful areas or procedures should be saved until the end of the examination. However, what constitutes invasive varies with age groups. For example, examining ears, mouth, and nose is invasive to toddlers, whereas genitourinary system and abdominal procedures are invasive to school-age children and adolescents. If the child refuses to cooperate, a firm approach should be used and the examination performed as quickly as possible. Regardless of the order in which the examination is performed, it needs to be charted in a logical head-to-toe format.

EQUIPMENT

Paper and pencil/pen
A general physical examination outline or the standard format used at the health care agency
Stethoscope
Tape measure
Pen light
Tongue blade
Otoscope/opthalmoscope

GENERAL GUIDELINES

1. Gather equipment. *Promotes organization and efficiency.*

2. Wash hands. *Reduces spread of microorganisms.*
3. Explain purpose of physical examination to parent/child. *Promotes cooperation and reduces anxiety and fear.*
4. Refer to information presented in introductory section above. *Helps ensure successful examination.*
5. Provide time for play and becoming acquainted (talk to child/parent, make eye contact, play with equipment, etc.). *Helps reduce child's anxiety, and increases cooperation.*

PROCEDURE

1. The child's first name, regardless of age, should be used throughout the examination. *Promotes trust.*
2. The child's weight and height/length should be obtained before the actual examination begins. The specific methods for weighing and measuring the child's height/length follow the physical examination guidelines. *Non-invasive procedures should be carried out first to assure cooperation.*
3. Vital signs (temperature, pulse, respirations, blood pressure) need to be obtained either right as the examination begins or during the examination. For example, it may be easier to obtain the temperature at the beginning of the examination, whereas it may be easier to count a child's pulse while listening to the child's heart, or count a child's respirations while listening to a child's lungs. It may also be easier to measure the blood pressure while examining the cardiovascular system. The specific methods of obtaining vital signs are listed after the weighing and measuring guidelines. *Non-invasive procedures should be carried out first to assure cooperation.*

Follow the physical examination guidelines listed below. *These are traditionally used in the pediatric setting but may be modified or shortened according to the situation.*

General Appearance

Note the overall appearance of the child. For example, is the child small, obese, well nourished, awake, alert, cooperative, developmentally appropriate for age, lethargic, or distressed? What is the client's state of consciousness?

Skin. Inspect and palpate the skin for color. (Remember that room color, gown color, and lighting affect observation. Evaluate for jaundice in natural lighting of a window; cyanosis blanches momentarily, bruises do not.) Also note pigmentation, temperature, texture, moisture, and turgor.

Note and describe all lesions for the following:

Location—exactly where on body
Pattern—clustered, confluent, evanescent, linear
Size—measured in centimeters
Color—red, pink, brown, white, hyperpigmented, or hypo-
  pigmented
Elevation—raised (papular), flat (macular), fluid-filled
  (vesicular)
Blanching—do they pale when pressure is applied?

Hair. Note color, texture, distribution, quality, and loss. Look in hair behind the ears for nits.

Nails. Note color, cyanosis, shape, and condition of nails. Clubbing is determined by checking nail angle. The normal angle is 160 degrees. An angle of 180 degrees or larger is seen in clubbing caused by hypoxia.

Head. Inspect and palpate, feeling for bogginess, sutures, and fontanels. In children under 2 years of age, measure anterior fontanel in two dimensions; usually is 4 to 5 cm by 3 to 4 cm, but should be at least 1 cm by 1 cm. Normally, the fontanels should feel flat. In states of dehydration, fontanels may be sunken. In states of increased intracranial pressure, fontanels may be bulging. Measure occipital frontal circumference (OFC) (see information at end of examination) until the child is 36 months old or if its size is important to the child's condition after 2 years of age. Always plot OFC and note size, shape, and symmetry of the head. Palpate the scalp for tenderness and lesions.

Neck. Inspect for swelling, webbing, nuchal fold, and vein distension. Palpate for swelling, carotid pulse, trachea, and thyroid.

Ears. Inspect for shape, color, symmetry, helix formation, and position. The top of the ear should go through an imaginary line from the inner canthus to the outer canthus of the eye to the occiput. Palpate for firmness and pain, and observe for and describe any discharge from the ear canal. Assess for gross hearing. Infants less than 4 months of age startle to sound. Older infants turn to localize the sound of jingling keys and other objects. Use the whisper test with verbal and cooperative children.

Eyes. Inspect for position, alignment, lid closure, inner canthal distance (average = 2.5 cm), epicanthal folds, and slant of fissure. Note dark circles under the eyes (usually present in children with allergies).

Brows—note separateness, nits
Lashes—note if they curve into eye
Lids—note color, swelling, lesions, discharge
Conjunctiva
  Palpebral (should be pink)—note redness, pallor
  Sclera and bulbar—note injection, redness, color (should
    be white; yellow in jaundice, blue in osteogenesis
    imperfecta)

Pupils—note shape, size, and briskness of reaction to light by constricting directly and consensually and accommodation for near and far vision
Iris—note color, roundness, any clefts or defects
Extraocular movements (EOMs)
  Six cardinal fields of gaze—Hold chin and have child's eyes follow your finger, moving in the shape of an H. Note asymmetric eye movement or nystagmus; a few beats of nystagmus in the far lateral gaze are normal.
  Corneal light reflex—Hold light 15 inches from bridge of nose and shine on bridge. It should reflect in the same place in each eye in normally aligned eyes.
  Cover—uncover test—Check for movement when one eye is covered and the other is gazing at a distant object. Remove cover and note movement of covered eye. Repeat using a near object.
Gross vision—Newborns blink and hyperextend their necks to light. Infants who can see fix on and follow objects. Grossly assess older children's vision by having them describe what they see on the wall or outside the window.

Face. Note color, symmetrical movement, expression, skin folds, and swelling.

Nose. Inspect for color of skin, any nasal crease, nasal mucosa, any discharge and its color, and patency. Flaring of nares may be a sign of respiratory distress. Assess turbinates by shining a light into the nares while pushing up gently on the tip of the nose (red and swollen indicates possible upper respiratory infection; pale and boggy indicates possible allergic rhinitis). Palpate sinuses for tenderness. Frontal sinuses are not developed completely until approximately 8 years of age.

Mouth. Inspect all areas. Note number and condition of teeth. Observe tonsils for swelling (grade 1+ indicates mild swelling; grade 4+ indicates touching, or "kissing," tonsils), color (should be same color as buccal mucosa), and discharge. Examine the hard and soft palate for color, patency, and lesions. The uvula should rise symmetrically; a bifid uvula could indicate a submucosal cleft. Note tongue shape, size, color, and movement, and inspect for any lesions (most common lesions are white and are thrush). Note breath odor.

Thorax and Lungs. Inspect for symmetry, movement, color, retractions, breast development, and type and effort of breathing. Count respirations (refer to vital signs section). Breathing is predominately abdominal until age 7 years. Note nasal flaring and use of accessory muscles. Retractions usually start subcostal and substernal, then progress to suprasternal and supraclavicular, and lastly intercostal, indicating severe distress. Palpate for tactile fremitus (increased in congestion and consolidation). Percuss for resonance (sound becomes dull with fluid or masses). Auscultate side to side for symmetry of sound. Infants breathe deeper when they cry; toddlers and preschoolers can breathe deeper when they blow bubbles or try to "blow out the light" of your pen light. Assess all fields. Listen to the back to assess the lower lobes in children younger than 8 years of age. Auscultate in the axillae to best hear crackles in children with suspected pneumonia. Normal sounds are vesicular or bronchovesicular. Infants' breath sounds are louder and more bronchial because they have thin chest walls.

Describe adventitious sounds as follows:

Rhonchi—a continuous, low-pitched sound with a snoring quality
Crackles—intermittent, brief, repetitive sounds caused by small collapsed airways popping open
   Fine crackles—soft, high-pitched and brief
   Coarse crackles—louder, lower-pitched and slightly longer than fine crackles
Wheezes—musical, more continuous sounds produced by rapid movement of air through narrowed passages. Usual progression of wheezing starts with expiratory wheezes only, then inspiratory wheezes with decreased expiratory wheezes, then inspiratory wheezes only (airways are collapsing on expiration), and finally no sounds because there is little air movement.
Stridor—inspiratory wheeze heard louder in neck than in chest, usually right over trachea

Infants with upper airway congestion can have sounds transmitted to lungs because they are obligate nose breathers. Listen to their lungs when they are crying and breathing through their mouths to decrease the amount of transmitted noise and better assess their breath sounds.

Cardiovascular System. Inspect for point of maximum impulse (PMI), cyanosis, mottling, edema, respiratory distress, clubbing, activity intolerance, and tiring with feeds. Palpate PMI and brachial, radial, femoral, and pedal pulses. (Refer to vital signs section.)

Auscultate the following areas with bell and diaphragm of the stethoscope:

Aortic area: Right second intercostal space (ICS) at right sternal border (SB)
Pulmonic area: Left second ICS at left SB
Erb's point: Left third ICS at left SB
Tricuspid: Left fifth ICS at left SB
Mitral: Left fifth ICS at left midclavicular line

S_1 correlates with the carotid pulse and is best heard at the apex of the heart. S_2 is best heard in the aortic and pulmonic areas (base of heart). Quality of sound should be crisp and clear. Heart rate should be normal for age and condition and synchronous with the radial pulse. Rhythm should be regular or may slow and speed up with respirations in young infants. Auscultate with the child in two positions if possible. Aus-

cultate for muffled or additional sounds and note where they are best heard.

Murmurs should be assessed for the following:

Location—where heard best on the chest wall
Timing in cardiac cycle—continuous, systolic, or diastolic
Grade—I/VI to VI/VI
   I/VI—very faint, have to listen carefully
   II/VI—quiet, but can hear soon after placing stethoscope on chest
   III/VI—moderately loud
   IV/VI—loud
   V/VI—very loud, may be heard with stethoscope partially off chest
   VI/VI—can hear without stethoscope
Pitch—high (best heard with the diaphragm), medium, or low (best heard with the bell)
Quality—harsh, blowing, machinery-like, musical
Radiation—does it radiate, and if so where (listen to back, axillae, and above clavicles)?

Abdomen. Inspect for pulsation, contour, symmetry, peristaltic waves, masses, and normal skin color. Auscultate before palpating so normal bowel sounds are not disturbed. Listen in all four quadrants for a full minute. Normal sounds should be heard every 10 to 30 seconds (4 to 5 sounds per minute). Less than 4 per minute indicates decreased bowel sounds. Listen for a full 5 minutes before concluding that they are absent.

Percuss for dullness over the client's liver and full bladder. The rest of the abdomen should percuss tympani. Palpate using light pressure first. Have the child bend the knees up while lying on his or her back to relax the abdomen. Use the child's hands under your hands if the child is very ticklish or tense. With deep palpation, support the child from the back, then palpate. Start in lower quadrants and move upward to detect an enlarged liver or spleen. Note areas of tenderness, pain, or any masses.

Anus. Inspect the skin and perineum for excoriation, bruising, discoloration, or tears.

Genitourinary System. Female genitalia—Note redness, excoriation, discharge, and odor.

Male genitalia—Note if circumcised or uncircumcised. (If uncircumcised, see if foreskin is retractable.) Note position of meatus. Close off the canals and feel for the testes or any masses in the scrotal sac. If you feel a mass other than the testes, transilluminate for fluid.

Lymphatic System. Nodes should be firm, small (1 cm or less), freely moveable, and nontender. Palpate preauricular, postauricular, anterior and posterior cervical chains, supraclavicular and subclavicular, axillary, and inguinal lymph nodes with pads of fingers.

Musculoskeletal System. Incorporate assessment into the examination. Observe walking, sitting, turning, and range of motion in all joints. Observe spinal curvature and mobility. Exaggerated lumbar curve is normal in toddlers. Note sacral dimples or tufts of hair at the base of the spinal column. Note symmetry and movement of the extremities.

Test muscle strength. Strength is graded on a 0 to 5 scale. Normal muscle strength is grade 5.

0—no contraction noted
1—barely a trace of contraction
2—active movement without gravity
3—active movement against gravity
4—active movement against gravity and resistance
5—active movement against full resistance without tiring

Note size, color, temperature, and mobility of joints. Examine palmar creases. Note extra digits and deformities.

Note stance and gait. Bowed legs (genu varum) are normal in toddlers until approximately age 2 years. Knock-knees (genu valgum) are normal from 2 until approximately 6 to 10 years. Note foot deformities. Stroke the side of the foot to see if it returns to a neutral position. Check for dislocatable hips using Barlow's test and Ortolani's maneuver in infants. Also look for uneven skin folds.

Neurological System. Observe grossly for speech and ability to follow directions in an older child. In an infant, observe activity and tone. In ambulatory patients, observe gait and balance.

Check deep tendon reflexes. These are graded from 0 to 4+.

4+—very brisk, hyperactive
3+—brisker than average
2+—normal
1+—decreased
0—absent

Use a percussion hammer or the side of the stethoscope diaphragm to elicit the following responses (Table III-1).

Test infant reflexes on children under 1 year of age (Table III-2).

Neurovascular System. Assess closely in children with intravenous (IV) lines in extremities and those in casts, restraints, or traction. Note color and size of extremity and compare with unaffected extremity. Check pulses bilaterally for equality of strength. Check capillary refill time by pinching a toe or finger and noting the time it takes for the color to return. They should have brisk, immediate blood return. Both congestive heart failure and dehydration can increase capillary refill time. Assess for any alterations in sensation or increased pain.

DOCUMENTATION

1. Time and date examination was performed.
2. Head to toe findings of examination.

⌛ **Estimated time to complete procedure:** *20–30 minutes or longer, depending on child's age and cooperation.*

Table III-1   Deep tendon reflexes

Deep Tendon Reflex	Procedure	Response
Biceps	Hit antecubital space	Forearm flexes
Triceps	Bend arm at elbow, hit triceps tendon above elbow	Forearm extends
Patellar	Strike patellar tendon	Lower leg extends
Achilles	Hold foot lightly, hit Achilles tendon	Foot flexes downward
Cranial nerves	Most are integrated into routine examination and are not specifically tested.	

Table III-2   Infant reflexes

Reflex	Age Reflex Is Elicited	Assessment
Babinski	Birth to 2 yr	Stroke bottom of foot; toes fan
Galant	Birth to 4–8 wk	Stroke infant's side; hips swing to that side
Moro	Birth to 3–4 mo	Arms extend, fingers fan (if asymmetrical, brachial plexus injury should be suspected); if Moro persists beyond 6 mo, brain damage should be suspected
Palmar grasp	Birth to 4 mo	Put your finger in infant's palm from ulnar side; infant closes fingers around your finger
Rooting	Birth to 4 mo (up to 12 mo during sleep)	Stroke infant's cheek and corner of mouth; infant's head turns in that direction
Sucking	Birth to 4 mo (7 mo during sleep)	Infant has reflexive sucking to stimuli

Growth Measurements

OVERVIEW

One of the most important areas in assessing children's health is physical growth, which includes weight, height/length, and head circumference. These measurements are plotted on growth charts to determine percentiles to compare an individual child's measurement with that of the general population. The National Center for Health Statistics (NCHS) has developed growth charts according to age and gender. One growth chart is to be used for children from birth to 36 months of age and another growth chart is to be used for children 2 to 18 years.

The NCHS uses the 5th and 95th percentile as the parameters for determining if children fall outside of the normal limits for growth. Those children below the 5th percentile are considered underweight and/or small in stature, and those above the 95th percentile are considered overweight and/or large in stature. Children falling outside normal limits should be followed closely, especially when genetic factors are not responsible for the discrepancy.

General Guidelines

1. Gather equipment. *Promotes organization and efficiency.*
2. Wash hands. *Reduces transmission of microorganisms.*
3. Explain to child and parents what you will be doing. *Promotes cooperation and reduces anxiety and fear.*

PROCEDURE 10

MEASURING WEIGHT

OVERVIEW

The type of scale and method of obtaining weight vary depending on the age of the child. Platform scales are used for infants and small children (Figure III-1); standing scales are used for children who are able to stand independently.

EQUIPMENT

Pen/pencil
Scale
    a. Stand-up scale for children
    b. Platform scale for children who are not able to stand up
Paper, if using the platform scale

PROCEDURE

1. Steps 1–3 of General Guidelines.
2. Balance the scale. *Ensures accurate reading.*
3. If using the platform scale
    a. Cover the scale with paper. *Assures cleanliness, decreases chance of child getting exposed to microorganisms from another child.*
    b. Zero scale according to manufacturer's instructions, if appropriate. *So weight obtained is accurate.*
    c. Remove the infant's clothes. *To obtain an accurate weight.*
    d. Lay or allow the child to sit on the scale. *So child is correctly positioned on scale.*
    e. Keep one hand close to but not touching the infant. *To protect from falling.*
    f. Press weigh button and read weight. *To obtain accurate weight.*
4. If using the standing scale
    a. Zero scale according to manufacturer's instructions, if appropriate. *So weight obtained is accurate.*
    b. Ask the child to remove all shoes and clothing except for underwear. *To obtain an accurate weight.*
    c. Ask the child to stand quietly in the center of the scale. *To obtain an accurate weight.*
5. Record the weight in both pounds and kilograms. *So permanent record of weight is recorded on child's chart.*

DOCUMENTATION

1. Time and date weight was obtained.
2. Actual weight obtained in both pounds and kilograms.
3. Plot measurement for child's age on standardized growth curve chart and date.

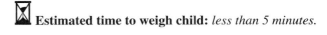

Estimated time to weigh child: *less than 5 minutes.*

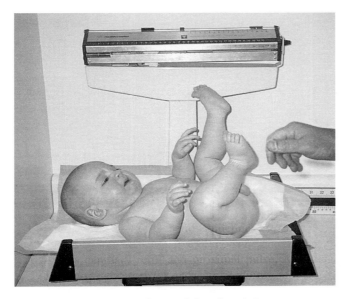

FIGURE III-1   Measuring weight of an infant.

PROCEDURE 11

MEASURING HEIGHT

OVERVIEW

Height for all children over the age of 2 years can be measured in the same fashion as for an adult (Figure III-2).

EQUIPMENT

Pen/pencil
Platform scale with stature-measuring device

PROCEDURE

1. Steps 1–3 of General Guidelines.
2. Move the headpiece of the stature-measuring device so it is as high as it can be moved. *So an accurate height is obtained.*
3. Ask child to remove shoes. *To obtain an accurate height.*
4. Ask child to stand up straight in the center of the scale with his/her back to the scale and his/her head looking straight ahead. Be sure the knees are not flexed, the child's head is in the midline, the shoulders are not slumped, and the heels are not raised. *So an accurate height is obtained.*
5. Move the headpiece down to touch the top of the child's head. *To accurately measure child's height.*
6. Ask the child to step off the scale. *So accurate height can be recorded.*
7. Read the height in both inches and centimeters. *To obtain accurate height in English and metric system.*
8. Record the height. *So an accurate permanent record of height is recorded in child's chart.*

DOCUMENTATION

1. Time and date height was obtained.
2. Actual height measured in both inches and centimeters.
3. Plot measurement for child's age on standardized growth curve chart

⊠ **Estimated time to obtain child's height:** *less than 5 minutes.*

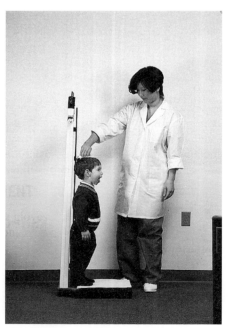

FIGURE III-2   Measuring height in preschooler.

PROCEDURE 12

MEASURING RECUMBENT LENGTH

OVERVIEW

Recumbent length is used to measure children younger than 2 years of age (Figure III-3). *Since an accurate measurement of height may not be possible if using a standing scale.*

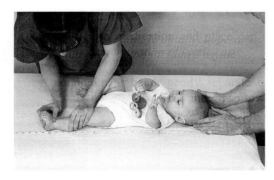

FIGURE III-3 Measuring recumbent length of infant.

EQUIPMENT

Pen/pencil
Paper tape measure
Paper covered surface

PROCEDURE

1. Steps 1–3 of General Guidelines.
2. Lay the child supine on the papered surface, making sure to fully extend the legs. *To obtain an accurate measurement.*
3. Mark where the top of the child's head and the bottom of the child's heel (with foot flexed) touch the paper. *To determine child's length.*
4. Measure the distance between the marks with the paper tape measure, noting distance in centimeters or inches. *To determine child's length.*

DOCUMENTATION

1. Time and date and method of obtaining height.
2. Actual measurement of recumbent length in both inches and centimeters.
3. Plot measurement for child's age on standardized growth curve chart.

⊠ **Estimated time to obtain recumbent length:** *less than 5 minutes.*

PROCEDURE 13

MEASURING HEAD CIRCUMFERENCE

OVERVIEW

Head circumference is measured in all children less than 2 years of age or in children with known or suspected hydrocephalus (Figure III-4).

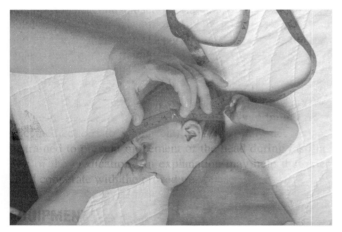

FIGURE III-4   Measuring infant head circumference.

EQUIPMENT

Paper tape measure

PROCEDURE

1. Place child in sitting or supine position. *So an accurate measurement can be obtained.*
2. Remove any hat or scarf the child is wearing. *So an accurate measurement of head circumference can be obtained.*
3. Measure anteriorly from just above the eyebrows and around posteriorly to the occipital protuberance over the ears. *This is the largest circumference of the head and the correct place on the head to measure the circumference.*

DOCUMENTATION

1. Time and date head circumference was obtained.
2. Actual circumference obtained in centimeters.
3. Plot measurement for child's age on standardized growth curve chart.

⊠ **Estimated time to measure head circumference:** *less than 2 minutes.*

Vital Signs

General Guidelines

1. Check record for baseline and factors (age, illness, medications, etc.) influencing vital signs. *Provides parameters and helps in device and site selection.*
2. Gather equipment, including paper and pen, for recording vital signs. *Promotes organization and efficiency.*
3. Wash hands. *Reduces transmission of microorganisms.*
4. Prepare child and family in a quiet and nonthreatening manner. *Enhances cooperation and participation; reduces anxiety and fear, which can affect readings.*

NOTE*: Infants and young children may be quiet and more cooperative if vitals signs are obtained while child is sitting on caregiver's lap.*

PROCEDURE 14

MEASURING A TEMPERATURE

OVERVIEW

Temperature assessment is the measurement of body temperature. When heat production exceeds heat loss and body temperature rises above the normal range, pyrexia (fever) occurs. Pyrexia can accompany any inflammatory response or prolonged exposure to high temperature. When the body is exposed to temperatures lower than normal for a prolonged period of time, hypothermia occurs. However, hypothermia can also accompany some neonatal and infant infections (i.e., meningitis). Hospitalized children are at risk for infection and accompanying fever. Therefore, accurate monitoring and recording of a child's temperature is essential for diagnosis and treatment.

EQUIPMENT

Thermometer appropriate for site (glass [mercury] or electronic) (Table III-3 and Figure III-5)
Lubricant (rectal)
Gloves, nonsterile (rectal)
Tissue

Table III-3   Centigrade and Fahrenheit temperature chart

Centigrade (C)	Fahrenheit (F)
36.0	96.8
36.5	97.7
37.0	**98.6**
37.5	99.5
38.0	100.4
38.3	101.0
39.0	102.2
39.5	103.1
40.0	104.0

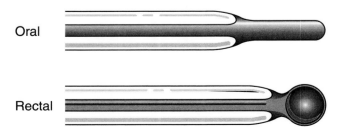

Oral

Rectal

FIGURE III-5   Oral and rectal thermometers.

NOTE: *Infants and young children may be more cooperative if oral temperature is obtained while child is sitting on caregiver's lap.*

Oral Temperature
SAFETY

1. Oral temperatures contraindicated in following circumstances: *temperature obtained would not be accurate*
   a. Uncooperative or unconscious children.
   b. Following oral surgery.
   c. Children under 2 years of age.
2. Oral temperatures are inaccurate in children receiving oxygen therapy. *Oxygen cools the mouth, and tachypnea leads to a low reading.*

PROCEDURE

1. Steps 1–4 of General Guidelines.
2. Select thermometer: glass with oral bulb (usually blue-tipped) or electronic. *These are appropriate oral thermometers.*
3. Prepare thermometer.
   a. Glass thermometer.
      1. If stored in a chemical solution, remove from storage container and rinse under cool water. *Removes disinfectant, which can irritate oral mucosa and have an objectionable taste. Cool water prevents the expansion of mercury.*
      2. Use tissue to dry from bulb end toward fingertips. *Wipe from least to most contaminated area.*
      3. Check mercury level. It should be 35° C (95° F) or below. *Must be below normal body temperature to ensure accurate reading.*
      4. If not below 35° C (95° F), grasp the nonbulb end of the thermometer firmly with thumb and forefinger and shake briskly by snapping the wrist in a downward motion. *To return temperature reading below body temperature.*
   b. Electronic thermometer.
      1. Remove from charger. *So can measure temperature.*
      2. Place disposable sheath over the probe. *Reduces transmission of microorganisms.*
      3. Grasp tip of probe stem, avoiding pressure on the ejection button. *Pressure on the ejection button releases the sheath from the probe.*

4. Place the tip of the thermometer under the tongue along the gumline to the posterior sublingual pocket. *Ensures contact with the large blood vessels under the tongue.*
5. Instruct the child to close mouth around the thermometer. *Maintains appropriate placement, decreases time needed to obtain accurate reading. Open-mouth breathing produces an abnormally low reading.*
6. If electronic, turn on scanner and follow manufacturer's instructions. *To obtain an accurate temperature reading.*
7. Leave under tongue required amount of time. Stay with child while thermometer in place. *Reduces risk of injury.*
   a. Glass thermometer: 3–5 minutes as specified by agency policy. *Allows sufficient time to register accurate results.*
   b. Electronic thermometer: Will sound tone or beep when finished recording temperature. *Allows sufficient time to register temperature.*
8. Remove thermometer and read temperature.
   a. Glass thermometer.
      1. Wipe with tissue away from fingers toward bulb end as necessary to read thermometer. *Wipe from least contaminated to most contaminated area.*
      2. Read at eye level. Rotate slowly until mercury level visualized. *Ensures accurate reading.*
   b. Electronic thermometer: read digital display.
9. Clean and store thermometer.
   a. Glass thermometer.
      1. Wipe toward bulb end of thermometer with soft tissue. Dispose of tissue in accordance with guidelines for handling body fluids. *Reduces spread of microorganisms; mucus on thermometer may interfere with effectiveness of disinfectant solution.*
      2. Cleanse with cool soapy water and rinse under cool water. Shake down the thermometer. *Mechanical cleansing removes secretions that promote growth of microorganisms. Hot water may cause coagulation of secretions and expansion of mercury in thermometer.*
      3. Store according to agency policy. *Prolongs life of thermometer.*
      4. Wash hands. *Reduces transmission of microorganisms.*
   b. Electronic thermometer.
      1. Push ejection button and discard disposable sheath into an appropriate receptacle. *Reduces transmission of microorganisms.*
      2. Return probe to storage well. *Prolongs life of thermometer.*
      3. Wash hands. *Reduces transmission of microorganisms.*
      4. Return electronic thermometer to storage unit. *Prolongs life of equipment, easy for other personnel to find in future.*

Rectal Temperature

SAFETY

1. Rectal temperature contraindicated in the following circumstances:
   a. Infants < 1 month of age.
   b. Premature infants.
   c. Prolapsed rectum.
   d. Following rectal surgery.
   e. Severe diarrhea.
   f. Bleeding tendency, e.g., leukemia, thrombocytopenia.
   g. Imperforate anus.

PROCEDURE

Taking a rectal temperature is an intrusive procedure representing an invasion of the child's body; may cause an increase in fear of body mutilation, especially in toddlers and preschoolers. Take a rectal temperature only when necessary.

1. Steps 1–4 of General Guidelines.
2. Select thermometer: glass with rectal bulb (usually red-tipped) or electronic. *These are appropriate rectal thermometers.*
3. Provide privacy for child. *Reduces anxiety and embarrassment.*
4. Prepare thermometer as in Oral Temperature, step 3 of Procedure.
5. Lubricate the tip of the thermometer with a water-soluble gel. *Reduces friction and promotes ease of insertion. Minimizes irritation of mucus membranes in the anal canal.*
6. Place tissues in easy reach. *To wipe anus after removal of thermometer.*
7. Put on nonsterile gloves. *Reduces transmission of microorganisms; protects nurse from contact with body fluids.*
8. Position child. *Ensures visualization of anus.*
   a. Infant: prone position or supine, grasping ankles with one hand and elevating the legs. *Promotes ease of insertion.*
   b. Older child: on side with upper knee flexed. *Flexing of the knee relaxes muscles and promotes ease of insertion.*
9. Separate buttocks to expose anal opening, and gently insert thermometer. Instruct older child to take a deep breath. *Gentle insertion decreases discomfort and prevents trauma to mucous membranes. Taking a deep breath relaxes the anal sphincter* (Figure III-6).

NOTE: *If resistance is felt, do not force. Remove thermometer and check temperature by another route.*

   a. Infant: insert ¼ to ½ inch. *Inserting more than ½ inch may cause rectal perforation.*
   b. Older child: insert 1–1½ inches. *Inserting more than 1–1½ inches may cause rectal perforation.*

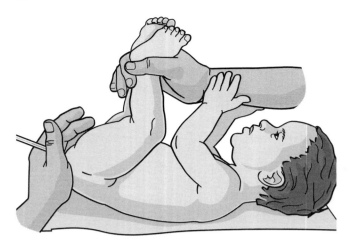

FIGURE III-6   Infant position when taking a rectal temperature.

10. If electronic, turn on scanner and follow manufacturer's instructions. *Assures accurate reading.*
11. Leave thermometer in place required amount of time. Hold thermometer in place and do not leave child alone. *Reduces risk of injury. Assures accurate reading.*
    a. Glass thermometer: 3–4 minutes as specified by agency policy. *Allowing sufficient time for the thermometer to register results in a more accurate assessment of body temperature.*
    b. Electronic thermometer: will sound a tone or beep when finished. *Allows sufficient time to register temperature.*
12. Remove thermometer gently in a straight line.
13. Wipe anal area to remove any lubricant and/or fecal material. *Reduces spread of microorganisms.*
14. Read temperature as in Oral Temperature, step 8 of Procedure. *Ensures accurate reading.*
15. Reposition child in a comfortable position. *Assures cooperation in the future.*
16. Clean and store thermometer as in Oral Temperature, step 9 of Procedure.

NOTE: *Need to remove gloves before washing hands.*

Axillary Temperature

SAFETY

1. There are no age restrictions for taking an axillary temperature.

PROCEDURE

1. Steps 1–4 of General Guidelines.
2. Select thermometer: glass or electronic. Follow agency guidelines regarding type of thermometer to use. *These*

are appropriate thermometers to use in obtaining axillary temperature.
3. Expose axillary area. *Assists correct placement.*
4. Make sure axillary skin is dry. Pat dry if necessary. *Prevents a false low reading.*
5. Prepare thermometer as in Oral Temperature, step 3 of Procedure. *Refer to earlier rationale.*
6. Place tip of thermometer under the child's arm, well up into the axilla. Bring the child's arm down close to the body and hold in place. *Ensures more accurate measurement; allows thermometer tip to rest against superficial blood vessels in axilla; brings skin surfaces together, thus reducing air around the tip of the thermometer that might affect temperature reading* (Figure III-7).
7. Leave in place required amount of time. *Allowing sufficient time for the thermometer to register results in a more accurate assessment of body temperature.*
    a. Glass thermometer: 6–10 minutes according to agency policy.
    b. Electronic thermometer: will sound a tone or beep when finished.
8. Remove thermometer and read as in Oral Temperature, step 8 of Procedure.
9. Clean and store thermometer as in Oral Temperature, step 9 of Procedure.

Tympanic Temperature
SAFETY

1. Do not use in infected or draining ear or if lesion or incision is adjacent to ear.

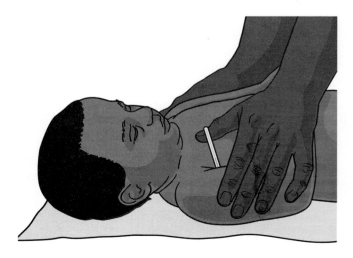

FIGURE III-7   Positioning when taking an axillary temperature.

2. Further study needed regarding accuracy of tympanic temperature with otitis media, sinusitis, or in premature infants with small ear canal.

PROCEDURE

1. Steps 1–4 of General Guidelines.
2. Select contact infrared tympanic thermometer. *Appropriate type to use.*
3. Remove probe cover from container and attach probe cover to probe tip. *Prevents contamination.*
4. Position child for access to ear. Turn head to one side. Pull pinna down and back for a child under 3 years of age and up and back for a child over 3 years of age. *Provides access to ear canal.*

NOTE: *Do not use ear on side child has been lying on. Ear in contact with a surface can build up heat and give abnormally high reading.*

5. Gently insert probe tip into the external ear canal. Use firm pressure to obtain an adequate seal. *Prevents trauma to the ear canal and ensures accurate temperature reading* (Figure III-8).

NOTE: *A better seal (thus a more accurate assessment of body temperature) is generally achieved using the right hand to take a temperature from the right ear and the left hand to take a temperature from the left ear.*

6. Quickly achieve a seal making sure the probe tip is aimed toward the tympanic membrane. As soon as the probe is in place, press the scan button. *Measures temperature by measuring infrared energy from tympanic membrane. Pressure of the probe in the ear canal can draw down the temperature, leading to an abnormally low reading.*
7. Remove probe after temperature is displayed. Read display. *Allows accurate reading of temperature.*
8. Remove probe cover and discard; replace probe in storage container. *Prevents probe damage.*
9. Return tympanic thermometer to charging unit.
10. Wash hands. *Reduces transmission of microorganisms.*

DOCUMENTATION

1. Temperature.
2. Route and for tympanic temperature which ear used.
3. Device used.
4. Who notified if finding of concern.

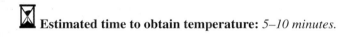 **Estimated time to obtain temperature:** *5–10 minutes.*

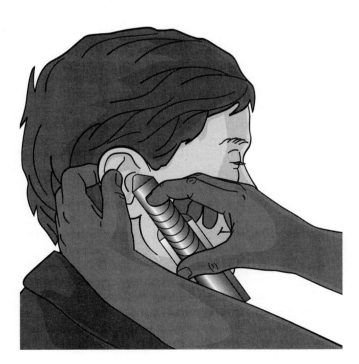

FIGURE III-8   Insertion of temperature probe into child's ear canal.

PROCEDURE 15

MEASURING A PULSE

OVERVIEW

Pulse assessment involves measuring a pressure pulsation created when the heart contracts and ejects blood into the aorta. Assessment of pulse characteristics provides clinical data regarding the heart's pumping action and the adequacy of peripheral artery blood flow.

EQUIPMENT

Stethoscope (for apical pulse)
Watch with a second hand

NOTE: *Infants and young children may be quiet and more cooperative if vital signs are obtained while child is sitting on caregiver's lap.*

Apical Pulse

PROCEDURE

Apical pulse should be the first vital sign assessed. *Other assessment procedures may be upsetting, leading to increased heart rate and crying, which makes hearing apical pulse difficult.*

An apical pulse should be taken on neonates, infants, and young children (under 2 years of age) and on all children with cardiac problems or receiving digitalis preparations. *Radial pulse is unreliable in neonates and infants due to their small size and normally rapid heart rate. Radial pulse is unreliable in children with cardiac problems or receiving digitalis preparations due to possibly irregular heart rhythm.*

1. Steps 1–4 of General Guidelines.
2. Cleanse earpieces and diaphragm of stethoscope with an alcohol wipe. *Reduces transmission of microorganisms from practitioner to practitioner and from client to client.*
3. Warm stethoscope in hand for 5–10 seconds. *Prevents client from being startled by cold bell; promotes client comfort.*
4. Raise client's gown to expose sternum and left chest. *Allows for proper placement of stethoscope.*
5. Place stethoscope over point of maximal impulse (PMI). *Enhances ability to clearly hear heart sounds.*
   a. For infant, PMI is at third to fourth intercostal space near the sternum (Figure III-9).
   b. For older child, PMI is at fifth left intercostal space in the midclavicular line.

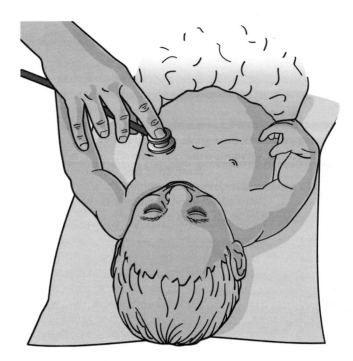

FIGURE III-9   Place stethoscope over point of maximum impulse to count heart rate.

6. Count pulse for one full minute. Each "lub-dub" sound is one beat. Assess apical pulse for rate, rhythm, and any abnormal heart sounds. If an irregular rhythm, determine if there is a regular pattern to the irregularity. *Counting for less than one minute may lead to inaccurate heart rate, especially in neonates, infants, and young children where arrhythmia is normal or in children with cardiac problems or receiving digitalis preparations.*
7. If appropriate, evaluate for pulse deficit between the apical pulse and peripheral pulse by simultaneously taking the apical and radial pulse. For the inexperienced nurse, this may be more accurately accomplished by using two nurses, one to count the apical pulse and one to count the radial pulse. Both nurses should use the same watch when performing this procedure. *Assures accurate pulse rate is read.*
8. Wash hands. *Reduces transmission of microorganisms.*

Radial Pulse

PROCEDURE

A radial pulse is reliable in children over 2 years of age except as specified under apical pulse above. Some agency policies require apical pulses on all children regardless of age or condition. Be familiar with the policy of your agency.

1. Steps 1–4 of General Guidelines.
2. Place index and middle finger along child's radial artery. *Fingertips are sensitive to touch. Use of thumb might lead to nurse feeling own pulse.*
3. Apply gentle pressure, enough to feel the pulsating artery. *Too firm a pressure obliterates the pulse. Too gentle a pressure does not allow one to feel the pulse.*
4. Count pulse rate for 30 seconds and multiply by 2 to get the rate per minute. If there are any abnormalities in the pulse, count the rate for one full minute. *Ensures sufficient time to count irregular beats.*
5. Assess the pulse for rate, rhythm, amplitude (strength), and elasticity of vessel (distention of vessel).
6. Wash hands. *Reduces transmission of microorganisms.*

Peripheral Pulses
PROCEDURE

1. Steps 1–4 of General Guidelines.
2. Assess peripheral pulses by placing index and middle finger against pulse site and applying gentle pressure. Pulse sites to be assessed generally include brachial, radial, femoral, popliteal, posterior tibial, and dorsalis pedis (pedal). See steps 2 and 3 of radial pulse procedure.
3. Assess equality of pulses, amplitude, and elasticity of vessels bilaterally (i.e., right side compared to left side). Assess for any pulse deficit between upper and lower extremities. *Assures accurate reading of pulse; determines bilateral pulse equality, amplitude, and vessel elasticity.*
4. Wash hands. *Reduces transmission of microorganisms.*

DOCUMENTATION

1. Pulse rate and site.
2. Rhythm, and, if applicable, number and character of irregular beats.
3. Sites, character, and quality of peripheral pulses. Note if bilateral equality and if deficits exist between upper and lower extremities.
4. Who notified if concerned about findings.

 Estimated time to obtain pulse: *5 minutes.*

PROCEDURE 16

COUNTING RESPIRATIONS

OVERVIEW

Respiratory assessment is the measurement of the breathing pattern and provides clinical data regarding the pH of arterial blood. Normal breathing is slightly observable, effortless, quiet, automatic, and regular. It can be easily assessed by observing chest wall expansion and bilateral symmetrical movement of the thorax, or by placing the back of the hand next to the child's nose and mouth to feel expired air.

When assessing respirations, it is important to ascertain the rate, depth, and rhythm of ventilatory movement. The rate is assessed by counting the number of breaths taken per minute; the depth and rhythm are assessed by observing the normal thoracic and abdominal movements and symmetry in chest wall movement. Normal respirations are characterized by a rate ranging from 12 to 20 breaths per minute.

One inspiration and expiration cycle is counted as one breath. Most respiratory rates are counted for 30 seconds and then multiplied by 2. If the child is experiencing respiratory difficulties, the respiratory rate should be counted for a full 60 seconds.

The movement of the chest wall should be even and regular without noise and effort. Different respiratory wave patterns are characterized by their rate, rhythm, and depth. Eupnea refers to easy respiration with a normal rate of breaths per minute that are age specific. Bradypnea is a respiratory rate of 10 or fewer breaths per minute. Hypoventilation is characterized by shallow respirations. Tachypnea is a respiratory rate greater than 24 breaths per minute. Hyperventilation is characterized by deep, rapid respirations. Hyperpnea occurs with exercise when respirations are increased in depth and rate. Sighing is a protective physiologic mechanism for expanding small airways not used with normal breathing.

Costal breathing occurs when the external intercostal muscles and other accessory muscles are used to move the chest upward and outward. Diaphragmatic (abdominal) breathing occurs when the diaphragm contracts and relaxes as observed by movement of the abdomen. Dysnea refers to difficulty in breathing as observed by labored or forced respirations through the use of accessory muscles in the chest and neck to breathe. Apnea is the cessation of breathing for several seconds.

EQUIPMENT

Stethoscope
Watch with a second hand

NOTE: *Infants and young children may be quiet and more cooperative if vitals signs are obtained while child is sitting on caregiver's lap.*

PROCEDURE

1. Steps 1–4 of General Guidelines.
2. Be sure light is adequate for the procedure. *Allows accurate counting of respirations.*
3. Place hand on chest or abdomen or observe rise and fall of chest or abdomen. Count respirations for one full minute for infants and younger children, because respirations are normally irregular. Count for one full minute for any child with irregular respirations. For older children with regular respirations, respirations may be counted for 30 seconds and multiplied by 2 to obtain the rate per minute. Respirations also may be counted by auscultation. *Counting for less than one minute may lead to inaccurate respiratory rate in infants, young children, and those with irregular respirations.*
   a. Respirations are diaphragmatic on children younger than 7 years of age—observe or place hand on abdomen. *Assures adequate observations/counting of respirations.*
   b. Respirations are thoracic in children older than 7 years of age—observe or place hand on chest. *Assures adequate observations/counting of respiratory rate.*
4. Observe movement of chest and abdomen.
   a. Assess chest movements for symmetry. *Helps determine chest innervation.*
   b. In infants observe movement of abdomen. *Paradoxical abdominal movement, i.e., abdomen rises on inspiration as chest retracts (seesaw movement), is abnormal except in premature infants.*
5. Observe for signs of respiratory distress (retractions, nasal flaring, grunting, use of accessory muscles). *Indicates child may have respiratory difficulties.*
6. Auscultate for normal, abnormal, and diminished and/or absent breath sounds on both back and chest; use a regular pattern; compare breath sounds side to side. *Assures adequate assessment of respiratory effort.*
7. Wash hands. *Reduces transmission of microorganisms.*

DOCUMENTATION

Document the following in the appropriate place in the client's chart:

1. Rate, depth, and character of respirations.
2. Breath sounds heard and placement of sounds.
3. Any signs and symptoms of respiratory distress.
4. Who notified if findings of concern.

 Estimated time to count respiration: *5 minutes.*

PROCEDURE 17

MEASURING A BLOOD PRESSURE

OVERVIEW

Blood pressure measurement is assessed in order to determine the pressure of the circulating blood against the walls of the blood vessels. Blood pressure in infants or children is usually measured by the indirect technique using a sphygmomanometer and stethoscope.

EQUIPMENT

Stethoscope and manual blood pressure cuff or
Electronic blood pressure machine

CUFF SIZE

The American Heart Association recommends:
1. Width: 40–50% of limb circumference.
2. Length: Bladder of cuff needs to completely or nearly completely encircle the arm without overlapping.

SAFETY

1. Do not take a blood pressure (BP) on an injured or painful extremity or one where there is an intravenous line (IV). *Cuff inflation can temporarily interrupt blood flow and compromise circulation in an extremity already impaired or a vein receiving IV fluids.*

Blood Pressure, Auscultation, or Palpation

PROCEDURE

1. Steps 1–4 of General Guidelines.
2. Cleanse earpieces and bell/diaphragm of stethoscope with an alcohol wipe. *Reduces transmission of microorganisms from practitioner to practitioner and from client to client.*
3. Position child.
   a. Arm: Sitting or recumbent position with forearm supinated and slightly flexed and supported at heart level. *If arm is below level of heart, BP reading is higher than normal; if it is above the level of the heart, BP reading is lower than normal.*
   b. Leg: Prone or if unable to lie prone, supine with knee slightly flexed to permit placing stethoscope over popliteal area. *Allows accurate reading.*

4. Remove clothing as necessary to expose extremity. *Allows accurate reading.*
5. Place correct size cuff around the extremity with the center of the bladder cuff over the artery. *Too narrow a cuff will give a false high reading; too wide a cuff will give a false low reading.*
   a. Arm: Cuff should be placed around upper arm with the lower edge about 3 cm above the antecubital fossa.
   b. Leg: Cuff should be placed around the midthigh with the lower edge about 2 cm above the popliteal space.
6. Locate the artery by palpation. *Allows for proper placement of stethoscope to hear BP.*
7. Palpate a pulse distal to the cuff, e.g., brachial or radial. Close air valve and rapidly inflate cuff to 30 mm Hg above where pulse no longer felt or above expected systolic blood pressure. *Ensures cuff is inflated to a pressure exceeding the child's systolic BP.*
8. Place stethoscope gently over artery. *Too firm a pressure will occlude blood vessel.*

NOTE: *While the diaphragm of the stethoscope is frequently used, the American Heart Association recommends using the bell of the stethoscope.*

NOTE: *To obtain a blood pressure reading by palpation, keep fingers on a distal pulse.*

9. Open the valve and slowly release the air, permitting the pressure to drop 2–3 mm Hg per heart beat while auscultating for BP sounds or palpating for a pulse. *Slower or faster deflation yields false readings.*

NOTE: *Do not reinflate cuff without letting cuff totally deflate. Reinflating cuff results in erroneously high readings.*

10. Obtain a blood pressure reading. *Following instructions assures accurate reading.*
    a. Auscultation.
       1. Systolic pressure: The pressure at which you first hear sounds.
       2. Diastolic pressure: The American Heart Association recommends the onset of muffling as the diastolic pressure in children up to 13 years of age; the pressure when sounds become inaudible is the diastolic pressure in children under 13 years of age.
    b. Palpation: Continue to slowly release pressure until a pulse is felt. This is the systolic pressure. The diastolic pressure is recorded as P, e.g., 100/P. The systolic pressure obtained by palpation is 5–10 mm Hg lower than that obtained by auscultation.

NOTE: *If using a mercury manometer, read at eye level to ensure accuracy.*

11. Do not leave the cuff inflated for a prolonged period. *Inflated cuff is uncomfortable.*
12. Deflate the cuff rapidly and completely, and remove from the arm. *Prevents discomfort (from numbness or tingling) and arterial occlusion.*
13. Wait two minutes before taking another blood pressure. *Releases blood trapped in vessels.*

Blood Pressure, Electronic

PROCEDURE

1. Steps 1–4 of General Guidelines.
2. Set up machine according to instructions *to obtain accurate measurement:*
   a. Plug in monitor/machine.
   b. Connect dual air hose to back of monitor.
   c. Connect correct size cuff by screwing the pressure cuff's tubing into the other end of the air hose.
3. Place cuff. (See step 5 of Blood Pressure, Auscultation, or Palpation.)
4. Turn machine on, and follow manufacturer's instructions.
5. Obtain reading.
6. Remove cuff.

Blood Pressure, Flush

Flush is used to obtain a BP reading on a newborn or small infant when BP is difficult or impossible to obtain by other means.

PROCEDURE

1. Place infant in a recumbent position. *To obtain accurate reading.*

2. Apply cuff snugly and smoothly to distal arm, with outer edge at the wrist or to the distal leg with the outer edge at the ankle. *Facilitates accurate reading.*
3. Elevate extremity above heart level. *Facilitates flow of blood out of extremity.*
4. Wrap the extremity distal to the cuff with an elastic bandage. Begin with the finger or toes and progress to the edge of the cuff. *Forces blood out of extremity.*
5. Inflate the cuff to 150–200 mm Hg.
6. Remove elastic bandage. The hand or foot should appear pale in color and exsanguinated.
7. Lower the pressure in the cuff by 5 mm Hg and leave there for 3–4 seconds. Repeat process until flushing observed in the pale extremity, i.e., a sudden pink color appears below the edge of the cuff and spreads distally.
8. Reading is taken at point flushing appears. This is the mean arterial pressure. To be accurate, an assistant is needed to observe for flushing while you monitor the pressure gauge.
9. Repeat the procedure at least twice to confirm the reading. *Ensures more accurate reading.*

DOCUMENTATION

1. Blood pressure reading.
2. Method used.
3. Site.
4. Size of cuff.
5. Who notified if findings of concern.

Estimated time to obtain blood pressure: *5 minutes.*

Standard Assessments

OVERVIEW

There is a variety of standard assessments that can be performed in pediatrics. The assessment depends on the child's condition and age.

PROCEDURE 18

NUTRITIONAL ASSESSMENT

OVERVIEW

Nutritional status affects the general health of a child and has a direct influence on growth, development, cognition, and learning. The nutritional assessment should contain information about dietary intake and include a clinical assessment of nutritional and biochemical status. Primary caregivers should be interviewed if the child is an infant or young child.

EQUIPMENT

Paper and pencil/pen
A general nutritional assessment outline or the standard format used at the health care agency

GENERAL GUIDELINES

1. Wash hands. *Prevents spread of infection.*
2. Explain purpose of nutritional assessment to parent/child. *Promotes cooperation and reduces anxiety and fear.*

PROCEDURE

1. Steps 1 and 2 of General Guidelines.
2. The child's first name, regardless of age, should be used throughout the assessment. *Allows trust to be established. Helps child feel more comfortable.*

3. The nutritional assessment questions listed below are traditionally used in the pediatric setting but may be modified or shortened according to the situation.
   a. What are usual mealtimes?
   b. Which family member is responsible for meal preparation and shopping?
   c. How much money is allotted for groceries each week?
   d. How are most foods prepared (e.g., baked, fried, broiled, microwaved)?
   e. How often does the family eat out (frequency of fast food restaurants)?
   f. Do family members eat together?
   g. What are the child's favorite foods, drinks, and snacks?
   h. What are the child's snacking habits?
   i. What foods does the child dislike?
   j. What vitamin and mineral supplements are taken?
   k. Has the child recently lost/gained weight?
   l. Does the child have any food allergies?
   m. Does the child have any feeding problems (colic, difficulty swallowing)?

DOCUMENTATION

1. Time and date assessment was performed.
2. Child/family responses to assessment topics.

⧗ **Estimated time to obtain nutritional assessment:** *5–10 minutes.*

PROCEDURE 19

DEVELOPMENTAL ASSESSMENT

OVERVIEW

Evaluation of developmental functioning is an essential component of any pediatric assessment. Purposes of the developmental assessment are to (1) validate a child is developing normally, (2) detect problems, (3) identify caregiver/child concerns, and (4) provide an opportunity for anticipatory guidance/teaching relative to expected and age-appropriate behaviors. The developmental assessment may be completed either before or after the physical examination.

A commonly used measure for assessing neuromuscular development of the child from birth through 6 years of age is the Denver Developmental Screening Test II (Denver II; Frankenburg, 1994; see Figure III-10). The test is composed of four sections: personal-social, fine motor-adaptive, language, and gross motor. There are a total of 125 items described on the test. Some items can be scored by simply observing the child. For instance, the child may be smiling spontaneously, saying words other than "mama" or "dada," or sitting with the head held steady. Certain items can be given an automatic pass mark if the caregiver indicates that the child is able to accomplish the corresponding item, such as drinking from a cup, washing and drying hands, or dressing without help. Documentation is reflected by using "P" for pass, "F" for fail, "R" for refuses, and "no" for no opportunity to observe the child. It is important to give the child three opportunities to attempt the item before documenting the item's score. A normal test consists of no delays and a max-

imum of one caution. A caution is a failure of the child to perform an item that had been achieved by 75–90% of children of the same age. A delay is a failure of any item to the left of the age line. A suspect test is one with one or more delays and/or two or more cautions. In these instances, the child should be retested within two to three weeks.

Several other assessment measures are listed in Table III-4. These measures evaluate a variety of aspects, including behavior, temperament, cognition, memory, and the child's home environment. Screening procedures using these measures quickly and reliably identify children whose development is below normal and may also be used to monitor developmental progress. Most measures can be administered in a variety of settings with a minimal amount of preparation. Although all measures listed are valid and reliable, some may not be standardized on children of lower socioeconomic status or of different ethnic groups. Caution should always be taken to guarantee that administration is accurate; directions and explanations to caregivers and children need to be clear and concise. Following administration, it would be helpful to ask caregivers if the child's performance was typical, since retesting/rescreening may be necessary if the behavior was atypical. All results should be carefully communicated to caregivers so that misunderstandings and misinterpretations are kept to a minimum. Before administering any measure, it is essential to read and follow instructions carefully.

⧗ **Estimated time to obtain developmental assessment:** *20–30 minutes depending on the measure used and child's cooperation.*

Table III-4   Developmental assessment measures for infants and children

Test Name	Ages	Features Evaluated
Carey-Revised Infant Temperament	4–8 months	Temperament, patterns of feeding, sleeping, elimination, responses to different situations
Denver Articulation Screening Exam	2.5–6 years	Intelligibility; articulation of 30 sound elements
Developmental Profile II	Birth–9 years	Physical, self-help, social, academic, communication skills
Early Language	Birth–3 years	Auditory expressive and receptive, visual components of speech
Goodnough-Harris Drawing Test	5–17 years	Child's drawing of a person: analyzed for body parts, clothing, proportion, perspective
HOME (Home Observation for Measurement of the Environment)	Birth–6 years	Organization, play materials, parental control, stimulation, punishment or restriction
McCarthy Scales of Children's Abilities	2.5–8.5 years	Intellectual and motor development, memory, quantitative, perceptual performance, general cognition

DIRECTIONS FOR ADMINISTRATION

1. Try to get child to smile by smiling, talking or waving. Do not touch him/her.
2. Child must stare at hand several seconds.
3. Parent may help guide toothbrush and put toothpaste on brush.
4. Child does not have to be able to tie shoes or button/zip in the back.
5. Move yarn slowly in an arc from one side to the other, about 8" above child's face.
6. Pass if child grasps rattle when it is touched to the backs or tips of fingers.
7. Pass if child tries to see where yarn went. Yarn should be dropped quickly from sight from tester's hand without arm movement.
8. Child must transfer cube from hand to hand without help of body, mouth, or table.
9. Pass if child picks up raisin with any part of thumb and finger.
10. Line can vary only 30 degrees or less from tester's line.
11. Make a fist with thumb pointing upward and wiggle only the thumb. Pass if child imitates and does not move any fingers other than the thumb.

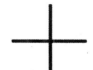
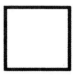

12. Pass any enclosed form. Fail continuous round motions.	13. Which line is longer? (Not bigger.) Turn paper upside down and repeat. (pass 3 of 3 or 5 of 6)	14. Pass any lines crossing near midpoint.	15. Have child copy first. If failed, demonstrate.

When giving items 12, 14, and 15, do not name the forms. Do not demonstrate 12 and 14.

16. When scoring, each pair (2 arms, 2 legs, etc.) counts as one part.
17. Place one cube in cup and shake gently near child's ear, but out of sight. Repeat for other ear.
18. Point to picture and have child name it. (No credit is given for sounds only.)
    If less than 4 pictures are named correctly, have child point to picture as each is named by tester.

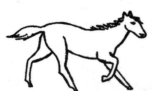

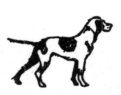
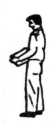

19. Using doll, tell child: Show me the nose, eyes, ears, mouth, hands, feet, tummy, hair. Pass 6 of 8.
20. Using pictures, ask child: Which one flies?... says meow?... talks?... barks?... gallops? Pass 2 of 5, 4 of 5.
21. Ask child: What do you do when you are cold?... tired?... hungry? Pass 2 of 3, 3 of 3.
22. Ask child: What do you do with a cup? What is a chair used for? What is a pencil used for?
    Action words must be included in answers.
23. Pass if child correctly places and says how many blocks are on paper. (1, 5).
24. Tell child: Put block on table; under table; in front of me, behind me. Pass 4 of 4.
    (Do not help child by pointing, moving head or eyes.)
25. Ask child: What is a ball?... lake?... desk?... house?... banana?... curtain?... fence?... ceiling? Pass if defined in terms of use, shape, what it is made of, or general category (such as banana is fruit, not just yellow). Pass 5 of 8, 7 of 8.
26. Ask child: If a horse is big, a mouse is __? If fire is hot, ice is __? If the sun shines during the day, the moon shines during the __? Pass 2 of 3.
27. Child may use wall or rail only, not person. May not crawl.
28. Child must throw ball overhand 3 feet to within arm's reach of tester.
29. Child must perform standing broad jump over width of test sheet (8 1/2 inches).
30. Tell child to walk forward, ⌒⌒⌒⌒→ heel within 1 inch of toe. Tester may demonstrate.
    Child must walk 4 consecutive steps.
31. In the second year, half of normal children are non-compliant.

OBSERVATIONS:

FIGURE III-10 Denver II. Reprinted with permission of Denver Developmental Materials, Denver, CO.

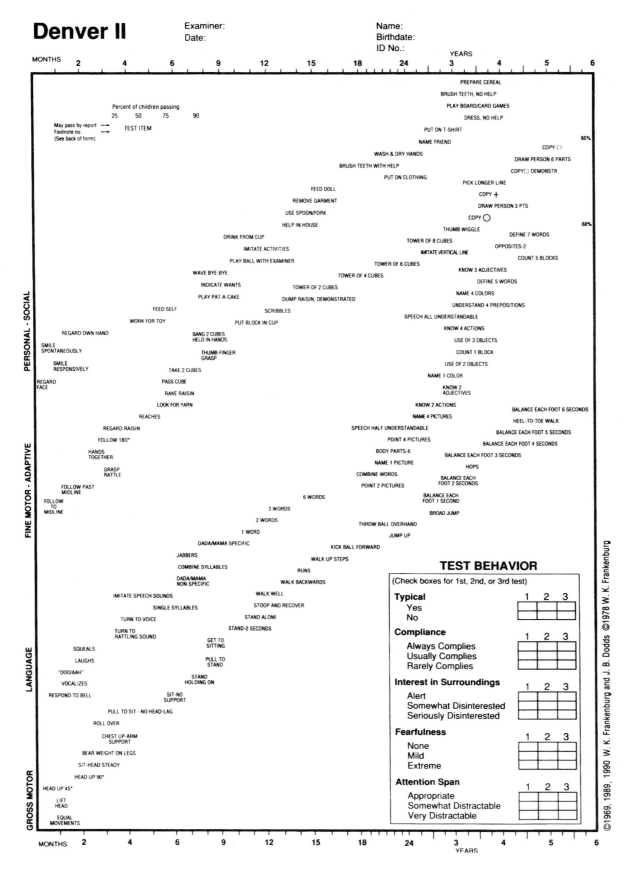

FIGURE III-10 (continued)

PROCEDURE 20

VISION SCREENING

OVERVIEW

Several screening tests are available to evaluate visual acuity in children, including the adult Snellen, Snellen E, and Allen. The child's age and developmental level determine the measures used. The adult Snellen chart can be used on children as young as 6 years of age provided they are able to read the alphabet. The Snellen E chart, which shows the letter "E" facing different directions, is used for children over 3 years of age or any child who cannot read the alphabet. If the child resists wearing an eye patch, make a game out of wearing the patch. The Allen test (a series of seven pictures on different cards) can be used with children as young as 3 years of age. Visual acuity screening should begin when the child is 3 years of age; children should be tested every one to two years through adolescence.

EQUIPMENT

Screening chart
Card or eye patch
Room or hall long enough to accommodate test (20 feet of length needed) with 20 feet marked off with tape

PROCEDURE

1. Gather equipment. *Improves organization and effectiveness.*
2. Prepare child and family. *Enhances cooperation and parental participation; reduces anxiety and fear.*
3. Ask child to place his/her heels at the 20-foot mark and stand up straight. *Allows accurate assessment of vision.*
4. Assess eyes separately and then both together. If child wears glasses, assess eyes with and without glasses. While one eye is being tested, cover the other eye with the card or patch. Ask child not to close eye not being tested. See information below regarding different tests. *Will detect differences in acuity of each eye; will determine if acuity different with and without corrective lenses.*
5. Observe child for squinting, tearing, excessive blinking, or moving of head toward chart. *May indicate problems with acuity and child's attempt to compensate.*

6. Record last line where child can read more than half the symbols or direction of the "E" on the line. *Determines the child's visual acuity.*
7. If results are abnormal, test again in two weeks; refer to ophthalmologist. *Needs another evaluation.*

Snellen E Chart

Ask the child to point an arm or a finger in the direction the "E" is pointing. Vision is 20/40 from 2 to 6 years of age, when it approaches the normal 20/20 acuity. The test is abnormal if results are 20/40 or greater in a child 3 years of age, or 20/30 or greater in a child 6 years or older, or if results are different for each eye.

Allen Test

With both of the child's eyes open, show each card to the child and elicit a name for each picture. Do not use any pictures with which the child is not familiar. Place the 2–3-year-old child 15 feet from where you will be standing. Place the 3–4-year-old child 20 feet from you. Ask the caregiver to cover one of the child's eyes. Show pictures one at a time, eliciting a response after each showing. Show the same pictures in different sequence for the other eye. To record findings, the denominator is always 30 because a normal child should see the picture on the card at 30 feet. To document the numerator, determine the greatest distance at which three of the pictures are recognized by each eye. The child should correctly identify three of the cards in three trials. Two- to three-year-old children should have 15/30 vision. Three- to four-year-old children should score 15/30 or 20/30. Each eye should have the same score.

DOCUMENTATION

1. Time and date of test.
2. Chart or test used.
3. Visual acuity.
4. Any noticeable squinting, tearing, excessive blinking, or moving of child's head toward chart.

 Estimated time to complete procedure: *10 minutes.*

Special Assessments

OVERVIEW

Occasionally, it is necessary to perform special assessments on infants and/or children because of circumstances related to their condition or an illness. These special assessments involve utilizing specialized equipment (apnea monitor, cardiac monitor, pulse oximeter) to assess/monitor the cardiorespiratory system.

PROCEDURE 21

APPLYING AN APNEA MONITOR

OVERVIEW

The apnea monitor is used to keep track of irregular or abnormal breathing in infants. Most commonly, the monitor is used when there is a need to monitor the infant's breathing pattern and heart rate. It is important to follow the manufacturer's instructions whenever setting up the monitor. The monitor sounds an alarm when the infant does not breathe for 20 seconds. If the alarm sounds, it is important to determine if the infant has stopped breathing or if the machine is not working properly.

EQUIPMENT

Apnea monitor
Electrodes
Straps to hold electrodes in place
Alcohol wipes

GENERAL GUIDELINES

1. Check order for placement of apnea monitor. *Ensures appropriate infant is monitored.*
2. Gather equipment. *Improves organization and effectiveness.*
3. Set high and low limits of machine (usually 15–20 seconds for the period of apnea). *Improves organization and effectiveness.*
4. Wash hands. *Reduces transmission of microorganisms.*
5. Prepare family. *Enhances cooperation and parental participation and reduces anxiety and fear.*

PROCEDURE

1. Steps 1–5 of General Guidelines.
2. Place infant/child in a supine position. *Helps placement of electrodes on chest.*
3. Clean with alcohol wipes the area where the electrodes are to be applied; allow the area to dry. *Removes oils from skin so electrodes will adhere.*
4. Place electrodes on infant's chest: one on the left, one on the right, and one on the abdomen according to manufacturer's instructions. *Assures accurate assessment.*
5. Turn machine on; if alarm sounds, check child and electrodes (placement on infant, connections with machine). *Allows accurate reading of child's breathing patterns.*

DOCUMENTATION

1. Time and date.
2. Sites of electrode placement.
3. How infant tolerated procedure.

Estimated time to complete procedure: *5 minutes.*

PROCEDURE 22

APPLYING A CARDIAC MONITOR

OVERVIEW

The cardiac monitor is used to keep track of the heart's electrical activity and rate. It is often used in conjunction with the apnea monitor when cardiorespiratory monitoring is needed for continuous assessment. It is important to follow the manufacturer's instructions whenever setting up the monitor. The monitor sounds an alarm when the infant's heart rate becomes higher or lower than the machine settings. If the alarm sounds, it is important to determine if the infant's heart rate is lower or higher than the machine settings or if the machine is not working properly.

EQUIPMENT

Cardiac monitor
Electrodes
Straps to hold electrodes in place
Alcohol wipes

GENERAL GUIDELINES

1. Check order for placement of cardiac monitor. *Ensures appropriate infant is monitored.*
2. Gather equipment. *Improves organization and effectiveness.*
3. Set high and low limits of machine. *Improves organization and effectiveness.*

4. Wash hands. *Reduces transmission of microorganisms.*
5. Prepare family. *Enhances cooperation and parental participation, and reduces anxiety and fear.*

PROCEDURE

1. Steps 1–5 of General Guidelines.
2. Place infant/child in a supine position. *Helps placement of electrodes on chest.*
3. Clean with alcohol wipes the area where the electrodes are to be applied; allow the area to dry. *Removes oils from skin so electrodes will adhere.*
4. Place electrodes on infant's chest: one on the left, one on the right, and one on the leg according to manufacturer's instructions. *Assures accurate reading of child's pulse.*
5. Turn machine on; if alarm sounds, check child and electrodes (placement on infant, connections with machine). *Assures accurate reading of child's pulse.*

DOCUMENTATION

1. Time and date.
2. Sites of electrode placement.
3. How infant tolerated procedure.

 Estimated time to complete procedure: *5–10 minutes.*

PROCEDURE 23

APPLYING A PULSE OXIMETER

OVERVIEW

Pulse oximetry is an easy, quick and fairly accurate method of assessing arterial blood oxygen saturation by using an external sensor. The most common site for placing the sensor in infants/children is either on the large toe or a finger. One side of the sensor contains light emitting diodes; the other side of the sensor contains a photo detector. As a beam of light passes through the finger/toe from the emitting diode to the photo detector, the amount of light absorbed by oxygenated and unoxygenated hemoglobin is measured. Unoxygenated hemoglobin absorbs more red light; oxygenated hemoglobin absorbs more infrared light. The arterial blood oxygen saturation is determined by the spectrum of light measured by the photo detector.

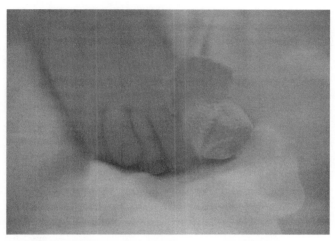

FIGURE III-11 Placement of pulse oximeter on toe.

EQUIPMENT

Pulse oximeter
Appropriate sensor probe

GENERAL GUIDELINES

1. Check order for placement of pulse oximeter. *Ensures appropriate patient is monitored.*
2. Gather equipment, including paper and pen, for recording vital signs. *Promotes organization and efficiency.*
3. Wash hands. *Reduces transmission of microorganisms.*
4. Prepare child and family in a quiet and nonthreatening manner. *Enhances cooperation and participation; reduces anxiety and fear, which can affect readings.*

PREPROCEDURE

1. Determine if the child has undergone a test that used an intravenous dye. *Intravenous dyes may interfere with pulse oximeter readings.*
2. Evaluate client status. *To determine client condition.*

PROCEDURE

1. Follow steps 1–4 of General Guidelines.
2. Select sensor site that is free of moisture and drainage. Assess capillary refill and proximal pulse. *Adequate perfusion necessary for accurate reading.*
   a. Infant: Big toe or foot (Figures III-11 and III-12).
   b. Toddler through adolescent: finger.

NOTE: *May also use earlobe.*

3. Cleanse site. Remove nail polish or artificial nails. *Nail polish and artificial nails alter results.*
4. Follow manufacturer's instructions for setting up oximeter. Connect sensor to oximeter, and set alarms as ordered. *Assures accurate reading.*
5. Position sensor with light-emitting diode (LED) and photosensor aligned on opposite sides of the selected site. *Prevents optical shunting, and ensures accurate results.*
6. Obtain reading. *Determines oxygen saturation.*
7. Watch pulse bar for pulse sensing. *To determine rate.*
8. Obtain arterial blood gas (ABG) if ordered. *Promotes confidence in oximetry readings.*
9. Cover sensor. *Ambient light can skew readings.*
10. Assess probe/sensor site every two to four hours. *Protects against skin breakdown; ensures correct placement.*
11. Rotate probe/sensor site every two hours for a spring-loaded sensor and every 4 hours for an adhesive sensor. *Maintains skin integrity. Assures accurate reading.*
12. Wash hands. *Reduces transmission of microorganisms.*

DOCUMENTATION

1. Pulse oximeter readings at regular intervals per agency policy.

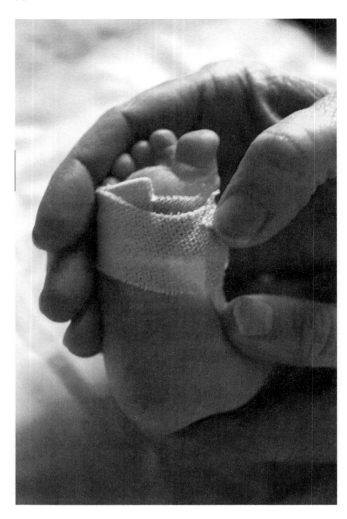

FIGURE III-12   Placement of pulse oximeter on foot.

2. Site sensor applied, when changed.
3. Skin condition at sensor site.
4. Setting of alarm limits.

 Estimated time to complete procedure: *5 minutes.*

UNIT IV

Specimen Collection

Specimen Collection

General Guidelines

1. Check physician's order. *Ensures appropriate specimen obtained from the correct child.*
2. Check child for allergies to any materials used, e.g., povidone-iodine. *To prevent allergic reaction.*
3. Prepare child and family. *Enhances cooperation/participation; reduces anxiety/fear.*

NOTE: *Have an assistant hold/comfort the child as necessary and in accordance with agency policy.*

4. Gather equipment. *Promotes organization and efficiency.*

5. Wash hands. Put on gloves. *Reduces transmission of microorganisms.*

Documentation

1. Time, source/site, specimen sent to lab (specify for what test).
2. Record results of any test performed on the unit.

Blood Drawing

OVERVIEW

Obtaining a blood sample is a common procedure for a variety of diagnostic tests. Blood test results are a source of valuable information to screen children for disease, to evaluate the progress of therapy, and to monitor the child's well-being. Commonly, it is the nurse who obtains the specimens.

There are three primary methods of obtaining blood specimens: venipuncture, skin puncture, or arterial stick. Venipuncture involves inserting a large bore needle into a vein and then attaching a syringe or Vacutainer tube for the collection of the specimen. Skin puncture (heel or finger stick) is the easiest and most common way to obtain a small specimen from the finger, toe, or heel. A lancet is used for the puncture, and a drop of blood is collected through a capillary tube. An arterial stick is the most complicated and requires special assessment skills and techniques.

PROCEDURE 24

PERFORMING CAPILLARY BLOOD DRAW
(HEEL AND FINGER STICK)

EQUIPMENT

Lancet
Cleansing solution
Cotton balls or 2 × 2 sponges, sterile
Gloves, nonsterile
Adhesive bandage
Appropriate sample container
Labels
Completed laboratory requisition forms

PROCEDURE

1. Steps 1–5 of General Guidelines.
2. Select site.
   a. Heel (infants younger than 1 year of age): Plantar surface beyond lateral and medial calcaneous. *Avoids arteries and veins; reduces risk of scar tissue formation, which may be painful when the infant begins to walk.*
   b. Great toe (children older than 1 year). Plantar surface; *avoids arteries and veins; reduced risk of scar tissue formation.*
   c. Finger: Side of ball of finger (third or fourth finger) across the fingerprint. *Avoids damage to nerve endings and calloused areas of the skin. If stick made along lines of fingerprint, blood will run down the finger.*
3. Apply moist compress to area for 5–15 minutes. *Facilitates blood supply to the area.*
4. Put on nonsterile gloves. *Reduces exposure to bloodborne pathogens.*
5. Remove compress and wash selected site with soap and water or antiseptic solution as specified by agency policy. *Reduces transmission of microorganisms.*

NOTE: *Use of alcohol for skin preparation may lead to rapid hemolysis. Povidone-iodine interferes with readings of Chemstrip and Dextrostix.*

6. Let area dry completely before puncture. *Damp area may dilute blood sample or hemolyze it, causing distorted values.*
7. Gently massage base of finger or heel, stroking toward selected puncture site. Do not touch the puncture site. *Massaging increases blood flow to the area. Excessive squeezing causes bruising, produces a sample that*

contains more plasma than cells, and can lead to hemolysis, causing falsely elevated potassium levels.
8. Isolate the puncture site using the nondominant hand to hold the child's hand or foot. Hold the selected site in a dependent position. *Increases blood supply to the puncture site* (Figures IV-1A and IV-1B).
   a. Heel: Support dorsum of foot with thumb and ankle with other fingers.
   b. Toe: Grasp foot across dorsum, support toe with thumb on plantar surface.
   c. Finger: Keep finger to be used extended and pointed downward.
9. Using the dominant hand, puncture the site at a 90° angle to the skin using a quick, forceful motion. Remove the lancet immediately. Do not use a slashing motion. *Provides blood sample with minimal discomfort to the child.*
10. Wipe away the first drop of blood using a sterile cotton ball or 2 × 2. *The first drop may contain*

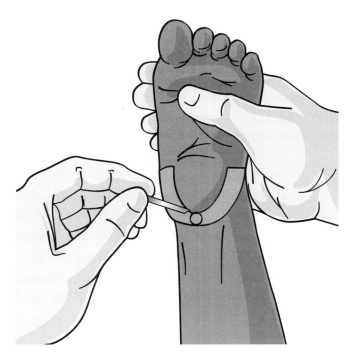

FIGURE IV-1A   U-shaped area denotes area to puncture with lancet.

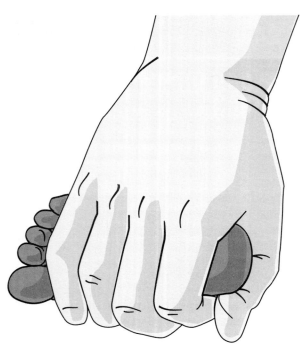

FIGURE IV-1B   Position that allows blood to drip.

traumatized blood cells and be contaminated by contact with the skin.

11. Allow blood to collect at puncture site. *To be sure there is adequate blood for the needed specimen.*

12. Allow blood to flow into the collecting tube (Figure IV-2). *Appropriate method of collecting capillary specimen.*

13. Wipe site with sterile cotton ball or 2 × 2 and apply pressure for two to three minutes. *Controls bleeding.*

14. Apply bandage if appropriate. *Prevents blood from getting on clothing.*

NOTE: *Use bandage with caution in infant and young children. Child may aspirate or swallow the bandage.*

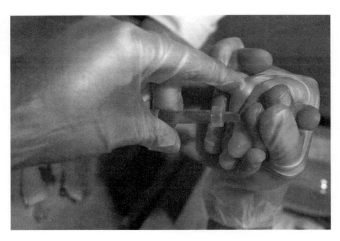

FIGURE IV-2   Position used when performing needle stick.

15. Discard equipment in appropriate container. *Consistent with handling of body fluids.*

16. Label specimen, place in appropriate bag or container along with laboratory requisition slips. *Ensures specimen is properly identified and appropriate test performed.*

17. Remove gloves. Wash hands. *Reduces transmission of microorganisms.*

18. Send specimens to laboratory. *To allow ordered tests to be conducted.*

DOCUMENTATION

1. Time, source/site, specimen sent to lab (specify for what test).
2. Record results of any test performed on the unit.

 Estimated time to complete procedure: *15 minutes.*

PROCEDURE 25

PERFORMING VENIPUNCTURE

EQUIPMENT

Syringe and needle (scalp vein or straight) or Vacutainer and needle
Appropriate blood collection tubes
Labels
Completed laboratory requisition forms
Tourniquet or rubber band
Adhesive bandage
Antiseptic pads (alcohol or povidone-iodine)
Gloves, nonsterile
Dry gauze pads (2 × 2 sponges, sterile)

PROCEDURE

1. Steps 1–5 of General Guidelines.
2. Prepare equipment so you are ready to obtain sample. *Promotes organization and efficiency.*
   a. Syringe method: Have syringe with appropriate needle attached. *A very small bore needle can damage red blood cells, leading to inaccurate results.*
   b. Vacutainer method: Attach double-ended needle to Vacutainer and have proper blood specimen tube resting inside the Vacutainer. Do not puncture the rubber stopper yet. *Vacuum is lost when stopper is punctured.*

NOTE: *Long end of needle punctures vein, short end punctures stopper.*

3. Raise or lower bed to a comfortable working height. *Maintains good body mechanics.*
4. Extend arm to form a straight line from shoulder to wrist; place a pillow or towel under upper arm to enhance extension; child should be in supine or semi-Fowler's position. *Protects against injury if child should become faint.*
5. Put on nonsterile gloves. *Protects from contact with blood-borne organisms.*
6. Apply tourniquet 3–4 inches above venipuncture site. *Provides improved visibility of veins as they dilate in response to decreased venous return from extremity to heart.*

NOTE: *Tourniquet should be able to be removed by pulling the end with a single motion.*

7. Check for distal pulse. If none, tourniquet is too tight and should be reapplied. *If too tight, arterial blood flow impeded.*

8. Have child open and close fist several times, leaving fist clenched prior to venipuncture. *Muscle contraction increases blood flow to the arm, increases venous distention, and enhances vein visibility.*

NOTE: *Vigorous motion may result in hemoconcentration of the specimen.*

9. Maintain tourniquet only one to two minutes. *Prolonged time may increase child's discomfort and alter some laboratory results, e.g., falsely high serum potassium.*
10. Identify best venipuncture site by palpation. Ideal site is straight, prominent vein that feels firm and slightly rebounds when palpated. *Straight, intact veins are easier to puncture. A thrombosed vein is rigid or rolls easily and is difficult to stick.*
11. Select site. If tourniquet has been on too long release it, wait one to two minutes and reapply. *Increases client comfort; ensures accuracy of results.*
12. Cleanse site with solution prescribed by the agency using circular motion at the site and extending 2 inches beyond the site. Allow to dry. *Cleans skin surface of bacteria that may cause site infection; allowing antiseptic to dry reduces stinging sensation.*
13. Remove needle cover and warn child will feel needle stick. *Child better able to control reactions when knows what to expect.*
14. Place thumb or forefinger of nondominant hand 1 inch below site and pull skin taut. *Helps stabilize the vein during insertion.*
15. Hold needle at 15°–30° angle from skin, bevel up. *Reduces chance of penetrating through vein on insertion. Causes less trauma to skin and vein.*
16. Slowly insert needle. *Prevents puncture through other side of vein.*
17. After entering vein, slowly lower needle toward skin. Thread needle along path of vein. *Decreases risk of penetrating other side of vein.*
18. Check for blood flow. *To be sure needle in vein.*
    a. Syringe method: Gently pull back on plunger and look for blood return. Obtain desired amount of blood. *Allows blood to flow into syringe.*
    b. Vacutainer method.
       1. Hold Vacutainer securely and advance specimen tube into needle of holder, being careful not to advance the needle further into the vein. Blood should flow into the collection tube. *Pushing the needle through the stopper breaks the vacuum*

and causes blood to flow into the collection tube. Failure of blood to appear in collection tube indicates that vacuum in tube has been lost or needle is not in vein.

   2. After collection tube full, grasp Vacutainer firmly and remove tube; insert additional collection tubes as needed. *To be able to conduct all tests ordered.*

19. After specimen collection complete, remove tourniquet. *Reduces bleeding from pressure when needle is removed.*

20. Apply 2 × 2 gauze over puncture site without applying pressure and quickly remove the needle from the vein. *Positions gauze for removal and helps to gently prevent skin from pulling with needle removal.*

21. Immediately apply pressure over venipuncture site with gauze for two to three minutes or until the bleeding has stopped. Hold arm straight. *Stops bleeding and minimizes formation of a hematoma. Bending the elbow can facilitate hematoma formation.*

22. If syringe method used to obtain sample, transfer blood to appropriate specimen tube.

   a. Carefully transfer blood to the appropriate specimen container. *If specimen not handled carefully, red blood cells can be destroyed and false readings may be obtained.*

   b. Using one hand, insert the needle into the appropriate collection tube and allow vacuum to fill the tube. *Allowing tube to fill slowly helps prevent hemolysis. Using one hand helps reduce chance of needle-stick injury.*

   c. Alternative method is to remove stopper from collection tube and needle from syringe. Fill the tube with the amount of blood needed and replace the stopper. *This method allows you to control speed and amount of fill in collection tubes.*

   d. If any specimen tubes contain additives, gently rotate back and forth 8–10 times. *Ensures additive is properly mixed throughout the specimen.*

23. Inspect the puncture site for bleeding. Reapply a clean tape and gauze if necessary. *Keeps site clean and dry.*

24. Assist child to a comfortable position. *Enhances cooperation in future.*

25. Check tubes for external blood. If any, wipe away with alcohol. *Prevents contamination of equipment and other personnel.*

26. Check tubes for proper labeling. Place tubes in appropriate bag or container along with laboratory requisition slips. *Ensures specimen properly identified and appropriate test performed.*

27. Dispose of equipment in appropriate manner. *Consistent with handling of body fluids.*

28. Remove gloves. Wash hands. *Reduces transmission of microorganisms.*

29. Send specimens to laboratory. *To allow ordered tests to be conducted.*

DOCUMENTATION

1. Time, source/site, specimen sent to lab (specify for what test).
2. Record results of any test performed on the unit.

⧖ **Estimated time to complete procedure:** *10–15 minutes.*

PROCEDURE 26

DRAWING BLOOD FROM A CENTRAL VENOUS CATHETER

EQUIPMENT

Povidone-iodine wipes
Alcohol wipes
10 cc syringes (4)
Heparin (10 u/cc)
Normal saline flush
Gloves, nonsterile
Povidone-iodine swabs or sticks (culture)
Mask (culture)
Gloves, sterile (culture)

PROCEDURE

1. Steps 1–5 of General Guidelines.
2. Position child as necessary to complete procedure. *So area is visible where blood drawn.*
3. Select lumen for blood withdrawal when child has multilumen catheter. *So correct lumen used.*
   a. Preferable to select largest lumen.
   b. Avoid using lumen where total parenteral nutrition (TPN) currently infusing if possible.
   c. Check for medication/serum sample interactions.
4. Turn off all infusions; clamp other infusions with multilumen catheters. *Avoids dilution or contamination of specimen with infusion solution.*
5. Put on nonsterile gloves. *Protects from contact with blood-borne organisms; reduces transmission of microorganisms.*
6. Prep end of injection port as specified by agency policy. One method is to wipe off injection port with three povidone-iodine wipes; allow to dry. Wipe with alcohol wipes. *Reduces transmission of microorganisms. Povidone-iodine must dry to be effective. Using alcohol removes povidone-iodine, which could be introduced into the central line.*

NOTE: *Agency policy may require removal of injection port when drawing blood for culture. When this is required, a new injection cap is placed after blood sample is obtained. When drawing blood for culture, wear sterile gloves. Put gloves on after cleansing injection port to maintain sterility of gloves.*

7. Wipe injection port with alcohol wipe. *Prevents povidone-iodine from being introduced into the central line.*

8. Attach syringe with saline flush to injection port. Flush with 5–10 cc, enough to equal two to three times the intraluminal volume of the catheter. *Clears the tubing of all infusion solution.*

NOTE: *Small amounts are used with neonates.*

9. Attach empty syringe to catheter. Withdraw blood equal to two to three times the intraluminal volume of the catheter. *Clears the catheter and prevents contamination of the blood sample with infusion solution.*

NOTE: *Policy regarding return of withdrawn blood varies from agency to agency. Discard or return in accordance with agency policy. If blood is to be returned, it must be drawn into a syringe that contains heparin, generally 1 cc of heparin (10 u/cc).*

10. Attach empty syringe onto injection port and withdraw volume of blood needed for ordered lab tests. *So have sufficient blood to conduct tests.*
11. Discard or return blood per agency policy. Discard in appropriate container. *Maintains body fluid precautions.*
12. Attach syringe and flush with normal saline. *Clears blood from catheter and prevents clotting in or blockage of catheter.*
13. Resume previous infusion(s) or heparin/saline flush per agency policy. *To maintain patency of line.*
14. Place blood into appropriate containers. *For transport to laboratory.*
15. Label containers and place specimen in appropriate bag or container along with laboratory requisition slips. *Ensures specimen is properly identified and appropriate test is performed.*
16. Remove gloves. Wash hands. *Reduces transmission of microorganisms.*

DOCUMENTATION

1. Time, source/site, specimen sent to lab (specify for what test).
2. Record results of any test performed on the unit.

 Estimated time to complete procedure: *10 minutes.*

PROCEDURE 27

MEASURING ARTERIAL BLOOD GASES

OVERVIEW

Arterial blood gases are measured to assess a client's oxygenation, ventilation, and acid-base balance. The blood sample is obtained from an artery and analyzed for arterial blood pH, partial pressure of oxygen (PaO2), partial pressure of carbon dioxide (paCO2), and arterial oxygen saturation (SaO2). Analysis provides information on the child's respiratory or metabolic status and response to disease process.

EQUIPMENT

Heparinized syringe with cap, 3 ml (check agency policy for heparin solution use)
23–25 gauge needle
Povidone-iodine and alcohol swabs
Gauze pad, 2 × 2
Heparin, 1:1000 solution
Cup with crushed ice
Label with date, time, and child's name
Laboratory requisition
Disposable gloves
Protective eyewear

PROCEDURE

1. Steps 1–5 of General Guidelines.
2. Put on protective eyewear. *Prevents exposure to microorganisms.*
3. Prepare syringe with heparin. *Needed if a heparinized syringe is not available.*
    a. Aspirate 0.5 ml sodium heparin (1000 U/ml) into syringe from vial. *Prevents blood from clotting before analysis is performed.*
    b. Withdraw plunger entire length of syringe and eject all heparin out of syringe. *Coats barrel of syringe with heparin. More than 0.25 ml of sodium heparin in 3 ml of blood may affect pH level.*
4. Select safest and most accessible site for arterial blood gas (ABG) sample. *Arterial puncture may result in spasm, clotting, or hematoma, which could reduce blood flow, so collateral circulation is essential.*
    a. Perform Allen's test. Have child make a tight fist, and apply direct pressure to both radial and ulnar arteries. When child opens hand, release pressure over ulnar artery and observe color of fingers, thumb, and hand. Fingers should flush within 15

seconds—this is a positive Allen's test. *Determines adequate blood flow to the hand by removing blood from hand, obstructing blood flow, then allowing blood to flow into hand through ulnar artery. Indicates that collateral flow is positive.*
    b. If Allen's test is positive, use the radial artery. *The radial artery is the safest and most accessible site.*
    c. Brachial artery should be used if radial artery is inaccessible or Allen's test is negative. *Has collateral blood flow but is less superficial and more difficult to palpate and stabilize, and has risk of damage to adjacent structures (brachial nerve or vein).*
    d. Femoral artery should be used only by specially trained personnel. *Has no collateral blood flow if obstructed below the inguinal ligament, is difficult to stabilize, and is adjacent to femoral vein. This is the best artery to use in emergency situations (cardiac arrest, shock).*
5. Wash hands. *Reduces number of organisms.*
6. Put on nonsterile gloves. *Reduces exposure to bloodborne pathogens.*
7. Palpate selected radial site with fingertips. *Determines area of maximal impulse for puncture site.*
8. Stabilize artery by slightly hyperextending wrist. *Facilitates successful insertion of needle.*
9. Wash selected site with alcohol in circular motion. *Reduces number of bacteria on skin surface.*
10. Let area dry completely before puncture. *Damp area may dilute blood sample or hemolyze it, causing distorted values.*
11. Hold alcohol swab in fingers of one hand while keeping a fingertip from the other hand on the artery. *Keeps swab accessible during procedure.*
12. Insert the needle with bevel up into artery at a 45° angle. *Allows for better arterial flow into needle. Oblique hole in artery seals more easily.*
13. Hold the needle and syringe still when blood appears in the syringe. *Prevents traversing needle through artery.*
14. Allow arterial pulsing to slowly pump 2–3 ml of blood into heparinzed syringe. *Prevents air bubbles from entering sample, which can alter results.*
15. When sample is collected, hold alcohol swab over puncture site and withdraw needle. *Swab minimizes pulling of skin as needle is withdrawn.*
16. Apply pressure with alcohol swab over site for 5 minutes or 10 minutes if child has bleeding disorder or is on anticoagulant therapy. *Ensures adequate coagulation at puncture site.*

17. Examine site for bleeding, change or disappearance of pulse, color of hand. *Determines need for further treatment (continue to exert pressure, which shows change in blood flow to hand; color indicates whether there is obstruction to blood flow to hand).*

18. Apply bandage if appropriate. *Protects site.*

NOTE: *Use bandage with caution in infant and young children. Child may aspirate or swallow the bandage.*

19. Discard equipment in appropriate container. *Consistent with handling of body fluids.*

20. Remove gloves. *Reduces transmission of organisms.*

21. Wash hands. *Reduces transmission of organisms.*

22. Prepare sample and send to laboratory. *So ordered test can be run.*

    a. Expel air bubbles from syringe. *Prevents false ABG results.*

    b. Label syringe with client identification. *Ensures results are correct for child.*

    c. Place syringe in cup of crushed ice. *Reduces blood cell metabolism.*

    d. Fill out requisition form, including amount of oxygen child is receiving (e.g., 2 liters O2 by nasal cannula, room air, 70% on ventilator). *Ensures proper identification and condition of child.*

DOCUMENTATION

1. Time, source/site, specimen sent to lab (specify for what test).

2. Record results of any test performed on the unit.

 Estimated time to complete procedure: *10–15 minutes.*

Nose, Throat, and Sputum Specimens

OVERVIEW

A nose, throat, or sputum specimen is a simple diagnostic tool for clients with signs or symptoms of upper respiratory or sinus infections. Nose and throat specimens are collected from the client using a sterile swab, whereas sputum specimens are collected in a sterile cup. Sputum specimens can also be obtained via a specimen trap connected to suction, which is then sent to the laboratory.

PROCEDURE 28

OBTAINING A NASOPHARYNGEAL SWAB

OVERVIEW

A nasopharyngeal swab is obtained if the client has signs and symptoms of an upper respiratory or sinus infection. A sterile swab is used to collect the specimen and then it is placed in a culture medium to allow any pathogens on the swab to grow.

EQUIPMENT

Gloves, nonsterile
Penlight
Nasopharyngeal applicator (swab or flexible wire) in sterile culture tube
Bulb syringe (for infant)

PROCEDURE

1. Steps 1–5 of General Guidelines.
2. Put on nonsterile gloves. *Protects the nurse from contact with respiratory secretions.*
3. Position child for easy access to nose. *To allow specimen to be obtained successfully.*
4. Prepare applicator for use by loosening the top of the container. *Avoids contamination of applicator.*
5. Have child blow nose. Use bulb syringe for an infant. *Clears nasal passage of mucus containing resident bacteria.*
6. Ask child to tilt head back. *Promotes visualization.*
7. Check nostrils for patency using the penlight, or ask child to occlude one nostril and then the other and exhale. *Determines which nasal passage is optimal for obtaining specimen.*
8. Bend nasopharyngeal applicator into a curve and remove from package. *Facilitates insertion of applicator from nares into pharyngeal area.*
9. Insert applicator into nostril gently until it reaches inflamed area. *Ensures collection of appropriate exudate* (Figure IV-3).
10. Rotate applicator quickly and remove without touching adjacent structures. *Minimizes child's discomfort. Prevents contamination with normal nasal flora resulting in erroneous culture results.*
11. Places applicator in culture tube. Crush ampule at the bottom. *Places applicator tip in culture medium to preserve bacteria.*

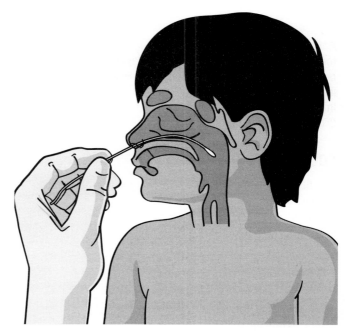

FIGURE IV-3 Obtaining a nasopharyngeal specimen.

12. Secure top to culture tube. Label specimen and place in appropriate bag or container along with laboratory requisition slips. *So specimen remains intact; so ordered tests can be carried out.*
13. Dispose of any used materials in appropriate container. *Is consistent with body fluid precautions.*
14. Remove gloves. Wash hands. *Reduces transmission of microorganisms.*
15. Send specimen to lab. *So ordered test can be carried out.*

DOCUMENTATION

1. Time, source/site, specimen sent to lab (specify for what test).
2. Record results of any test performed on the unit.

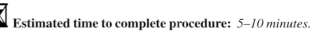 **Estimated time to complete procedure:** *5–10 minutes.*

PROCEDURE 29

OBTAINING A THROAT CULTURE

OVERVIEW

A throat culture is obtained if the client has signs and symptoms of a sore throat which may or may not be accompanied by an upper respiratory infection. A sterile swab is used to collect the specimen from the back of the throat. It is then placed in a culture medium to allow any pathogens on the swab to grow, or examined under a microscope for microorganisms.

EQUIPMENT

Applicator (swab or flexible wire) in sterile culture tube
Tongue blade
Penlight
Gloves, nonsterile

PROCEDURE

1. Steps 1–5 of General Guidelines.
2. Position child for access to throat. *So can successfully obtain specimen.*
3. Prepare applicator for use by loosening the top of the container. *Avoids contamination of applicator.*
4. Ask child to tilt head back, open mouth, and say "ah." *Promotes visualization, relaxes throat muscles, and minimizes gag reflex.*
5. Depress anterior third of tongue with tongue blade. *Promotes visualization.*

NOTE: *May induce gag reflex; be careful.*

6. Insert swab without touching lips, teeth, or tongue. *Prevents contamination with oral flora.*

7. Swab tonsillar area from side to side with quick, gentle motion. *Ensures collection of microorganisms for testing and minimizes child's discomfort.*

NOTE: *Swab only one side. Check agency policy regarding obtaining a second specimen from the other side.*

8. Withdraw swab without touching adjacent structure. *Avoids contamination of the specimen.*
9. Place applicator in culture tube. Crush ampule at the bottom. *Places applicator tip in culture medium to preserve bacteria.*
10. Secure top to culture tube. Label specimen and place in appropriate bag or container along with laboratory requisition slips. *So specimen remains intact; so ordered tests can be conducted.*
11. Dispose of any used materials in appropriate container. *Is consistent with body fluid precautions.*
12. Remove gloves. Wash hands. *Reduces transmission of microorganisms.*
13. Send specimen to lab. *So ordered tests can be conducted on specimen.*

DOCUMENTATION

1. Time, source/site, specimen sent to lab (specify for what test).
2. Record results of any test performed on the unit.

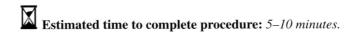 **Estimated time to complete procedure:** *5–10 minutes.*

PROCEDURE 30

COLLECTING SPUTUM

OVERVIEW

When given appropriate directions, older children and adolescents are able to cough deeply and provide adequate sputum specimens. Sputum specimens can be obtained from infants and younger children by nasopharyngeal suctioning.

EQUIPMENT

Gloves, nonsterile
Sterile specimen container

PROCEDURE

1. Steps 1–5 of General Guidelines.
2. Emphasize to child that the specimen must be sputum, coughed up from the back of the throat or lungs. *Promotes client cooperation; assumes adequate specimen.*
3. Put on nonsterile gloves. *Protects the nurse from contact with respiratory secretions.*
4. Remove the lid from the sterile specimen container. *Specimen is to be collected in a sterile cup to prevent contamination; opening the lid facilitates easy access when the specimen is ready to be placed in the container.*
5. Encourage child to take several deep breaths and then cough deeply. *Helps loosen secretions so a specimen can be obtained.*
6. Ask child to cough sputum up and spit it directly into the sterile specimen container without touching the inside of the container. *Prevents contamination of the specimen.*
7. Close the lid of the container without touching the inside of the lid or the container. *Prevents contamination of the specimen.*
8. Provide child with tissue and make him/her comfortable. *Promotes comfort; enhances future cooperation.*
9. Remove gloves. *Reduces transmission of organisms.*
10. Wash hands. *Reduces transmission of microorganisms.*
11. Label specimen container. *Identifies child's specimen.*
12. Send specimen to lab. *So appropriate tests can be conducted on specimens.*

DOCUMENTATION

1. Time, source/site, specimen sent to lab (specify for what test).
2. Record results of any test performed on the unit.

▧ **Estimated time to complete procedure:** *5–10 minutes.*

Stool Specimens

PROCEDURE 31

COLLECTING STOOL SPECIMENS

OVERVIEW

Stool specimens are obtained to detect the presence of occult blood as well as bacteria or other organisms in the intestinal tract. Both tests require a small amount of stool and are easy to conduct. Stool samples can be obtained from stool collected in a diaper or a cup, or from a rectal swab. However, the test for parasites requires larger size samples and is usually submitted in a stool specimen container.

Collecting Stool Specimens

EQUIPMENT

Diaper (nontoilet-trained child)
Plastic liner for diaper (if stool watery)
Bedpan or "hat" (older child)
Tongue blade
Specimen container
Gloves, nonsterile

PROCEDURE

1. Steps 1–5 of General Guidelines.
2. If stool is watery, line diaper with plastic. *Allows watery stool to be collected rather than absorbed into diaper.*
3. Check diaper for stool at frequent intervals. Wear exam gloves as for any diaper change. *To determine if specimen obtained; to reduce transmission of microorganisms.*

NOTE: *Stool may be obtained from bedpan or "hat" of older child.*

4. Put on nonsterile gloves. *Protects nurse from contact with body fluids.*
5. Remove diaper. Set soiled diaper aside. Clean perineum and put on a clean diaper. *Prevents skin irritation.*
6. Remove small amount of stool from diaper, bedpan, or hat with a tongue blade. *Only need a small amount for specimen sent to laboratory.*
7. Place specimen in container. *For transport to laboratory for examination and testing; to reduce transmission of microorganisms.*

8. Label specimen and place in appropriate bag or container along with the laboratory requisition slip. *Ensures specimen properly identified and the appropriate test is done.*
9. Remove gloves. Wash hands. *Reduces transmission of microorganisms.*

NOTE: *To obtain a swab stool specimen, insert swab ½–¾ inch into rectum. Place swab in culture tube as described under nasopharyngeal specimens (Figure IV-4).*

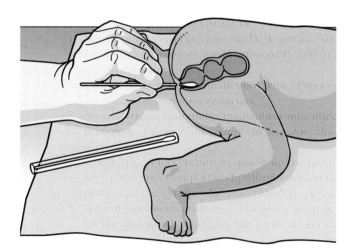

FIGURE IV-4   Using a rectal swab to obtain a stool specimen.

DOCUMENTATION

1. Time specimen collected.
2. Color and consistency of stool.
3. Test collected for.
4. Condition of skin.

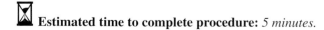

Estimated time to complete procedure: *5 minutes.*

PROCEDURE 32

OBTAINING A STOOL SPECIMEN
FOR THE FECAL OCCULT BLOOD TEST (FOBT)

EQUIPMENT NEEDED

Diaper (untoilet-trained child)
Plastic liner for diaper (if stool watery)
Bedpan or "hat" (older child)
Tongue blade
Occult blood test kit
Gloves, nonsterile

PROCEDURE

1. Steps 1–5 of General Guidelines.
2. If stool is watery, line diaper with plastic. *Allows watery stool to be collected rather than absorbed into diaper.*
3. Check diaper for stool at frequent intervals. Wear exam gloves as for any diaper change. *To determine if specimen obtained; to reduce transmission of microorganisms.*

NOTE: *Stool may be obtained from bedpan or "hat" of older child.*

4. Put on nonsterile gloves. *Protects nurse from contact with body fluids.*
5. Remove diaper. Set soiled diaper aside. Clean perineum and put on a clean diaper. *Prevents skin irritation.*
6. Remove small amount of stool from diaper, bedpan, or "hat" with a tongue blade. *Only need a small amount for specimen sent to lab; to reduce transmission of microorganisms.*
7. Read and follow the manufacturer's instructions. *Ensures accurate results.*

8. Open flap of slide and smear thin sample of feces on paper in first box. *Guiac-impregnated paper is sensitive to fecal blood.*
9. Apply feces from a different area or the specimen to the second box. *Occult blood from upper GI tract is not always equally dispersed throughout the stool.*
10. Close slide cover and turn to reverse side. Open flap and apply two drops of developing solution to each sample box and on each control box according to the manufacturer's instructions. *Developing solution penetrates fecal specimen through the paper.*
11. Note color change after 60 seconds or according to manufacturer's instructions. *Bluish color indicates the presence of occult blood. Control box color can be used for comparison. No change in color is negative.*
12. Dispose of slide and applicator wrapped in paper towel in proper receptacle. *Reduces transfer of microorganisms.*
13. Remove gloves. *Reduces transfer of microorganisms.*
14. Wash hands. *Reduces transfer of microorganisms.*

DOCUMENTATION

1. Time specimen collected.
2. Color and consistency of stool.
3. Test collected for.
4. Results of test.

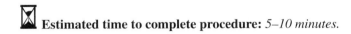 **Estimated time to complete procedure:** *5–10 minutes.*

Urine Specimens

OVERVIEW

Urine specimens are obtained to determine the levels of glucose, blood, acetone, bilirubin, protein, drugs, hormones, metals, and electrolytes, and to determine whether or not the child has an infection. Urine is also evaluated for pH, specific gravity, crystals, or other substances.

Urine specimens are collected from infants and young children who are not toilet trained by using a urine collecting bag. A clean-catch urine specimen is often obtained if the child is older or is an adolescent.

PROCEDURE 33

COLLECTING A URINE SPECIMEN WITH INFANT OR YOUNG CHILD

EQUIPMENT

Urine collector/bag (newborn or pediatric size as appropriate)
Specimen container
Gloves, nonsterile
Sterile water
Antiseptic solution or soap
Sterile cotton balls or 4 × 4s

PROCEDURE

1. Steps 1–5 of General Guidelines.
2. Put on nonsterile gloves. *Protects nurse from contact with body fluids and microorganisms.*
3. Position child on back with legs in froglike position to expose the genitalia. *Facilitates cleansing and allows proper placement of collection bag.*
4. Cleanse genitalia. *To wash off possible contaminants.*
   a. Male.
      1. Wipe the tip of the penis with a cotton ball soaked with soap solution. Use a circular motion going from the tip of the penis toward the scrotum. If not circumcised, retract the foreskin. *Cleans from least contaminated to most contaminated area. Retraction of the foreskin allows cleaning at the meatus.*

   NOTE: *If the foreskin does not retract easily, do not force.*

      2. Repeat cleansing process with a cotton ball soaked with sterile water. *Rinses soap solution from the area and prevents contamination of the specimen with the soap solution.*
      3. Let air dry. *So collection bag will stick to skin.*
      4. Replace foreskin if necessary. *Prevents swelling or injury, which may make it difficult to replace the foreskin later and could interfere with urinary elimination.*
   b. Female.
      1. Wipe labia majora with sterile cotton ball and soap solution from front to back (clitoris to anus). Wash only once with each cotton ball. *Prevents contamination of genitalia from anus and prevents contamination of urine specimen.*
      2. Spread labia apart with one hand, using other hand to wipe labia minora as described above. *Allows cleaning the area around the meatus.*

3. Repeat procedure with sterile cotton ball saturated with sterile water. *Rinses soap from area and prevents contamination of the specimen with soap solution.*
4. Let air dry. *So collection bag will stick to skin.*
5. Remove paper backing from adhesive surface of collection bag. *So adhesive surface will come in contact with skin.*
6. Apply collection bag and press adhesive firmly against skin. *Proper placement decreases possibility of needing to repeat procedure. Prevents leakage of urine* (Figure IV-5).
   a. Male: Insert penis through opening in bag. *So urine will flow into bag.*
   b. Female: Apply opening over vulva and beneath urethral orifice. *So urine will flow into bag.*
7. Diaper child and make him or her comfortable. *So anxiety is reduced.*
8. Remove gloves. Wash hands. *Reduces transmission of microorganisms.*
9. Check every 30–60 minutes for appearance of urine in bag. *Lessens likelihood of losing specimen.*

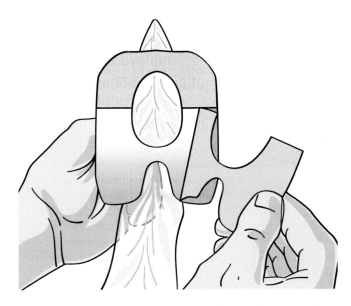

FIGURE IV-5 Urine collection. A. Protective paper is removed from bottom half.

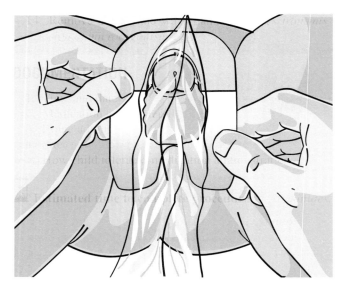

FIGURE IV-5   B. Place bag over penis and scrotum (or vagina). Press adhesive to skin. Work outward pressing adhesive firmly. Remove backing from top half, press firmly, and keep wrinkle-free.

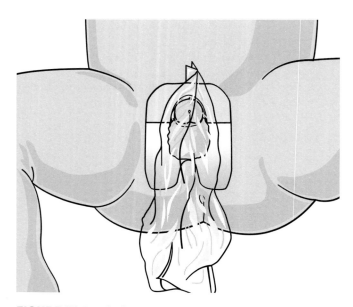

FIGURE IV-5   C. Secured urine collection bag.

10. When child has voided, put on nonsterile gloves, gently remove bag, and place urine in specimen container. *Protects nurse from contact with body fluids and microorganisms.*

11. Cleanse and dry area and rediaper. *Prevents skin irritation.*

12. Remove gloves. Wash hands. *Reduces transmission of microorganisms.*

13. Label specimen and place in appropriate bag or container along with the laboratory requisition slip. *Ensures specimen is properly identified and appropriate test is performed.*

14. Remove gloves. Wash hands. *Reduces transmission of microorganisms.*

15. Send specimen to laboratory. *So appropriate tests can be conducted on specimen.*

DOCUMENTATION

1. Time specimen collected.
2. Amount of urine collected.
3. Color of urine.
4. Type of test to be performed.
5. Condition of skin of perineal area.

Estimated time to complete procedure: *10–15 minutes.*

PROCEDURE 34

COLLECTING A MIDSTREAM, CLEAN-CATCH URINE SPECIMEN WITH OLDER CHILD

EQUIPMENT

Urine specimen container, sterile
Washcloths, cotton balls, or softnets
Antiseptic solution or soap
Sterile water
Bedpan or urinal if child on bedrest
Gloves, nonsterile

PROCEDURE

1. Steps 1–5 of General Guidelines.
2. Moisten half of washcloths, cotton balls, or softnets with soap solution and half with water. *Half used to wash area; half used to rinse area.*
3. Put on nonsterile gloves. *Protects from contact with body fluids.*
4. Cleanse area. *To remove microorganisms.*
   a. Male.
      1. Wipe tip of penis in circular motion downward toward shaft. Wipe only once with each cloth or cotton ball. Repeat until comes away clean. If uncircumcised, retract foreskin before cleansing. Retract only if it retracts easily, and replace foreskin after cleansing. *Maintains asepsis by cleaning from least to most contaminated area.*
2. Repeat process using water to rinse away all soap. *Removes soap or antiseptic solution, which could contaminate the specimen.*
   b. Female.
      1. Spread the labia major with one hand and wipe from front to back once with each cloth or cotton ball. Repeat until comes away clean. *Maintains asepsis by cleaning from least contaminated to most contaminated area.*

2. Repeat process with water to rinse away all soap. *Removes soap or antiseptic solution, which could contaminate the specimen.*

NOTE: *Older children can clean themselves. They should be instructed to wash their hands and then clean in manner as described above.*

5. Have child start to void into a receptacle (e.g., bedpan, "hat"); after a few drops, stop flow, then urinate into sterile container. Collect enough urine for a specimen, approximately 30–50 cc. *Avoids contamination of urine by bacteria at urinary oriface.*
6. Allow child to finish voiding in receptacle. *Avoids contamination of urine.*
7. Label specimen and place in appropriate bag or container along with laboratory requisition slip. *Ensures specimen is properly identified and correct test is performed.*
8. Remove gloves. Wash hands. *Reduces transmission of microorganisms.*
9. Send specimen to lab. *So appropriate tests can be conducted on specimen.*

DOCUMENTATION

1. Time specimen collected.
2. Amount of urine collected.
3. Color of urine.
4. Type of test to be performed.
5. Condition of skin of perineal area.

⧗ **Estimated time to complete procedure:** *10–15 minutes.*

Wound Culture

OVERVIEW

Altered wound healing is often the result of bacterial contamination. If the amount of bacteria in the wound is sufficient or the child's immune defenses are compromised, infection may result and become apparent within a few days. Infection slows healing by prolonging the inflammatory phase of healing, competing for nutrients, and producing chemicals and enzymes that are damaging to the tissues. Identification of the infectious agent is an important step in wound healing.

PROCEDURE 35

OBTAINING A WOUND CULTURE

EQUIPMENT

Nonsterile gloves
Sterile gloves
Dressing supplies
Normal saline and irrigation tray
Culture tube
Sterile swab
Moisture-proof container or bag

PROCEDURE

1. Steps 1–5 of General Guidelines.
2. Put on nonsterile gloves. *Protects nurse from contact with body fluids and microorganisms.*
3. Remove old dressing. Place old dressing in moisture-proof container, and remove and discard gloves *Reduces transmission of microorganisms; makes wound accessible for culture.*
4. Wash hands again. *Reduces transmission of microorganisms.*
5. Open dressing supplies using sterile technique. *Maintains sterile environment.*
6. Apply sterile gloves. *Maintains sterile environment.*
7. Assess wound's appearance; note quality, quantity, color, and odor of discharge. *Provides information about the amount and character of the wound's drainage before irrigation. Reddened areas and heavy drainage suggest infection.*
8. Irrigate wound with normal saline prior to culturing; do not irrigate with antiseptic. *Irrigation decreases the risk of culturing normal flora and other exudates such as protein; irrigating with an antiseptic prior to culturing destroys microorganisms.*
9. Using a sterile gauze pad, absorb the excess saline, then discard the pad. *Removal of excess irrigant prevents maceration of tissue due to excess moisture.*
10. Remove the culture tube from the packaging; remove the culture swab from the culture tube and gently roll the swab over the granulation tissue. Avoid eschar and wound edges. *Decreases chance of collecting superficial skin microorganisms.*
11. Replace the swab into the culture tube, being careful not to touch the swab to the outside of the tube; recap the tube; crush the ampule of medium located in the bottom of cap of the tube. *Avoids contaminating with microorganisms; releases medium to surround the swab.*
12. Remove gloves, wash hands, apply sterile gloves. Dress the wound with sterile dressing. *Prevents wound contamination.*
13. Label specimen container. *So specimen can be traced to correct client.*
14. Remove gloves. *Reduces transmission of microorganisms.*
15. Wash hands. *Reduces transmission of microorganisms.*
16. Label specimen container. *Identifies child's specimen.*
17. Send specimen to lab. *So appropriate tests can be conducted on specimen.*

DOCUMENTATION

1. Time and date specimen collected/dressing changed.
2. Wound and drainage appearance.
3. What was done with specimen.
4. Kind of dressing reapplied.

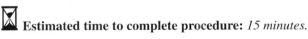 **Estimated time to complete procedure:** *15 minutes.*

Diagnostic Tests

Diagnostic tests

OVERVIEW

The child's history and presenting symptoms determine which diagnostic procedures are needed to formulate a medical diagnosis and the appropriate treatment. The role of the nurse in diagnostic testing is to teach the child/family about the procedures involved in diagnostic testing, the steps taken in preparation for the specific test, and the care following the procedure. The nurse may also assist in performing some of the invasive and noninvasive procedures.

General Guidelines

1. Explain procedure to child and family. *Enhances cooperation and participation and reduces anxiety and fear.*
2. Obtain signed consent from parent or legal guardian. *Legally and ethically needed before carrying out an invasive procedure.*
3. Gather equipment. *Promotes organization and efficiency.*
4. If possible, have child void before procedure. *Promotes comfort and avoids interruption of procedure.*
5. Wash hands. *Reduces transmission of microorganisms.*

PROCEDURE 36

ASSISTING DURING LUMBAR PUNCTURE

EQUIPMENT

Spinal tap (lumbar puncture) tray:
    Antiseptic solution
    Sterile drape
    3-way stopcock
    Spinal fluid pressure manometer
    Lumbar puncture needle (various sizes)
    Fluid collection tubes (3 or 4)
Gloves, sterile (physician)
Gloves, nonsterile (nurse)
Local anesthetic
Band-Aid or 2 × 2 gauze
Adhesive bandage
Gauze sponges

PROCEDURE

1. Steps 1–5 of General Guidelines.
2. Place child in a knee-to-chest position, either recumbent or seated, with neck flexed toward knees. *Provides maximal separation of vertebral bodies and allows access to spinal canal.*
   a. Recumbent position (lateral recumbent) (Figure V-1).
      1. Infant or young child.
         a. Restrain by placing one arm under child's flexed knees and grasping child's wrists. *Restrains both upper and lower extremities.*
         b. Place other arm posteriorly around child's neck and shoulders. *Restrains upper extremities.*

2. Older child.
   a. Child may grasp knees with hands. *Restrains lower extremities.*
   b. May place a pillow between the knees. *Prevents the upper leg from rolling forward.*
   c. Nurse helps hold arms and legs in flexed position. *Restrains both upper and lower extremities.*

NOTE: *It may require someone with strength to safely restrain the child during the procedure.*

   b. Sitting position.
      1. Older child.
         a. Sit on table with elbows resting on knees.
         b. Place pillow in front of child and instruct child to grab it. *Helps prevent child from moving.*
      2. Small infant (Figure V-2).
         a. Hold in sitting position. *Helps restrain child.*
         b. Flex thighs on abdomen and grab elbows and knees with hands. *Flexes spine at appropriate angle.*

NOTE: *This position is possible only with a small infant who is unable to struggle or with an older child who will cooperate without restraint.*

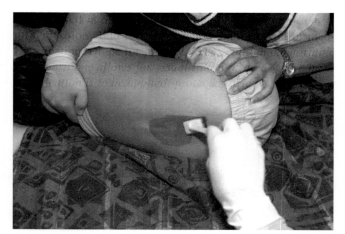

FIGURE V-1   Side-lying position for lumbar puncture.

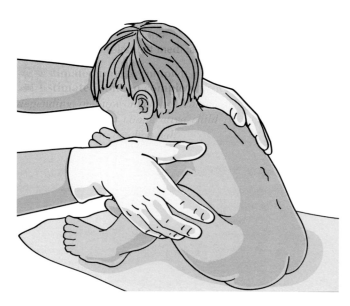

FIGURE V-2   Sitting position for lumbar puncture.

3. Once child is positioned, the physician drapes the back, identifies and cleanses the puncture area, infiltrates the area around the puncture site with local anesthetic, and carries out the procedure. Strict aseptic technique is maintained throughout. *Procedure for collecting spinal fluid.*

4. See Specimen Collection.

5. During the procedure, remind the child not to cough and to breathe slowly and deeply. *Coughing or changes in breathing increase cerebrospinal fluid (CSF) pressure, giving a false reading.*

6. Monitor for complications throughout the procedure; changes in level of consciousness (LOC); pupil size and reactivity; respiratory status; vital signs (VS); numbness, tingling, or pain radiating down the legs. *These are signs of complications.*

7. After the procedure, continue to observe/monitor for complications as well as:
   a. VS, LOC, and motor activity every 15 minutes for 1 hour, then every 30 minutes for 1 hour or according to agency policy. *To determine if complications occurring.*
   b. Bleeding or CSF leakage at puncture site every 4 hours for 24 hours or according to agency policy. *To determine if complications occurring.*
   c. Severe headache. *Leakage of CSF through puncture hole in meninges causes the headache pain.*

8. Keep child flat after procedure for 1–24 hours depending on agency policy. *Reduces the risk of spinal headache.*

9. Encourage child to take fluid by mouth unless contraindicated. *Replaces fluid lost during the procedure and reduces chance of spinal headache.*

⧗ **Estimated time to assist with procedure:** *20–30 minutes.*

PROCEDURE 37

ASSISTING DURING BONE MARROW ASPIRATION AND BIOPSY

EQUIPMENT

Bone marrow aspiration tray:
   Antiseptic solution
   Sterile drape
   Gauze sponges
   Sterile syringes, various sizes
   Needles, 23–25 gauge
   Bone marrow needle
Gloves, sterile (physician)
Gloves, nonsterile (nurse)
Local anesthetic
Test tubes or glass slides
Gauze
Tape
Antiseptic ointment
Mask and goggles (physician and nurse per agency policy)

PROCEDURE

1. Steps 1–5 of General Guidelines.
2. Premedicate per physician's order. *Reduces discomfort during the procedure.*
3. Wash hands. *Reduces transmission of microorganisms.*
4. Set up tray, open supplies for physician. *Promotes organization and efficiency.*
5. Position child according to site of aspiration. (Site determined by physician) (Figure V-3). *For visualization of area needed to obtain biopsy.*

   a. Anterior iliac crest: lateral recumbent or supine.
   b. Posterior iliac crest: prone or lateral recumbent with head flexed and knees drawn up to abdomen.
   c. Distal third of thigh: supine with sandbag underneath.
   d. Sternum: supine with small pillow beneath shoulders. Arms at sides, feet together. *Elevates chest and lowers head.*
   e. Tibia: supine with sandbag under proximal third of lower leg.
   f. Vertebral process: prone with feet together and arms at side.
6. Restrain child as necessary. *So child is not injured during procedure.*
7. Physician will cleanse site, drape, infiltrate area with local anesthetic and obtain specimen using sterile technique. *Procedure to follow to collect specimen.*
8. Hold pressure on puncture site for 5–15 minutes. *Prevents bleeding and hematoma formation, especially if child thrombocytopenic.*
9. Cover puncture site with sterile pressure dressing. *Protects site.*
10. Help child to comfortable position. *So able to rest.*
11. Put on nonsterile gloves. *Reduces transmission of microorganisms.*
12. Label specimens and place in appropriate bag or container along with laboratory requisition slips. *Ensures specimen is properly identified and appropriate test is performed.*

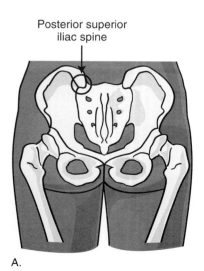

Posterior superior iliac spine

A.

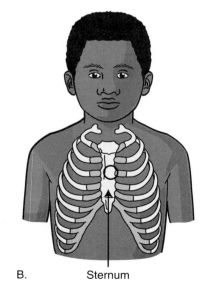

B.   Sternum

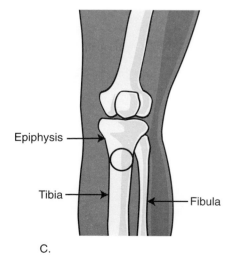

Epiphysis

Tibia   Fibula

C.

FIGURE V-3   Common sites used for bone marrow aspiration.

13. Dispose of equipment in appropriate container. *Consistent with body fluid precautions.*
14. Remove gloves. Wash hands. *Reduces transmission of microorganisms.*
15. Send specimen to lab. *So appropriate lab tests can be carried out.*
16. Monitor child for complications (hemorrhage, infection) according to agency policy. *So treatment can be provided.*
    a. Vital signs may be checked as often as every 15 minutes for 2 hours. *Changes in vital signs may indicate complications.*
    b. Observe puncture site for drainage, edema, and pain. *Complications associated with biopsy.*

DOCUMENTATION

1. Bone marrow aspiration performed, site, time, physician's name.
2. How procedure tolerated.
3. Specimens obtained and sent.
4. Vital signs, pain, bleeding, drainage.
5. Type of dressing over puncture site.

Estimated time to assist with procedure: *20–30 minutes.*

UNIT VI

Medication Administration

Medication Administration

Medication Administration

OVERVIEW

Assuring safe administration of medications to children is an important part of providing appropriate pediatric nursing care. In general, physiologic differences between children and adults make children more sensitive to drugs and increase the risk of adverse drug reactions. Differences in body size and composition and the immaturity of various organ systems account for these differences. Of particular significance are body fluid composition and differences in cardiovascular, gastrointestinal, renal, and neurological system functioning.

Administering medications to children also requires an understanding of all aspects of growth and development and their impact on the approach to giving medications. Of particular importance is the child's psychosocial and cognitive development. Physical and motor development are also important (e.g., ability to swallow tablets, size of muscles) and will be discussed in relation to their impact on the various routes of administration of medication.

Calculating Dosages

Appropriate drug dosages in children are most commonly calculated on the basis of unit of drug per kilogram of body weight or unit of drug per body surface area (BSA). When calculating drug dosages for an individual child, it is essential that the correct recommended dosage for the specific medication be used in the calculation since recommendations differ based on medication, route of administration, purpose, and age of child. Most dosage recommendations are for a 24-hour period (mg/Kg/24 hours). However, some dosage recommendations are for a single dose (mg/Kg/dose). It is essential to differentiate between these two methods when calculating dosages. Whether weight or BSA is used to compute recommended dose, the pediatric dose should not exceed the minimum recommended adult dose as a general rule. Once the child weighs 40 Kg or more, weight is not generally used to compute the recommended dose.

General Guidelines

1. Check for the six rights throughout medication preparation and administration. (See to Table VI-1). *To protect against medication errors.*
2. Identify any known drug allergies child may have. *Helps prevent allergic reaction child may have to the medication.*
3. Know action of drug. *Ensures that appropriate medication is ordered.*
4. Be aware of and watch for potential side effects of medication. *Ensures that side effects will be recognized if they develop.*
5. Wash hands. *Reduces transmission of microorganisms.*
6. Prepare medication. *Promotes organization and efficiency.*
7. Explain to child and family using minimally threatening language why medication is to be given, what child will experience, what is expected of child, and how parents/family can participate in what you will be doing. *Promotes cooperation and reduces anxiety and fear.*
8. Answer any questions child/parent may have about the medication. *Promotes cooperation and reduces anxiety and fear.*

PROCEDURE 38

ADMINISTERING A MEDICATION

EQUIPMENT

Physician's order for medication
Medication administration record (MAR)
Medication ordered

DOCUMENTATION

1. Time and date
2. Medication administered
3. Route administered
4. Site, if appropriate
5. Response to medication

Table VI-1   Six Rights of Administering Medications

Right Medication: Before administering the medication, compare the medication listed on the medication administration record (MAR) with the physician order, and check the label on the medication with the MAR.

Right Dosage: Calculate the dose of the medication the child should receive according to the child's weight. Compare that calculation with the dosage ordered. If the dosage ordered is inappropriate, check with the physician before administering the medication.

Right Route: Compare the route recommended for the medication with the route ordered. If the route ordered is not the route recommended, contact the physician. If there is no route written, contact the physician.

Right Time: Medications are usually ordered to be administered on a particular time schedule. Medications should always be administered within 20–30 minutes of the time ordered. If the medication is ordered to be administered p.r.n. (as necessary), check the last time the medication was administered to be sure enough time has passed since the child received the last medication. Then, check to see how often the child has been receiving the medication over the last 24 hours to be sure the child can receive another dose as requested.

Right Client: Check the child's identification band with the MAR. If the child does not have an identification band, ask the parent to state the child's name.

Right Approach: Check to see how nurses have talked to child about taking/receiving the medication (i.e., does pill need to be crushed and given with flavored syrup? Does child take liquid medication from a cup or syringe?) Implement these recommendations.

 Estimated time to complete procedure: *10 minutes*

PROCEDURE 39

ADMINISTERING AN ORAL MEDICATION

OVERVIEW

PREPARATION

Oral medications come in several forms: liquid, powder, tablets, and capsules. Liquid medications include syrups and elixirs, in which the medication is dissolved and distributed throughout the liquid, and suspensions, which contain undissolved particles of the drug suspended in the liquid. Suspensions require shaking before administration to distribute the medication evenly throughout the liquid so an appropriate dose is administered.

Since children under 5 years of age generally are unable to swallow tablets or capsules, it may be necessary to crush tablets or open capsules and remove the powder or liquid if a liquid form of the medication is not available. Before crushing a tablet or opening a capsule, it is essential to determine if this will interfere with the pharmacokinetics of the drug; for example, enteric-coated or timed-release tablets should not be crushed. Since crushed tablets or capsule contents generally have a bitter taste, the medication can be mixed with a pleasant-tasting liquid or nonessential food to make it more palatable. Common vehicles include flavored syrups provided by the pharmacy, jelly, pudding, ice cream, or applesauce. The medication should not be mixed with formula or other essential foods, since the child may associate the medicine taste with the food.

ADMINISTRATION

The administration of oral medications in the pediatric population may be a challenge since the appearance, smell, or taste of the medication may make children reluctant to accept it. Therefore, a firm, matter-of-fact approach, based on the child's developmental level and ability, usually results in cooperation. For example, asking children to administer the oral drug themselves or using the syringe to squirt the medicine into the child's mouth often is successful.

Liquid medication can be administered in a medicine cup, a measured medicine spoon, an oral syringe, or a dropper or through a nipple without the bottle attached. For some pediatric clients, oral medications are administered via a nasogastric, a gastrostomy, or a nasojejunal tube, but medications that act directly on the stomach (e.g. liquid antacids) will be ineffective if given via a nasojejunal tube. Before administering oral medications in this manner, it is essential to determine proper placement of the tube. (Refer to Procedure 71, Inserting a Nasogastric Tube.) A syringe with water is used to flush the tube before administering the medication. The medication is then put through the tube using a syringe, followed by enough water to ensure that the medication enters the gastrointestinal system rather than remaining in the tube.

EQUIPMENT

Infants (one of the items listed below):
   a. Syringe
   b. Dropper
   c. Measured medicine spoon
   d. Nipple
Children (one of the items listed below):
   a. Medicine cup
   b. Syringe
   c. Measured medicine spoon
Medication
Liquid (water, etc.)

PROCEDURE

1. Steps 1–8 of General Guidelines.

Note: *Preparation of medications for infants and young children may require crushing tablet and then mixing with a medium (pudding, flavored syrup, etc.) so that the medicine is easier for the child to swallow.*

2. Infants
   a. Position appropriately. *Helps prevent aspiration.*
      1. Semisitting in crib
      2. Semisitting held on lap of nurse or parent
   b. Place syringe, measured medicine, or dropper containing medication along side of mouth. Administer small amount of liquid at a time, waiting for infant to swallow. *Minimizes amount of medication child will spit up.*
   c. Place nipple containing medication in mouth. Allow infant to suck medication. *Minimizes amount of medication child will spit up.*
3. Young child (toddler, preschooler)
   a. Position appropriately. *Helps prevent aspiration.*
      1. Held on lap of nurse or parent
      2. Sitting in crib or chair
   b. Medicine cup
      1. Give cup to child. *Encourages child's independence and cooperation.*

2. Ask child to take pill.
3. Ask child to put pill in mouth.
4. Give child cup of liquid.
5. Ask child to take a drink of liquid and swallow pill.

  c. Syringe
1. Squirt syringe filled with liquid medicine to side and back of child's mouth. *Minimizes amount of medication child will spit up.*
2. Give syringe filled with liquid medicine to child and ask child to squirt medicine into back and side of mouth. *Minimizes amount of medication child will spit up.*

  d. Give child glass of liquid and ask child to swallow some liquid to wash the medicine down.

4. Child or adolescent
  a. See procedure for medicine cup above.

DOCUMENTATION

1. Time and date.
2. Medication administered.
3. Route administered.
4. How child tolerated medication administration.

 Estimated time to complete procedure: *5–10 minutes.*

PROCEDURE 40

ADMINISTERING AN INTRAVENOUS (IV) MEDICATION

OVERVIEW

Intravenous administration improves the therapeutic blood level of the medication and eliminates the discomfort associated with repeated intramuscular or subcutaneous injections. Since the medication is placed directly into the bloodstream where it can have an immediate effect, it is important to follow guidelines related to the concentration of medication, rate of delivery, and compatibility of solutions to help ensure the safety of the client.

ADMINISTRATION

Intravenous medication can be administered in several ways: syringe infusion pump, volume control mechanism (buritrol, metriset, soluset), IV push, or retrograde. Factors to consider when selecting an appropriate method of delivery include volume of solution necessary to dilute the medication, volume of solution tolerated by child, and hospital policies and procedures. Whatever method is used, the amount of fluid used for the medication and flushes must be included in the child's daily fluid intake.

Syringe infusion pumps allow medications to be delivered in a small volume of fluid over a prescribed period of time and are appropriate when larger fluid volumes are contraindicated. Tubing used with syringe infusion pumps is generally low volume (less than 5 cc, some as small as 0.5 cc), so only a small amount of solution is needed to flush the medication through the tubing in order for the client to receive the entire dose.

Medications that can be placed in a larger volume of solution may be administered via a volume control mechanism (buritrol, metriset, soluset), which allows the medication to be diluted in a small to moderate quantity of IV fluid in a calibrated chamber. The drip rate is then adjusted using the roller clamp or a dial-a-flow to deliver a set volume over a set time. This makes it easier to accurately regulate and manage the intermittent infusion of the IV medication.

Some medications may be delivered by direct, slow IV push into the injection port closest to the child. The IV push (bolus) is used when a rapid response to a drug is required, such as in a cardiac emergency. This method of administering medications carries with it the highest risk of side effects due to the immediate response of the medication and the inability to correct a medication error. Some medications can be irritating to the lining of blood vessels, and others, if injected into a vein that has become infiltrated, will injure the tissue. Medications delivered by IV push are generally of small volume and can be administered over a period of several minutes (e.g., three to five minutes). The nurse must carefully time the administration of the medication to be evenly spaced over the recommended time frame. For example, when giving 5 cc over a period of five minutes, each 1 cc should be administered slowly over a one-minute period of time. It is important to follow institutional guidelines to determine which medications may be administered by direct IV push.

A final method for administering IV medication is the retrograde method. The IV line to the client is clamped off, and the medication is injected into an injection port that has been cleaned with an alcohol or antiseptic wipe. The medication goes up the tubing toward the IV bag. The line is then opened, and the medication flows into the client with the IV solution. Tubing should be labeled to indicate the presence of medication in the IV line.

EQUIPMENT

Nonsterile gloves, if indicated
Medication
Syringe with appropriately sized needle attached
Syringe pump, metriset, or IV tubing, depending on method of administration
Alcohol wipes (IV push, IV retrograde, volume control mechanism)
Antiseptic swab or wipe (IV push, heparin lock)
Heparin flush (IV push)
Two labeled syringes with saline flush (IV push, IV retrograde)
Watch with second hand (IV push)

PROCEDURE

1. Steps 1–8 of General Guidelines.
2. Be sure the drug is completely dissolved and does not contain any particles. *Ensures delivery of medication ordered.*
3. Consult pharmacologic references for recommended time of infusion, maximum concentration of the drug in solution, and compatibility of the drug with IV solutions and other IV medications administered concurrently. *Ensures medication is appropriate for IV administration and proper administration techniques are followed.*
4. Check the IV site just before giving the medication. *Ensures the medication is given intravenously and not into the surrounding tissue.*

5. Prepare necessary labels. *Ensures care providers are aware an IV medication is being administered.*
6. Put on gloves. *Reduces exposure to body fluids and medications.*
7. Administer IV medication (refer to specific procedures below).
8. Attach label to appropriate equipment (tubing, metriset, etc.). *Ensures that others know a medication is being administered.*
9. Remove gloves and dispose in appropriate container. *Reduces transmission of microorganisms.*
10. Wash hands. *Reduces transmission of microorganisms.*
11. Check on child frequently during administration of medication. *Ensures that side effects or infiltrated IV will be discovered.*

Syringe Pump

1. Draw medication into syringe. *Allows for smooth and accurate medicating procedure.*
2. Prime tubing for the syringe infusion pump with IV solution or normal saline. *To prevent air from entering the tubing.*
3. Attach syringe containing medication to tubing. *So medication in syringe can be pushed into tubing.*
4. Place syringe in the infusion pump. *So infusion pump will push syringe plunger down and medication will enter tubing.*
5. Program pump to deliver medication in the prescribed amount of time. *So correct amount of medication is delivered in correct time frame.*
6. Attach tubing to child's IV through one of the ports in the child's IV tubing. *So child will receive medication.*
7. Turn on machine. *So syringe pump machine delivers ordered medication.*
8. When medication has been delivered, flush tubing with normal saline. *Allows medication to be completely infused.*
9. When flush has been delivered, disconnect infusion pump tubing. *No longer needed.*
10. Turn off infusion pump. *No longer needed.*
11. Reset IV flow rate to prescribed IV infusion rate. *Allows for resumption of IV therapy.*

Note: *Always read instructions accompanying the syringe pump, as there may be individual differences according to manufacturer specifications.*

Volume Control Mechanism

1. Draw medication into syringe. *Allows for smooth and accurate medication administration procedure.*
2. Fill chamber with appropriate amount of IV fluid; appropriate amount depends on child's age and weight as well as dose of medication to be administered. Contact pharmacy for information. *Fills chamber so that medication can be diluted.*

3. Close clamp; open air vent. *Prevents buildup of negative pressure in volume control set, allowing solution to flow out of chamber.*
4. Clean injection port with alcohol wipe. *Reduces transmission of microorganisms.*
5. Inject medication into chamber through port and gently mix. *Dilutes medication in chamber.*
6. Adjust flow rate to infuse medication over prescribed time frame. *Allows infusion of desired dosage strength in desired amount of time.*
7. When volume in chamber has infused, drop more fluid into chamber (10–20 ml or so) to flush chamber and tubing. *Allows medication to be completely infused.*
8. When flush has infused, close air vent and reset flow rate to prescribed IV infusion rate. *Allows for resumption of IV therapy.*
9. Dispose of syringe in appropriate container. *Prevents spread of microorganisms and injury to personnel.*

Direct, Slow IV Push

1. Draw medication into syringe. *Allows for smooth and accurate medication administration procedure.*
   a. Using injection port on existing IV:
      1. Select injection port close to IV Insertion site. *Decreases amount of medication in IV line if a reaction occurs.*
      2. Clean injection port with alcohol wipe. *Prevents transmission of microorganisms.*
      3. Insert syringe containing medication into injection port. *Correct procedure to use for slow, direct IV push.*
      4. Check for a blood return by pinching the tubing above the injection port and pulling back on the plunger of the syringe. *Ensures that IV is patent.*
      5. Administer medication by continuing to pinch tubing and slowly injecting the medication over the prescribed time period. *Each medication has a recommended infusion rate.*
      6. After administering the bolus of medication, clear the tubing by releasing the pinched tubing and allowing the infusion rate of the IV to resume. (If the medication is not compatible with the IV solution, a saline flush may be necessary before and after administering the bolus of IV medication. Check with pharmacy if you have questions.) *Ensures that entire dose of medication has been infused.*
      7. Dispose of syringe in appropriate container. *Reduces transmission of microorganisms and injury to personnel.*
   b. Using a heparin lock:
      1. Clean injection port with alcohol wipe or other appropriate antiseptic solution. *Reduces transmission of microorganisms.*
      2. Insert syringe with saline into port. *Correct procedure for using a heparin lock.*

3. Check for blood return by pulling back gently on the plunger of the syringe. *Ensures that IV is patent.*
4. Flush with saline. *Ensures that IV is patent.*
5. Remove syringe. *No longer needed for procedure.*
6. Clean port with antiseptic swab. *Reduces transmission of microorganisms.*
7. Insert syringe with medication into port. *So medication can be administered.*
8. Slowly inject medication over the prescribed time period. *Each medication has a recommended infusion rate.*
9. Remove syringe. *No longer needed for procedure.*
10. Clean port with antiseptic swab. *Reduces transmission of microorganisms.*
11. Insert another syringe with saline into the port and slowly inject. *Ensures that entire dose of medication has been infused.*
12. Insert syringe with heparinized saline into injection port and slowly flush. *Ensures that IV remains patent.*
13. Remove syringe. *No longer needed for procedure.*
14. Dispose of syringes in appropriate container. *Reduces transmission of microorganisms and injury to personnel.*

Note: *Always check with institutional policy and procedures before administering any IV medication through a heparin lock.*

Retrograde

1. Draw medication into syringe. *Allows for smooth and accurate medication administration procedure.*
2. Select injection port. *Decreases amount of medication in IV line if a reaction occurs.*
3. Clean injection port with alcohol wipe. *Prevents transmission of microorganisms.*

4. Insert syringe containing medication into injection port. *So medication can be administered through the port.*
5. Check for a blood return by pinching the tubing above the injection port and pulling back on the plunger of the syringe. *Ensures that IV is patent.*
6. Release pinched tubing. *Pinched tubing above port will result in medication administration that is IV push, not IV retrograde.*
7. Pinch tubing below injection port. *Allows medication to flow up IV tubing (retrograde).*
8. Administer medication by slowly injecting the medication over the prescribed time period. *Each medication has a recommended infusion rate.*
9. After administering the bolus of medication, clear the tubing by releasing the pinched tubing and allowing the infusion rate of the IV to resume. (If the medication is not compatible with the IV solution, a saline flush may be necessary before and after administering the bolus of IV medication. Check with pharmacy if you have questions.) *Ensures that entire dose of medication has been infused.*
10. Dispose of syringes in appropriate container. *Reduces transmission of microorganisms and injury to personnel.*

DOCUMENTATION

1. Time and date medication administered.
2. Route administered.
3. Method of administration (volume control, retrograde, IV push).
4. Appearance of IV site.
5. Response to medication.

 Estimated time to complete procedure: *5–10 minutes.*

PROCEDURE 41

ADMINISTERING AN INTRAMUSCULAR (IM) MEDICATION

OVERVIEW

Intramuscular injections are used to administer medications deep into the muscle, where they will be absorbed quickly due to the rich supply of blood vessels found in the muscles. Most aqueous medications are absorbed in 10–30 minutes.

Due to associated discomfort and psychological distress, intramuscular injections are not recommended for the pediatric population. However, at times it may be necessary to administer medication by this route. Selection of needle size and injection sites as well as techniques of administration are important considerations whenever administering medications intramuscularly.

SELECTING NEEDLE SIZE

Needle length and gauge are selected based on the child's size, amount of subcutaneous fat over the injection site, and viscosity of the medication. Age-based guidelines for selecting needle length and gauge are given in Table VI-2, although each child and situation must be assessed individually.

Table VI-2   Age-based guidelines for selecting needle length and gauge

Age Group	Needle Length	Needle Gauge
Infant	five-eighth inch	25–27
Toddler/Preschool	1 inch	22–23
School-age/Adolescent	1–1 1/2 inch	22–23

Viscosity of the solution to be injected must also be considered when selecting the needle gauge, since more viscous solutions require a larger gauge needle (smaller gauge number). The nurse should use the smallest gauge needle that will effectively deposit the medication in the muscle.

INJECTION SITES

Injection sites are determined primarily on muscle development and the amount of fluid to be injected. The preferred injection site for infants is the vastus lateralis. The rectus femoris is also an acceptable site and may be used as an alternative or to rotate injection sites. For the toddler, the vastus lateralis or rectus femoris are still the preferred sites for injection. The dorsogluteal site may be used for the child who has been walking for at least one full year. The ventrogluteal muscle may be used for children older than 3 years of age who have been walking for several years. The deltoid muscle is generally used only in children over 4–5 years of age due to the small muscle mass. However, the deltoid muscle may be used for immunizations in the child over 1 1/2 years of age since only a small amount of fluid is injected. Figure VI-1 illustrates injection sites.

The amount of solution that can be safely injected intramuscularly varies according to the age of the child and the specific muscle. Age-based guidelines for the amount of solution that can be injected are given in Table VI-3.

EQUIPMENT

Syringe filled with medication
Correct needle (size and length)
Alcohol wipe
Gauze pad or cotton ball
Nonsterile gloves
Small adhesive bandage

Table VI-3   Age-based guidelines for amount of solution to be injected intramuscularly

	Age Group				
Muscle	Infant	Toddler	Preschooler	School-age	Adolescent
	0–1½ yrs	1 ½ –3 yrs	3–6 yrs	6–15 yrs	≥ 15 yrs
Vastus lateralis	0.5–1 cc	1 cc	1.5 cc	1.5–2 cc	2–2.5 cc
Rectus femoris	0.5–1 cc	1 cc	1.5 cc	1.5–2 cc	2–2.5 cc
Dorsogluteal	*	1 cc**	1.5 cc	1.5–2 cc	2–2.5 cc
Ventrogluteal	*	1 cc**	1.5 cc	1.5–2 cc	2–2.5 cc
Deltoid	*	0.5 cc**	0.5 cc	0.5 cc	1 cc

*Not recommended.
**Not recommended unless other sites are not available.

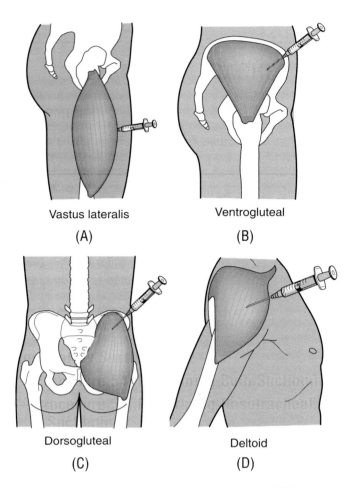

Vastus lateralis
(A)

Ventrogluteal
(B)

Dorsogluteal
(C)

Deltoid
(D)

FIGURE VI-1 Intramuscular injection sites. (A) Vastus lateralis: Identify the greater trochanter. Place hand at the lateral femoral condyle. The injection site is in the middle third and anterior to the lateral aspect. (B) Ventrogluteal: Place palm of left hand on right greater trochanter so the index finger points toward the anterosuperior iliac spine. When middle finger is spread to form a V, the injection site is in the middle of the V. (C) Dorsogluteal: Place hand on iliac crest and locate the posterosuperior iliac spine. The injection site is the outer quadrant when an imaginary line is drawn between the trochanter and the iliac spine. (D) Deltoid: Locate the lateral side of the humerus. One finger width below the acromion process is the deltoid.

PROCEDURE

1. Steps 1–8 of General Guidelines.
2. Wash hands and put on nonsterile gloves. *Reduces the number of microorganisms on skin; prevents transmission of microorganisms.*

3. Ask another person to help restrain the child while the injection is given. *Ensures that injection will be given appropriately; avoids injury due to a broken needle or giving the injection at the wrong site.*
4. Select injection site; inspect for bruises, inflammation, edema, masses, tenderness, and sites of previous injections; use anatomic landmarks. *Injection site should be free of lesions; repeated daily injections should be rotated; avoids injury to underlying nerves, bones, or blood vessels.*
5. Assist child into comfortable position; relax restrained arm or leg; distract child by talking about an interesting subject or explaining what you are doing step by step (depends on child's age). *Relaxation minimizes discomfort; distraction reduces anxiety.*
6. Clean site with alcohol wipe. *Removes microorganisms.*
7. Pull cap from needle while holding wipe between thumb and forefinger of dominant hand. *Swab remains accessible during procedure; prevents needle contamination.*
8. Administer injection:
   a. Hold syringe between thumb and forefinger of dominant hand like a dart. *Quick, smooth injection is easier with proper position of syringe.*
   b. Pinch skin with nondominant hand. *Needle penetrates tight skin easier than loose skin. Pinching elevates tissue.*
   c. Inject needle quickly and firmly (like a dart) at a 90° angle. *Quick, firm injection minimizes discomfort; 90° angle assures entry into muscle.*
   d. Grasp lower end of syringe with nondominant hand, and position dominant hand to the end of the plunger. Do not remove the syringe. *Injection requires smooth manipulation of syringe parts. Movement of syringe may cause discomfort.*
   e. Pull back on plunger to ascertain that the needle is not in a vein. If no blood appears, slowly inject the medication. *Aspiration of blood indicates intravenous placement of needle, so procedure needs to be abandoned.*
9. Quickly withdraw needle while applying pressure with alcohol wipe. *Pushing down on needle with wipe while withdrawing it will cause pain.*
10. Gently massage the site. Some medications should not be massaged; ask pharmacy if you do not know. *Stimulates circulation and improves drug distribution and absorption.*
11. Apply adhesive bandage. *Prevents any blood that is present from soiling clothes or linen. Children often like to have injection site covered by a bandage.*
12. Assist child to comfortable position. *Promotes comfort.*
13. Discard uncapped needle and syringe in a disposable needle receptacle. *Decreases risk of needle stick.*

14. Remove gloves and wash hands. *Reduces transmission of microorganisms.*

DOCUMENTATION

1. Time and date
2. Medication administered
3. Route administered
4. Site
5. How child tolerated medication administration

 Estimated time to complete procedure: *5–10 minutes.*

PROCEDURE 42

ADMINISTERING A SUBCUTANEOUS (SC) MEDICATION

OVERVIEW

A subcutaneous injection is used to administer medications into the loose connective tissues just below the dermis of the skin. Medications that do not need to be absorbed as quickly as those given intramuscularly are given this route because of the less richly supplied blood vessels in the subcutaneous (SC) tissue. However, children may respond more rapidly to an SC injection than an oral medication and should be monitored for potential side effects, allergic reactions, risk of infection, or bleeding.

Only small (.05 to 1 ml) doses of isotonic, nonirritating, nonviscous, and water soluble medications should be given subcutaneously. If larger volumes of medications remain in the SC tissue, a sterile abscess could form.

The most common sites for SC injections are the vascular areas around the outer aspect of the upper arms, the abdomen, and the anterior aspect of the thighs. Pinching up the subcutaneous layer isolates the site and prevents injection into a muscle, especially when the infant or child has little subcutaneous tissue. The infant or child should be restrained as necessary.

For an SC injection, a 2 to 3 ml syringe or a 1 ml syringe is recommended. The most common needle for a SC injection is a ⅝-inch 25-gauge needle.

EQUIPMENT

Syringe filled with medication
Alcohol wipe
Gauze pad or cotton ball
Nonsterile gloves
Small band aid

PROCEDURE

1. Steps 1–8 of General Guidelines.
2. Wash hands and put on nonsterile gloves. *Reduces the number of microorganisms on skin; prevents transmission of microorganisms.*
3. Ask another person to help restrain the child while the injection is given. *Ensures that injection will be given appropriately; avoids injury due to a broken needle or giving the injection at the wrong site.*
4. Select injection site; inspect for bruises, inflammation, edema, masses, tenderness, and sites of previous injections; use anatomic landmarks. *Injection site should be free of lesions; repeated daily injections should be rotated; avoids injury to underlying nerves, bones, or blood vessels.*
5. Assist child into comfortable position; relax restrained arm, leg, or abdomen; distract child by talking about an interesting subject or explaining what you are doing step by step (depends on child's age). *Relaxation minimizes discomfort; distraction reduces anxiety.*
6. Clean site with alcohol wipe. *Removes microorganisms.*
7. Pull cap from needle while holding wipe between thumb and forefinger of dominant hand. *Swab remains accessible during procedure; prevents needle contamination.*
8. Administer injection:
   a. Hold syringe between thumb and forefinger of dominant hand like a dart. *Quick, smooth injection is easier with proper position of syringe.*
   b. Pinch skin with nondominant hand. *Needle penetrates tight skin easier than loose skin. Pinching elevates SC tissue.*
   c. Inject needle quickly and firmly (like a dart) at a 45° angle. *Quick, firm injection minimizes discomfort; 45° angle ensures administering medication in SC tissue.*
   d. Grasp lower end of syringe with nondominant hand, and position dominant hand to the end of the plunger. Do not remove the syringe. *Injection requires smooth manipulation of syringe parts. Movement of syringe may cause discomfort.*
   e. Pull back on plunger to ascertain that the needle is not in a vein. If no blood appears, slowly inject the medication. *Aspiration of blood indicates intravenous placement of needle, so procedure probably needs to be abandoned.*
9. Quickly withdraw needle while applying pressure with alcohol wipe. *Pressure causes pain.*
10. Gently massage the site. Some medications should not be massaged; ask pharmacy if you do not know. *Stimulates circulation and improves drug distribution and absorption.*
11. Apply adhesive bandage. *Prevents any blood that is present from soiling clothes or linen. Children often like to have injection site covered by a bandage.*
12. Assist child to comfortable position. *Promotes comfort.*
13. Discard uncapped needle and syringe in a disposable needle receptacle. *Decreases risk of needle stick.*

14. Remove gloves and wash hands. *Reduces transmission of microorganisms.*

DOCUMENTATION

1. Time and date
2. Medication administered
3. Route administered
4. Site
5. How child tolerated medication administration

 Estimated time to complete procedure: *5–10 minutes.*

PROCEDURE 43

ADMINISTERING A RECTAL MEDICATION

OVERVIEW

Rectal suppositories (medications) are administered for their local or systemic effects. Suppositories producing local effects include laxatives; suppositories producing systemic effects include medications given to relieve pain, nausea, fever, or bladder spasm. However, rectally administered drugs may be erratic and unpredictable in their absorption and are not the most desirable route of medication administration for pediatric patients. Nonetheless, this route of administration may occasionally become the route of choice if the child is vomiting or is receiving nothing by mouth (NPO). This invasive procedure may be extremely upsetting to toddlers and preschoolers because of age-related fears; school-age children and adolescents may be embarrassed by this procedure. Therefore, age-appropriate explanation and reassurance are needed, as is proper restraint.

EQUIPMENT

Medication
Nonsterile gloves
Water-soluble lubricant

PROCEDURE

1. Steps 1–8 of General Guidelines.
2. Position child on left side or prone. *Descending colon is on left side.*
3. Put on gloves. *Prevents contact with fecal material.*
4. Lubricate tapered end of suppository. *Decreases friction and discomfort.*
5. Retract buttocks with nondominant hand, visualizing the anus. *Assists in correctly visualizing and inserting suppository.*
6. Slowly and gently insert the suppository into the child's rectum just beyond the internal sphincter using either the index finger in children over 3 years of age or the little finger in infants and toddlers. *Slow insertion with small finger minimizes pain; correct placement ensures adequate absorption and less chance for expulsion.*
7. Hold child's buttocks together for 5–10 minutes or until child loses the urge to defecate. *Keeps suppository in place so that medication can be absorbed.*
8. Remove gloves. *Reduces transfer of microorganisms.*
9. Wash hands. *Reduces transfer of microorganisms.*

DOCUMENTATION

1. Time and date
2. Medication administered
3. Route administered
4. How child tolerated medication administration

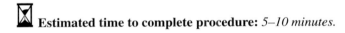 **Estimated time to complete procedure:** *5–10 minutes.*

PROCEDURE 44

ADMINISTERING AN OPHTHALMIC MEDICATION

OVERVIEW

Ophthalmic medications refer to drops and ointments that are used for diagnostic and therapeutic purposes. Most administered to pediatric clients are to treat eye conditions or infections. Diagnostically, eyedrops can be used to anesthetize the eye, dilate the pupil, and stain the cornea to identify abrasions and scars.

Whenever administering ophthalmic medications, the following safety measures should be followed:

Each child should have his/her own bottle of eyedrops.
Any solution remaining in the dropper after instillation should be discarded.
If the tip of the dropper is contaminated (touches the bottle or any part of the child's eye), the dropper should be discarded.

Administering ophthalmic medication requires special consideration in the pediatric population. Age-related concerns cause young children to fear having anything placed in their eyes, and even infants may close their eyelids so tightly that it is difficult to open them. Proper restraint is necessary to control the head, keep the child's hands from interfering, and prevent injury to the eye. This may require the help of more than one person, especially with infants and toddlers. Children who are old enough to comprehend the procedure should be given an age-appropriate explanation, which may help gain their cooperation. If possible, avoid giving ophthalmic medications when the child is crying, since this limits contact of medication with the eye and decreases its therapeutic value.

EQUIPMENT

Nonsterile gloves
Medication
Tissue

PROCEDURE

Eye Drops

1. Steps 1–8 of General Guidelines.
2. Wash hands again; put on nonsterile gloves if needed. *Decreases contact with bodily fluids and medication. Reduces transmission of microorganisms.*

3. Place child in supine position with head slightly hyperextended (refer to Figure VI-2). *Minimizes drainage of medication through tear duct.*
4. Remove cap from medication and place cap on its side. *Prevents contamination of bottle cap.*
5. Squeeze the prescribed amount of medication into the eyedropper. *Ensures correct dose.*
6. Place a tissue below the lower lid. *Absorbs the medication that flows from the eye.*
7. With dominant hand, hold eye dropper ½–¾ inch above the eyeball. Rest hand on child's forehead to stabilize. *Reduces risk of dropper touching eye structure, and prevents injury to eye.*
8. Place hand on cheekbone and expose lower conjunctival sac by pulling down on cheek. *Stabilizes hand and prevents systemic absorption of eye medication.*
9. Instruct child to look up; drop prescribed number of drops into center of conjunctival sac. *Reduces stimulation of blink reflex; prevents injury to cornea.*

Note: *An infant or young child may not be able to look up as directed.*

10. Instruct child to gently close eyes and move eyes. Place finger on either side of the child's nose to close the tear ducts and prevent medication from draining

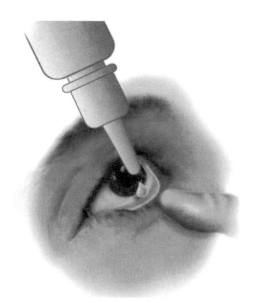

FIGURE VI-2   When administering an eye medication, gently press the lower lid down and have the child look upward while you instill the drops into the lower conjunctival sac.

out of the eye. *Distributes solution over conjunctival surface and anterior eyeball.*

Note: *An infant or young child may not be able to follow these instructions.*

11. Remove gloves; wash hands. *Reduces transmission of microorganisms.*

Eye Ointment

1. Steps 1–8 of General Guidelines.
2. Wash hands again; put on nonsterile gloves if needed. *Decreases contact with bodily fluids, reduces transmission of microorganisms.*
3. Place child in supine position with head slightly hyperextended. *Minimizes drainage of medication through tear duct.*
4. Remove cap from medication and place cap on its side. *Prevents contamination of bottle cap.*
5. Lower lid:
   a. With nondominant hand, gently separate child's eyelids with thumb and finger and grasp lower lid near margin immediately below the lashes; exert pressure downward over the bony prominence of the cheek. *Provides access to the lower lid.*
   b. Ask child to look up. *Reduces stimulation of the blink reflex and keeps the cornea out of the way of the medication.*
   c. Apply eye ointment along the inside edge of the entire lower eyelid from the inner to outer canthus. *Ensures drug is applied to entire lid.*
6. Upper lid:
   a. Instruct child to look down. *Keeps cornea out of way of medication.*
   b. With nondominant hand, gently grasp child's lashes near center of upper lid with thumb and index finger, and draw lid up and away from eyeball. *Keeps cornea out of way of medication.*
7. Squeeze ointment along upper lid, starting at inner canthus. *Ensures medication is applied to entire length of lid.*
8. Remove gloves; wash hands. *Reduces transmission of microorganisms.*

DOCUMENTATION

1. Time and date
2. Medication administered
3. Route administered
4. Site (which eye)
5. How child tolerated medication administration

 Estimated time to complete procedure: *5–10 minutes.*

PROCEDURE 45

ADMINISTERING AN OTIC MEDICATION

OVERVIEW

Solutions ordered to treat the ear are referred to as otic (pertaining to the ear) drops or irrigation. Eardrops may be instilled to soften ear wax, produce anesthesia, treat infection or inflammation, or facilitate removal of a foreign body such as food or an insect. External auditory canal irrigations are usually performed for cleaning purposes and less frequently for applying heat and antiseptic solutions. Before instilling any solution into the ear, it is important to inspect the ear for signs of drainage, an indication of a perforated tympanic membrane. Unless the tympanic membrane is ruptured, the instillation of otic medication is not a sterile procedure.

Age-related fears may be a concern when administering otic medications to young children, who may need to be restrained to prevent movement of the head during instillation of the medication. An explanation may help the older child cooperate with the procedure.

EQUIPMENT

Medication
Cotton ball

PROCEDURE

1. Steps 1–8 of General Guidelines.
2. Place child in side-lying position with the affected ear up; obtain assistance if appropriate. *Facilitates administration of medication.*
3. Straighten ear canal by pulling the pinna down and back for children under 3 years of age and up and back for children over 3 years of age. *Opens the canal and facilitates introduction of medication* (See Figure VI-3).
4. Instill drops into canal by holding the dropper at least ½-inch above the ear canal. *Prevents injury to ear canal.*

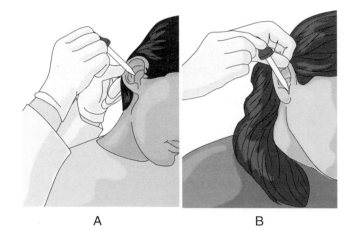

FIGURE VI-3   A. for a child under 3 years of age, pull pinna down and back. B. For an older child, pull the pinna up and back.

5. Ask child to maintain this position for at least two to three minutes. *Allows for distribution of medication.*
6. Loosely place a cotton ball on the outermost part of the canal. *Prevents medication from escaping when the child changes positions.*
7. Wash hands. *Reduces the transmission of microorganisms.*

DOCUMENTATION

1. Time and date
2. Medication administered
3. Route administered
4. Site (which ear)
5. How child tolerated medication administration

⧗ **Estimated time to complete procedure:** *5 minutes or less.*

PROCEDURE 46

ADMINISTERING A NASAL MEDICATION

OVERVIEW

Nasal medications may be administered by drops or sprays and are used to achieve local effects on the nasal mucosa, indirect effects on the sinuses, or a systemic effect. Although the nose is not considered a clean or sterile cavity, because of its connection with the sinuses medical asepsis should be used whenever instilling any nasal medication.

The infant and young child may react negatively to instillation of nose drops; proper restraint may be necessary to safely accomplish the procedure.

EQUIPMENT

Medication
Nonsterile gloves
Tissues as needed

PROCEDURE

1. Steps 1–8 of General Guidelines.
2. Place child supine; obtain assistance if appropriate. *Facilitates administration of medication.*
3. Hyperextend child's head (Figure VI-4). *Facilitates administration of medication.*
4. Instill drops into nose by holding the dropper ⅜ inch into the nostril, keeping the tip of the dropper away from the sides of the nostril. Insert the prescribed dosage of medication into the nostril. Discard any unused medication in the dropper to prevent contamination of medication when dropper is returned to bottle. *Prevents injury to nasal mucosa. Droppers should be kept away from the nostril to avoid inserting bacteria into the medication bottle.*
5. Blot excess drainage from nostril. *Avoids discomfort.*
6. Repeat procedure in other nostril. *Most of the time, both nostrils need to be treated.*

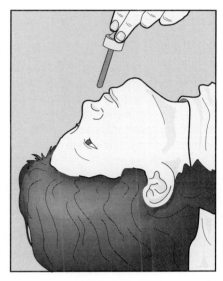

FIGURE VI-4   When instilling nose drops, the child should be placed on his/her back with the head tilted down or over the side of the bed. This will allow the medication to reach the back of the nose.

7. Maintain child's position for at least one minute. *Allows medication to reach desired areas.*
8. Wash hands. *Reduces the transmission of micro-organisms.*

DOCUMENTATION

1. Time and date
2. Medication administered
3. Route administered
4. Site
5. How child tolerated medication administration

⧗ **Estimated time to complete procedure:** *5 minutes or less.*

PROCEDURE 47

ADMINISTERING A TOPICAL MEDICATION

OVERVIEW

Topical medications are applied directly to the skin or mucus membranes. These medications are used for their local effect or to produce systemic effects by absorption. Topical medications include creams, ointments, and lotions. Medications applied to the skin are commonly used to relieve itching, prevent local infections, or moisten the skin or for vasodilatation. Most topical medications in pediatrics are used for their local effects.

Administering topical medication to children is the same as for an adult. If the skin is broken, sterile technique is required. The biggest challenge for the nurse administering topical medication to infants and children may be preventing the child from scratching an irritated or infected area. The child's nails should be kept short and clean, and his or her hands may need to be covered or restrained.

EQUIPMENT

Medication
Gloves
Applicator (tongue blade, cotton applicator, etc.)
Mild soap and water
Washcloth and towel
Drape

PROCEDURE

1. Steps 1–8 of General Guidelines.
2. Position child for appropriate administration of medication. Drape for privacy. *Keeps child in comfortable position; allows for visualization of area where medication is to be applied; protects privacy.*

3. Put on gloves. *Decreases contact with microorganisms.*
4. Remove old medication if present with mild soap and water. *Absorption of newly applied medication can be affected by residue from old medication.*
5. Assess area covered by topical medication. *Provides information about effect of medication.*
6. Change gloves. *Prevents spread of microorganisms and avoids absorption of medication by caregiver.*
7. Apply medication according to label or physician's order. *Dosages recommended according to standards.*
   a. If aerosol spray, shake container and administer according to directions. Spray evenly over affected area; avoid spraying close to child's face. *Aerosol may need to be mixed to be effective; avoid inhalation, since aerosol may have adverse effects on mucous membranes and lungs.*
   b. If gel or paste, applicator may be needed. Apply evenly. *Apply evenly, as excess gel or paste will be wasted because absorption can only occur at skin level. Inhalation can cause untoward effects on lungs and mucous membranes.*
8. Remove gloves; wash hands. *Reduces transmission of microorganisms.*

DOCUMENTATION

1. Time and date
2. Medication administered
3. Route administered
4. Site
5. How child tolerated medication administration

⊠ **Estimated time to complete procedure:** *5–15 minutes depending on how much topical medication needs to be administered, how cooperative child is, whether or not a dressing needs to be changed.*

PROCEDURE 48

ADMINISTERING A NEBULIZED MEDICATION

OVERVIEW

A nebulizer is a device used to aerosolize medications into a fine mist for delivery directly into the lungs, where it is absorbed immediately into the mucosa and bloodstream and becomes available to the body within minutes. This route is one of the fastest, most noninvasive methods of medication delivery. Even though this route can be used for a variety of medications, it is primarily used in pediatrics to ease respiratory distress.

There are two kinds of nebulizers: single-dose nebulizers and metered-dose inhalers. The single-dose nebulizer delivers smaller droplets and can be filled with any type of medication that is ordered. The metered-dose inhaler is small and portable and can be carried around in the child's pocket.

EQUIPMENT

Nebulizer
Mouthpiece
Medication

PROCEDURE (HAND-HELD NEBULIZER)

1. Steps 1–8 of General Guidelines.
2. Wash hands. *Reduces transmission of microorganisms.*
3. Ask child to sit in an upright position. *Promotes better expansion of lungs.*
4. Pour medication into nebulizer cap; avoid touching medication while pouring into cap. *Determines correct amount of medicine; assures accurate dosage; reduces transmission of microorganisms.*
5. Cover cup and fasten it. *Prevents spillage of medication.*
6. Fasten T-piece to the top of cap. *Provides connector for mouthpiece.*

7. Fasten a short length of tubing to one end of the T-piece. *Provides dead space to prevent room air from entering the system and medicated aerosol from escaping.*
8. Fasten mouthpiece and mask to other end of T-piece; avoid touching nebulizer mouthpiece of the interior part of the mask. *Provides portal for client to inhale aerosolized medication; reduces transmission of microorganisms.*
9. Attach tubing to bottom of nebulizer cup and attach other end to air compressor. *Provides conduit for compressed air.*
10. Adjust wall oxygen valve to 6 liters/minute or less (per order). *Drives medication into a mist or wet aerosol form.*
11. Instruct child to breathe in and out slowly and deeply through the mouthpiece and mask for about 10 minutes or until the medication has been nebulized; child's lips should be sealed tightly around mouthpiece. *Promotes better deposition and efficacy of medication in airways.*
12. Remain with child long enough to observe the proper inhalation-exhalation technique. *Ensures correct use of nebulizer to get the full effect from the medication administered.*

DOCUMENTATION

1. Time and date
2. Medication administered
3. Route administered
4. How child tolerated medication administration

 Estimated time to complete procedure: *15–20 minutes.*

UNIT VII

Intravenous Access

Intravenous Access

OVERVIEW

Performing venipuncture in order to establish venous access is a priority for children who are critically ill, NPO, have fluid and electrolyte disturbances, or for some other reason are not able to take food or fluids by mouth. Venous access is also used in children for infusion of IV fluids, parenteral nutrition, routine IV medications, emergency medications, or blood products.

Over the needle catheters (ONC) are most commonly used for infants and children and are available in 19 to 27 gauge sizes. These flexible catheters are made of plastic, Teflon, or other materials and have a metal stylet that is used to pierce the skin and vein and a plastic catheter that is threaded into the vein and attached to the IV tubing after the stylet has been removed. The straight steel needle is also used in children to obtain IV access, but the butterfly needle (23 gauge) may be used in infants or small children to gain access via a scalp vein.

The Centers for Disease Control and Prevention (CDC) guidelines, including changing the IV solution every 24 hours, changing the IV site and catheter every 24–72 hours, and changing the IV tubing every 48 hours should be followed whenever a child has an IV in order to decrease the risk of infection. Occupational Safety and Health Administration (OSHA) standards should also be followed in order to prevent exposure to blood-borne pathogens: use gloves, puncture-resistant containers for sharps, and special training for health care workers.

Sites

Peripheral veins (antaecubital fossa, forearm) are typically the best venous sites in children and adolescents because of their high visibility and easy access. It is not uncommon, however, to use veins of the dorsum of the foot and hand as well, especially in young children. Scalp veins are often used in infants when other sites are difficult to access (Figure VII-1). Whenever using a scalp vein, however, it is important to protect the

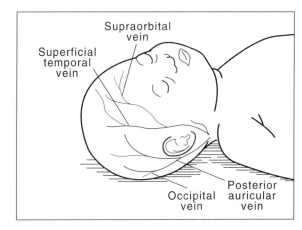

FIGURE VII-1   Scalp veins are frequently used for peripheral vascular access in infants.

area by covering it with a plastic medication cup that has been cut in half and taped in place.

General Guidelines

1. Check physician's order. *Ensures appropriate administration of prescribed intravenous therapy.*
2. Prepare child and family. *Enhances cooperation and participation and reduces anxiety and fear.*
3. Check child for allergies, especially allergies to tape, latex, and povidone-iodine. *Prevents allergic reaction.*
4. Gather equipment. *Promotes organization and efficiency.*
5. Wash hands. *Reduces transmission of microorganisms.*
6. Choose site and type of device.
   a. Use most distal portion of vein found. *Proximal site is still usable if needed.*
   b. Avoid using dominant hand if possible. *Interferes less with the child's usual activities.*
   c. Avoid bony prominences. *Difficult to access and maintain.*
   d. Avoid inserting IV through an infection or rash. *Reduces risk for IV-associated bacteremia.*

e. Use a padded armboard as a splint to *decrease mobility in an extremity where there is an IV.*

f. Attach a piece of tape to the sticky side of another piece of tape that is used to immobilize the child's extremity to the armboard to *decrease skin contact with tape.*

g. Avoid using two different antecubital veins if the child needs two IVs. *Would immobilize child's two extremities if two were used.*

h. Refrain from using foot veins in children who are walking. *Would not be able to ambulate.*

7. Apply a warm compress over the area if needed. *Helps distend the vein.*

8. Put on gloves. *Protects from contact with body fluids.*

9. Position child. *For easy access to vein.*

a. For scalp vein insertion, use a mummy restraint.

b. For infants and children who are unable to fully cooperate, have a second nurse restrain as necessary.

10. Cleanse the insertion site by using povidone-iodine or alcohol; use a circular motion moving outward from the puncture site. *Reduces the transmission of microorganisms and carries microorganisms away from site of entry.*

a. If using povidone-iodine, allow to dry for one to two minutes. *Povidone-iodine must dry to be effective.*

b. If povidone-iodine makes it difficult to visualize the vein, it can be wiped off with alcohol. *Povidone-iodine may stain skin.*

c. If using alcohol alone, scrub site until last applicator is visually clean. *Indicates site is clean.*

 Estimated time to complete procedure: *15–25 minutes.*

PROCEDURE 49

INSERTING A PERIPHERAL IV LINE

EQUIPMENT

Needle, scalp vein, or angiocath
Antiseptic solution (povidone-iodine and/or alcohol)
Tourniquet
Gloves, nonsterile

Insertion of Scalp Vein Needle

PROCEDURE

1. Steps 1–10 of General Guidelines.
2. Apply a rubber band tourniquet if using a scalp vein, or a tourniquet if using an extremity. *Distends vein and makes it easier to enter.*
3. Prepare needle by attaching a syringe with normal saline to the needle and forcing out a few drops of saline. *Determines patency of needle and removes air from needle.*
4. Select a fairly straight segment of vein; place the needle in the direction of the blood flow. *Easier to access vein.*
5. Grasp the needle by the winged tabs, bevel up and at a 23°–30° angle. *Produces less trauma to the skin and vein.*

6. Anchor the vein with a finger of the free hand by stretching the skin. *Applying traction to the skin helps to stabilize the vein.*
7. Hold the needle parallel to the long axis of the vein. *Decreases the risk of thrusting the needle through the wall of the vein as the skin is entered.*
8. Gently advance the needle into the vein until blood appears in the tubing. Do not advance the needle once blood is seen. *Reduces risk of piercing the distal wall of the vein. Increased venous pressure from the tourniquet increases backflow of blood.*
9. Release the tourniquet. *Permits venous flow of blood. Reduces backflow of blood.*
10. Infuse 2–3 ml of saline from the syringe into the vein. *Checks patency of the system.*
11. Secure IV by taping. *Reduces risk of needle becoming dislodged from the vein* (Figure VII-2A).
12. Attach hub of needle to adapter of the infusion tubing. *So child will receive ordered infusion.*
13. Set appropriate rate on infusion pump and begin infusion. *So infusion will be delivered at ordered rate.*
14. Place medicine cup or drinking cup cut in half and padded over IV site. (Commercial devices are also available.) *Protects site* (Figure VII-2B).

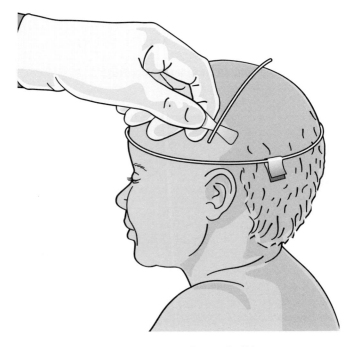

FIGURE VII-2A   Placement of a scalp IV.

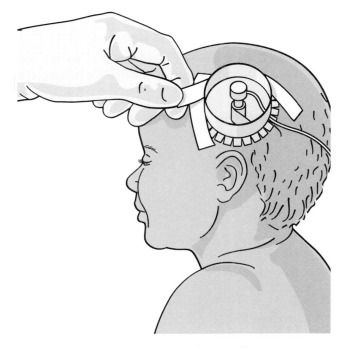

FIGURE VII-2B   Securing a scalp vein IV site.

15. Dispose of used equipment in appropriate container. *Consistent with body fluid precautions.*
16. Remove gloves. Wash hands. *Reduces transmission of microorganisms.*

Insertion of Angiocath
PROCEDURE

1. Steps 1–10 of General Guidelines.
2. Apply tourniquet above insertion site. Tourniquet should be tight enough to impede venous flow but not arterial flow. Check pressure of distal pulse. *Distends vein and makes it easier to enter. Decreased arterial flow prevents venous filling.*
3. With free hand, pull skin taut about 2 inches from insertion site. *Stabilizes vein and extremity.*
4. Select straightest portion of vein. Align needle in same direction as blood flow. *Is easier to access vein.*
5. Hold needle bevel up at a 10°–30° angle. Enter the skin. Do not enter the vein at this time. *Decreases risk of penetrating other side of vein. Causes less trauma to skin and vein.*
6. Decrease the angle of the needle depending on the depth of the vein and enter the vessel. Blood will enter the flash chamber. You may feel catheter "release" as it enters the vein. *Increased venous pressure from tourniquet decreases backflow of blood.*
7. Decrease the angle of the needle and slightly advance further into vein, ⅟₁₆ to ⅛ inch. *Ensures that plastic catheter has entered the vein.*
8. Hold needle hub, stabilize flash chamber, and advance catheter off needle into the vein. *Reinsertion of needle can cause catheter breakage in vein.*

NOTE: *Never reinsert the needle into the catheter.*

9. Release the tourniquet. Apply pressure on vein just beyond the catheter tip and slowly remove the needle while holding the catheter in place. *Permits venous blood flow. Reduces backflow of blood.*
10. Connect the primed extension tubing with the injection cap. Flush catheter slowly. *Checks for proper placement and infiltration.*
11. Place transparent dressing over insertion site and secure catheter and tubing. *Protects IV site and reduces risk of catheter becoming dislodged from the vein.*
12. Attach extension tubing to the infusion set tubing. *So child will receive ordered infusion.*
13. Set appropriate rate on infusion pump and begin infusion or heplock as ordered. *So infusion will be delivered at ordered rate.*
14. Place a label on the dressing with date, time, gauge, and name of person who started IV. *So caregivers know when IV started and who started IV.*
15. Immobilize area if needed (Figures VII-3A and VII-3B).
16. Place medicine cup or drinking cup cut in half and padded over IV site. (Commercial devices are also available.) *Protects site.*
17. Dispose of used equipment in appropriate container. *Reduces transmission of microorganisms and maintains body fluid precautions.*
18. Remove gloves. Wash hands. *Reduces transmission of microorganisms.*

DOCUMENTATION

1. Insertion site.
2. Type and gauge of needle or catheter used.
3. Date and time.
4. Person who placed the IV.
5. IV solution started and rate of infusion.
6. Type of dressing over site.

⧗ **Estimated time to complete procedure:** *5–10 minutes.*

![Footboard used to secure IV placement]

FIGURE VII-3A   Footboard used to secure IV placement.

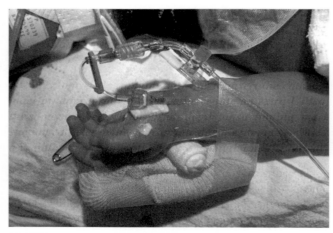

FIGURE VII-3B   Handboard used to secure IV placement.

PROCEDURE 50

APPLYING AN INTERMITTENT INFUSION DEVICE

OVERVIEW

The intermittent infusion device (also known as a heparin lock) is a small plastic device with a resealing rubber entry that is screwed onto the hub of the existing IV catheter or butterfly tubing. It maintains patency of the IV site when it is not hooked up to a running IV. The fluid used (saline or heparin) in the device depends on agency policy. The device is used more often with older children or adolescents than with infants. The intermittent infusion device is regularly flushed with a heparin solution or normal saline to prevent clotting. The device is used to deliver IV medications into the vein and can be quickly reattached to IV tubing.

EQUIPMENT

Nonsterile gloves
Syringe filled with 1 ml of heparin flush (10 U/ml) (optional; depends on agency policy)
Syringe with 2 ml of sterile normal saline
Intermittent infusion device adapter

PROCEDURE

1. Steps 1–10 of General Guidelines.
2. Prime the adapter with as much heparin or saline flush as is needed, using sterile technique. *Prevents air from entering the vein.*
3. Put on gloves. *Protects from contact with body fluids.*
4. Check IV site for infiltration and IV for patency by flushing normal saline through injection port. *Assures that IV is patent so heparin lock can function.*
5. Identify tubing where IV catheter or scalp vein connects to IV tubing. *Promotes organization and efficiency.*
6. Clamp tubing of catheter or scalp vein with T connecter. *Prevents blood from flowing out of IV.*
7. Separate IV tubing from scalp vein or IV catheter, and quickly place primed adapter on catheter tip. *So infusion continues with minimal interruption; to prevent air from entering scalp vein.*
8. Open the clamp and insert the syringe with normal saline through port on adapter. Slowly flush catheter. *Ensures patency.*
9. Remove syringe; clamp catheter tubing. *Syringe not needed; so blood does not flow into tubing.*
10. Tape adapter in place so that access is possible. *Allows easy access for IV.*
11. Remove gloves; wash hands. *Reduces transmission of microorganisms.*

DOCUMENTATION

1. Time and date
2. Site where adapter placed
3. Condition of IV site
4. Fluid type and amount used for flush

 Estimated time to complete procedure: *5–10 minutes.*

PROCEDURE 51

CHANGING THE IV BAG AND TUBING

OVERVIEW

The IV solution and tubing are changed at least every 24–48 hours depending on agency policy and the type of solution ordered, in order to decrease the risk of infection. This is a clean procedure.

EQUIPMENT

Nonsterile gloves
IV solution
IV tubing
Alcohol wipes
Label
Additives as indicated
Volume control mechanism (Metriset)

PROCEDURE

1. Steps 1–10 of General Guidelines.
2. Put on nonsterile gloves. *Reduces number of microorganisms.*
3. Prepare new IV bag with additives according to physician's order. *Ensures accurate administration of solution.*
4. Attach volume control mechanism (Metriset) to IV bag. *Promotes organization and efficiency.*
5. Attach IV tubing to volume control mechanism (Metriset). *Promotes organization and efficiency.*
6. Close air vent to volume control mechanism. *Allows fluid to drip into chamber.*
7. Open clamp from IV bag to volume control mechanism and drop IV solution into chamber (about 25–50 ccs); be sure drip chamber is at least half full. *Allows fluid to drip into chamber.*

8. Open air vent to volume control mechanism, close clamp from volume control mechanism to IV bag, remove tubing cap at end of tubing, and open roller clamp on IV tubing. *Allows fluid to flow through IV tubing.*
9. Allow solution to drip into and prime entire length of IV tubing. *Prepares equipment.*
10. When tubing is filled with IV solution, close roller clamp; recap end of tubing, and check tubing for air; if any found, allow to drip out end of tubing. *Reduces risk of air embolus.*
11. Remove old bag from IV pole and hang new bag. *Old bag no longer needed.*
12. Disconnect old tubing from catheter or scalp vein tubing; quickly connect new tubing and reestablish flow rate. *Maintains sterility of new tubing.*

Note: *Some agency policies may recommend wiping the area where IV tubing connects to IV catheter with alcohol wipe.*

13. Remove gloves; wash hands. *Reduces transmission from microorganisms.*
14. Attach label to IV bag with time and date, person who changed bag, and any additives. *Allows for planning of next IV tubing and solution changed; documents who hung IV, when IV was hung, and when the tubing was changed.*

DOCUMENTATION

1. Time and date
2. Fluid type, amount, and rate
3. Condition of IV site

⧗ **Estimated time to complete procedure:** *5–10 minutes.*

PROCEDURE 52

MONITORING INTRAVENOUS INFUSIONS AND FLOW RATES

OVERVIEW

Setting up the IV as well as the rate of an IV infusion is the nurse's responsibility after establishing that the IV is patent and checking with the physician orders. Most IV rates in pediatrics are controlled by an infusion pump or a syringe pump, which are electronic devices used to deliver a prescribed amount of fluid over a period of time in millimeters per hour. Pumps often have drop sensors that count each drop of fluid and sound an alarm if the flow rate differs from what is programmed. An alarm will also sound if the IV bag is empty or when pressure increases in the system, as when the IV has infiltrated. Before setting up any infusion pump, it is important to read the accompanying instructions and follow organizational policies. While setting up the infusion pump, it is important to set the controls for the rate of the infusion as well as the amount of fluid to be administered.

The rate of the IV is based on the child's weight and physical condition, and it is important that the IV rate be accurate in order to prevent complications in fluid balance. A rate that is too high may result in fluid overload. If the infusion rate is too slow, the vein could clot off or result in a more serious complication if the patient is seriously ill or at risk for becoming dehydrated.

EQUIPMENT

Nonsterile gloves
IV solution
IV tubing
Alcohol wipes
Label
Additives as indicated
Volume control mechanism (Metriset)
IV infusion pump

PROCEDURE

1. Check physician's order for type of fluid and infusion rate. *Ensures appropriate administration of prescribed intravenous therapy.*
2. Gather equipment. *Promotes organization and efficiency.*
3. Wash hands. *Reduces transmission of microorganisms.*
4. Check IV bag and tubing for leaks, color changes (unless additives may explain color changes), and expiration dates. *Ensures that IV equipment has remained sterile and is still guaranteed by manufacturer.*

5. Put on nonsterile gloves. *Reduces number of microorganisms.*
6. Attach volume control mechanism (Metriset) to IV bag. *Promotes organization and efficiency.*
7. Attach IV tubing to volume control mechanism (Metriset). *Promotes organization and efficiency.*
8. Close air vent to volume control mechanism. *Allows fluid to drip into chamber.*
9. Open clamp from IV bag to volume control mechanism and drop IV solution into chamber (about 25–50 ccs); be sure drip chamber is at least half full. *Allows fluid to drip into chamber. Provides enough fluid to administer in alotted time.*
10. Open air vent to volume control mechanism, close clamp from volume control mechanism to IV bag, remove tubing cap at end of tubing, and open roller clamp on IV tubing. *Allows fluid to flow through IV tubing.*
11. Allow solution to drip into and prime entire length of IV tubing. *Prepares equipment.*
12. When tubing is filled with IV solution, close roller clamp, recap end of tubing, and check tubing for air; if any found, allow to drip out end of tubing. *Reduces risk of air embolus.*
13. Thread IV tubing through pump according to manufacturer's directions. *So pump will function correctly.*
14. Check child's IV site for pain, redness, swelling, and infiltration. *Assures IV is patent.*
15. Remove cover from end of new IV tubing and place into catheter or scalp vein tubing at child's IV site. *So fluid in new IV tubing can flow into catheter or scalp vein.*
16. Turn on IV pump. *So child will receive ordered infusion.*
17. Remove gloves; wash hands. *Reduces transmission from microorganisms.*
18. Attach label to IV bag with time and date, person who changed bag, and any additives. *Documents who hung IV, when it was hung, and when tubing was changed.*

DOCUMENTATION

1. Time and date.
2. Fluid type and amount.
3. Rate of IV.
4. Type of infusion pump.
5. Condition of IV site.

 Estimated time to complete procedure: *10–15 minutes.*

Central Venous Catheter

OVERVIEW

The central venous catheter (CVC) is an IV catheter surgically inserted into a large central vein, with the catheter terminus in or near the right atrium. CVC insertion can be done on an outpatient basis and can remain in place from a few months to a few years.

Children need a central venous catheter placed for long-term IV therapy, total parenteral nutrition administration, chemotherapy administration, dialysis, or central venous pressure monitoring. The Broviac catheter, often used with children, can have a single, double, or triple lumen. The Hickman catheter may be used with older children and adolescents. Peripherally inserted central catheter (PICC) lines are commonly used in pediatrics as well as CVCs. All catheter lines require flushing, usually with heparinized saline, but institutional policies always need to be followed. The catheter site is usually covered with a clear occlusive dressing that is changed under sterile conditions every two or three days depending on agency policy.

PROCEDURE 53

CHANGING DRESSING ON A CENTRAL VENOUS LINE (TUNNELED, PERCUTANEOUS, AND IMPLANTED)

EQUIPMENT

Masks (for self and assistant)
Cleansing solution(s) for IV site
Gloves, nonsterile (exam)
Dressing materials (as prescribed by agency procedure)
Gloves, sterile
Sterile scissors (if necessary)

NOTE: *Some of the materials may come in a prepackaged kit.*

SAFETY

1. Assess for any allergies to tape or cleansing solution. *To reduce chance of allergic reaction.*
2. For infant, young child, or child unable to cooperate, use an assistant to help restrain the child. *Protects the integrity of the central line.*

PROCEDURE

1. Gather equipment; clean bedside stand. *Promotes organization and efficiency.*
2. Prepare child and family. Consider having someone to support or comfort the child during the procedure. *Enhances cooperation and participation and reduces anxiety and fear.*
3. Wash hands. *Reduces transmission of microorganisms.*
4. Position child as needed to perform the procedure. *So area can be visualized.*
5. Put on mask and nonsterile gloves. (Assistant should also wear a mask.) Carefully remove old dressing including any Steri-Strips. *Reduces transmission of microorganisms and protects nurse from contact with body fluids. Protects integrity of central line.*
6. Assess site. Examine for redness, swelling, and drainage. *To determine if inflamed or infected.*
7. Remove nonsterile gloves. Wash hands. *Reduces transmission of microorganisms.*
8. Open supplies and set up sterile field. *Promotes organization and efficiency.*
9. Put on sterile gloves. *Reduces transmission of microorganism, which could lead to infection of central line or sepsis.*
10. Cleanse insertion site and surrounding area with solution(s) prescribed by agency procedures. With each swab, begin at the catheter exit site and cleanse outward in a circular pattern without returning to the center. *Maintains asepsis by cleansing from least contaminated area to most contaminated area* (Figure VII-4A).
    a. A number of solutions may be used, singly or in combination, for cleansing the site. These include 10% povidone-iodine (or other iodophor), 70% alcohol, 0.5% chlorhexidine in 70% alcohol, 4% chlorhexidine in a detergent base (Hibiclens), and alcohol-acetone. *Povidone-iodine must be allowed to dry to be effective. If Hibiclens is used, it is recommended that it be removed from the skin using sterile water (Freiberger, 1994).*
    b. One procedure is to cleanse the site with 70% alcohol followed by 10% povidone-iodine. *Alcohol applied after povidone-iodine negates the fungicidal effects of the povidone-iodine.*
11. Clean catheter last, moving from insertion site up catheter by rolling swab (Figure VII-4B). *To prevent microorganism from entering insertion site.*

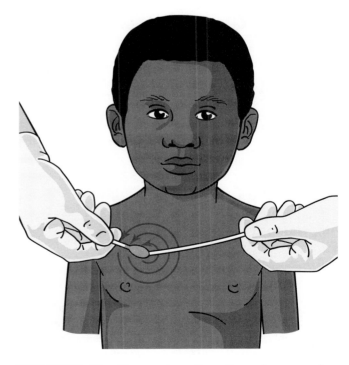

FIGURE VII-4A Cleanse insertion site and surrounding area by beginning at the catheter exit and moving outward in a circular pattern without returning to the center.

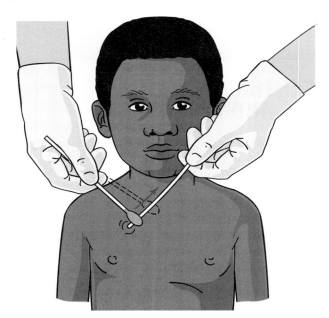

FIGURE VII-4B   Catheter is cleaned using upward strokes.

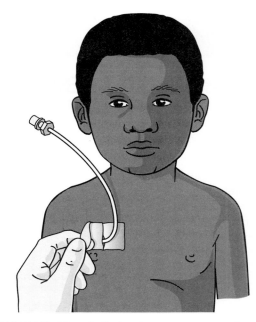

FIGURE VII-4D   Split 2 x 2 gauze surrounds catheter at site.

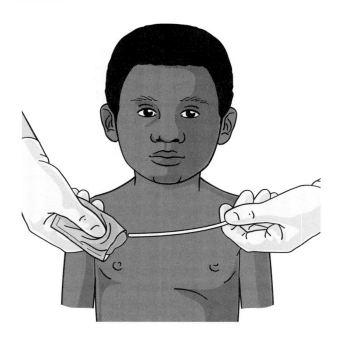

FIGURE VII-4C   Ointment is applied to site (per agency protocol).

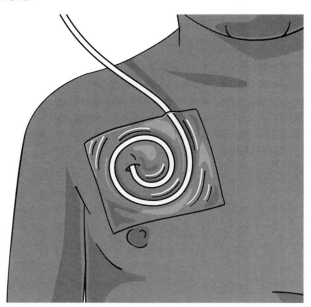

FIGURE VII-4E   Clear occlusive dressing is applied.

NOTE: *Type of dressing specified for peripherally inserted central catheters (PICC) and tunneled catheters may differ (Figures VII-4D and VII-4E).*

DOCUMENTATION

1. Dressing change and time.
2. Condition of site.

 Estimated time to complete procedure: *15–30 minutes.*

12. Apply skin prep to area avoiding ½-inch area around the catheter exit site. *To protect skin under dressing.*
13. Apply ointment as prescribed or per agency procedure (Figure VII-4C). *To help prevent infection at insertion site.*
14. Apply new sterile dressing as specified in agency policy. *To help prevent infection at insertion site.*

Respiratory System

Respiratory Suctioning

OVERVIEW

Suctioning secretions from the respiratory tract is necessary to maintain the airway for clients who are unable to effectively cough up the secretions. The procedure may be either a sterile procedure or a clean procedure.

PROCEDURE 54

PERFORMING BULB SUCTIONING

OVERVIEW

Secretions from the nose or mouth of an infant are removed by using a bulb syringe. This is a clean procedure.

EQUIPMENT

Bulb syringe
Normal saline drops
Gloves
Clean towel or paper towel

SAFETY

1. Avoid stimulating gag reflex, which may result in vomiting.

PROCEDURE

1. Gather equipment. *Improves organization and effectiveness.*
2. Prepare child and family. Consider having someone support or comfort the child. This may include having someone assist in holding child. *Enhances cooperation and parental participation, and reduces anxiety and fear.*
3. Wash hands. *Reduces transmission of microorganisms.*
4. Position child with head flat or slightly elevated. *So nares/mouth can be accessed easily.*
5. Assess respiratory status, including respiratory rate, color, and effort. *To determine if infant is in respiratory distress.*
6. If desired or if secretions are very thick, drop normal saline drops into nares before suctioning. *Helps loosen secretions.*
7. Deflate bulb prior to inserting tip into infant's nares or mouth by squeezing bulb (Figure VIII-1A). *Removes air from bulb.*
8. Insert tip into infant's nares or mouth (Figure VIII-1B). *Provides access to nares/mouth.*
9. Allow bulb to inflate and remove syringe from nares or mouth (Figure VIII-1C). *As bulb inflates a suction is formed that will remove secretions.*
10. Expel secretions into proper receptacle (cloth or paper towel). *Prevents transmission of microorganisms.*
11. Repeat as necessary. *More than one suctioning may be required to remove secretions.*

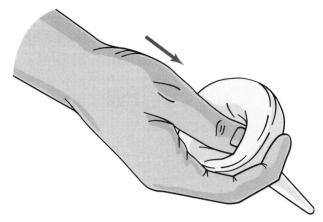

FIGURE VIII-1A   Deflate bulb prior to inserting tip into infant's nares or mouth by squeezing bulb.

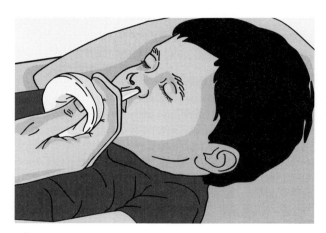

FIGURE VIII-1B   Insert tip into infant's nares or mouth.

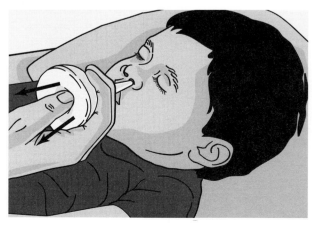

FIGURE VIII-1C   Allow bulb to inflate and remove syringe from nares or mouth.

12. Repeat assessment of respiratory status. *To determine if more suctioning needed.*

DOCUMENTATION

1. Color, consistency, and amount of secretions.
2. How well the child tolerated the procedure, and whether or not saline was used.
3. Respiratory status.
4. Frequency required to clear nares or mouth of secretions.

⊠ **Estimated time to complete procedure:** *less than 5 minutes.*

PROCEDURE 55

PERFORMING NASOTRACHEAL SUCTIONING

OVERVIEW

Secretions are removed from an older child's nose by using a catheter. This is a sterile procedure.

EQUIPMENT

Appropriately sized resuscitation equipment (mask, valve, bag)

Appropriately sized suction catheter pack (#8 to #10 French for children, #5 to #8 French for infants)

Mask, gloves, and goggle

Suction source (wall suction or portable suction machine)

Suction source canister and connecting tubing

Oxygen source and delivery source

Normal saline and container

K-Y Jelly

Moisture-resistant disposable bag

NOTE: *Requires order from physician to implement procedure. Suction only when assessment indicates need. Coordinate suctioning with other pulmonary hygiene interventions, e.g., inhaled bronchodilators, chest physiotherapy. Provide adequate hydration to minimize mucosal drying and promote ciliary action.*

SAFETY

1. Be prepared to maintain airway and initiate resuscitation measures should the child exhibit progressive signs of respiratory or cardiac distress.
2. Initiate "Code Blue" and provide resuscitation if child experiences respiratory or cardiac failure.
3. If both the oropharynx and nasopharynx are to be suctioned, use separate sterile catheters to prevent transmission of microorganisms.

PROCEDURE

1. Gather equipment. *Improves organization and effectiveness.*
2. Assemble suction canister and connecting tubing to suction source. Set suction levels as follows: 80–100 mm Hg for infants and children under 10–12 years, 100–120 mm Hg for older children. Ensure that appropriate resuscitation equipment (mask, valve, bag) is at bedside. *Improves organization and efficiency.*

3. Wash hands. *Reduces transmission of microorganisms.*
4. Identify an assistant to help position, hold, and comfort child as necessary. *Promotes organization and efficiency.*
5. Prepare child and family. Consider having someone support or comfort the child. *Enhances cooperation and parental participation; reduces anxiety and fear.*
6. Perform baseline respiratory assessment. *To determine if child's condition changes after suctioning.*
7. Open and prepare suction pack and normal saline container, maintaining clean technique. *Promotes organization and efficiency.*
8. Position child as needed to complete procedure using least restrictive immobilizing techniques (use assistant as necessary). *To provide access to nares.*
9. Oxygenate child above baseline oxygen saturation. *Suctioning may cause hypoxia.*
10. Wear mask, gloves, goggles, and gown (as needed). Observe standard and droplet precautions according to policy. *Prevents transmission of microorganisms.*
11. Using dominant hand, remove protective covering, pick up suction catheter, and connect it to the suction tubing with nondominant hand. Check suction pressures once the suction catheter is connected. *Promotes organization and efficiency; determines if connection is effective.*
12. Encourage the child to cough. *Helps pool secretions in hypopharynx; may prevent need for deep suctioning.*
13. Determine the correct distance to advance suction catheter. This is done by measuring from the tip of the child's nose to the opening of the ear; note position on the catheter. *If suction catheter is advanced more than necessary, may cause injury to child's treachea/lungs.*
14. Moisten the suction catheter using normal saline or K-Y Jelly. Using a downward motion, aiming toward midline, advance the catheter into the nare no farther than the premeasured distance. (For oropharyngeal suction, pull the tongue forward using gauze. Advance the catheter about 10–15 cm along one side of the mouth.) *Moisture enhances passage of catheter; downward motion allows catheter to follow anatomy of nasopharynx.*
15. Apply intermittent suctioning by covering the suction control hole with thumb. Gently rotate the catheter while withdrawing the catheter. Limit continuous suction within the airway to no more than 5 seconds (infants) to 15 seconds (child). *Rotating catheter assures that hole in catheter tip has better access to secretions.*

16. Reoxygenate the child to baseline oxygenation saturation. *Improves child's oxygen status if hypoxia developed.*

17. Clean the catheter by wiping with sterile gauze and flushing tubing with normal saline. *Removes secretions that may be on inside or outside of catheter.*

18. Repeat steps 13–15 as needed to clear the nasopharynx of secretions, alternating nares. Allow 20–30-second intervals between each episode of suctioning. Limit suctioning to a total of 5 minutes. *Procedure may need to be repeated to remove sufficient secretions to improve child's respiratory status.*

19. Assess respiratory status, including respiratory rate, color, and effort. Auscultate breath sounds. *To determine if there are any changes from assessment prior to suctioning.*

20. Comfort and praise child. *To obtain cooperation in the future if child needs to be suctioned again.*

DOCUMENTATION

Assess and document the following prior to and following the procedure:

1. Child's general condition.

2. Client assessment prior to and immediately following administration of oxygen. Include oxygen saturation, respiratory rate and effort, color, breath sounds, and heart rate. Complete appropriate scoring tool (bronchiolitis score or croup score) as indicated.

3. Color, consistency, and amount of secretions.

4. Note oxygen requirements, type of oxygen delivery device, and flow rate immediately and every four hours (if using a hood, FiO$_2$, flow rate, and temperature every four hours) or more frequently as needed.

5. Any complications that occurred.

6. Notify doctor should complications or unexpected responses occur.

7. Check cardiorespiratory assessment every four hours, or more frequently if needed; type and flow rate of oxygen on follow-up visits.

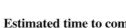 **Estimated time to complete procedure:** *5–10 minutes.*

Administering Oxygen

OVERVIEW

Oxygen is a drug and must be administered only as prescribed by the physician or qualified practitioner. Children unable to maintain adequate PO2 and O2 saturation levels on room air are candidates for oxygen therapy, and an adequate airway is important for the therapy to be effective.

The physician or qualified practitioner will order the oxygen delivery system and flow rate; the nurse will monitor the child's response. Even though in some acute care settings the respiratory therapy department is responsible for setting up oxygen equipment, it is important for the nurse to understand the basic reasons for oxygen therapy and know how to manage equipment.

Oxygen is delivered via mask, nasal cannula, hood, tent, or blow-by cannula. Method of delivery is selected based on:

Concentration of inspired oxygen needed

Ability of child to cooperate

PROCEDURE 56

ADMINISTERING OXYGEN VIA NASAL CANNULA, MASK, HOOD, TENT, BLOW-BY CANNULA

EQUIPMENT

Pulse oximeter
Stethoscope
Oxygen source
Flow meter
Sterile water container
Connecting tubing
Oxygen delivery device:
    Nasal cannula
    Simple face mask or nonrebreather mask
    Hood
    Tent
    Blow-by cannula

NOTE: *Oxygen is considered a medication. Delivery device, flow rate, and concentration must be ordered by a physician and checked frequently. However, in emergency situations administer oxygen in amounts necessary to provide immediate oxygenation. Humidification is needed when administering oxygen to prevent nasal passages from drying out. To provide this, attach a sterile, water-filled container to the oxygen or flow meter with a connecting tube.*

SAFETY

1. Place "Oxygen in Use" signs at the bedside and door of hospital room.
2. Verify use of hospital-approved electrical equipment in room. Check for frayed electrical cords of bed and other equipment in use.
3. Do not permit use of matches or lighters in room.
4. Keep flammable or volatile solutions outside the room.
5. Maintain temperature in tent or hood at 68°–75° F.
6. Do not allow toys in the tent that are metal, electrical, battery operated, or that use friction to operate.
7. Keep call light outside the tent.
8. Monitor for substernal pain and oxygen toxicity.

PROCEDURE

1. Gather equipment. *Improves organization and effectiveness.*
2. Wash hands. *Reduces transmission of microorganisms.*
3. Assemble equipment. Attach flow meter to oxygen outlet, ensure that tubing is not kinked, secure oxygen delivery device to flow meter, and attach humidification container (with connecting tubing if needed). *Improves organization and efficiency.*
4. Prepare child and family. Consider having someone support or comfort the child. This may include having someone assist in placing the nasal cannula or mask on the child. *Enhances cooperation and parental participation; reduces anxiety and fear.*
5. Position child as needed. *So procedure can be carried out successfully.*
6. Adjust flow meter *to ensure delivery of appropriate oxygen concentration per physician's order.*
7. Place oxygen delivery device on child. (If using the nasal cannula, place prongs of the cannula in the anterior nares. If using a mask, determine correct size. The mask should extend from the bridge of the nose to the cleft of the chin. It should fit snugly but not put pressure on the eyes, which could stimulate a vagal response. With either the cannula or the mask, place the elastic band around the child's head. If using a blow-by cannula, the caregiver may hold the child in his or her lap and direct the tubing toward the child's face. The cannula may also be placed next to the child's head and directed toward the child's face) (Figures VIII-2 and VIII-3). *So child receives oxygen as ordered.*
8. Observe child's response. Assess respiratory rate, effort, color, heart rate, and mental status. Auscultate

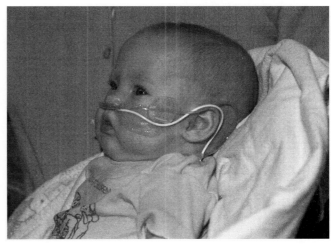

FIGURE VIII-2   O$_2$ per nasal cannula.

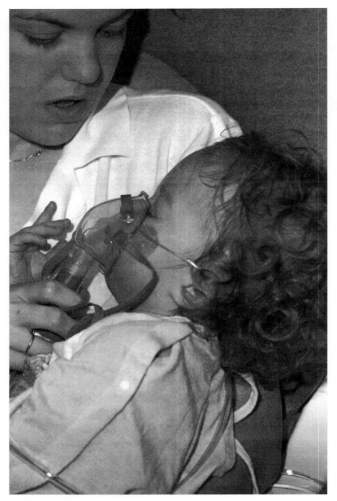

FIGURE VIII-3   O$_2$ per face mask.

breath sounds for symmetry and adventitious sounds. Continue to monitor as needed. *To determine effect of oxygen being delivered.*

NOTE: *Access to visual assessment of a child in a tent is difficult.*

9. Analyze inspired oxygen concentration using pulse oximeter. Analyze the oxygen concentration in the hood. Continue to monitor oxygen concentration hourly or continuously depending on the child's condition and/or physician's orders. If using a tent, determine oxygen concentration with an oxygen analyzer. *To determine level of oxygen child receives.*
10. Notify doctor of clinical changes. *In case oxygen order needs to be changed.*
11. Assess potential pressure sites at least every two hours (nares, ears, sides of the neck) for irritation if using nasal cannula. *Cannula may cause pressure on child's skin.*
12. Monitor sterile water container *to ensure adequate amount.*
13. Change gowns and linens frequently when using a hood or tent *to decrease dampness and ensure warmth.* Place additional clothing on children, or use additional linens, *to maintain a stable temperature.* Wipe sides of the hood or tent *to lessen moisture buildup to allow visualization of check.* Secure edges of tent with blankets *to avoid air leakage.*

DOCUMENTATION

1. Client assessment prior to and immediately following oxygen administration, including oxygen saturation, respiratory rate, effort, color, breath sounds, and heart rate.
2. Type of oxygen delivery device and flow rate every four hours (if using a hood, FiO$_2$, flow rate, and temperature every four hours).
3. Client cardiorespiratory assessment every four hours while oxygen administered. Note any changes in skin condition due to irritation of nasal cannula, mask, elastic band, or hood.

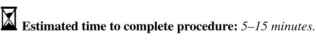 **Estimated time to complete procedure:** *5–15 minutes.*

Artificial Airways

OVERVIEW

Artificial airways are used in children to maintain an airway if the child is unconscious or needs assistance in ventilation. There are several types of artificial airways: oropharyngeal, nasopharyngeal, endotracheal, and tracheostomy.

PROCEDURE 57

ASSISTING IN PLACEMENT OF OROPHARYNGEAL OR NASOPHARYNGEAL AIRWAY

OVERVIEW

The oropharyngeal or nasopharyngeal airway is used when the child is unconscious. The airways are designed to prevent the tongue from falling into the posterior pharynx; they provide an open passageway past the lips and teeth, so air can flow around or through it and so a suction catheter can be passed into the laryngopharynx. The airways must be the correct size (airways range in size from 4 to 10 cm in length) and are placed by a physician or qualified practitioner. The nurse's role is to assist and monitor the child during the procedure and to care for the child after the procedure (Figures VIII-4A and VIII-4B).

EQUIPMENT

Oropharyngeal or nasopharyngeal airway
Airway suction equipment

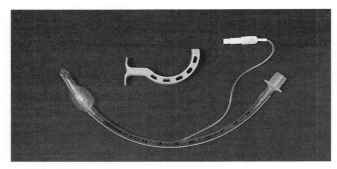

FIGURE VIII-4A   Oropharyngeal airway.

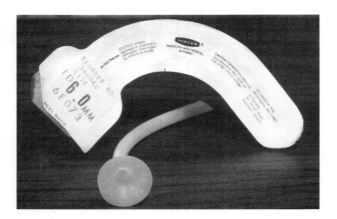

FIGURE VIII-4B   Nasopharyngeal airway.

Oxygen and humidity delivery source
Water-soluble lubricant
Gloves, mask, goggles, gown (as appropriate)

PROCEDURE

1. Gather equipment. *Improves organization and effectiveness.*
2. Wash hands. *Reduces transmission of microorganisms.*
3. Prepare child and family. Consider having someone support or comfort the child. *Enhances cooperation and parental participation; reduces anxiety and fear.*
4. Ensure that mouth and pharynx are cleared of secretions, blood, or vomit by using a suction catheter. *Reduces potential for aspiration.*
5. Assess child and assist physician or qualified practitioner during procedure. *To be sure child's condition doesn't worsen.*
6. After airway has been placed, maintain child's head and jaw in correct position (should be neutral, neither extended or flexed). *Keeps the trachea open.*
7. Dispose of all soiled materials and wash hands. *Reduces transmission of microorganisms.*

DOCUMENTATION

1. Time and date
2. Type of airway
3. Name of person who placed airway
4. Condition of child during procedure
5. Size of airway

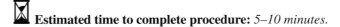 **Estimated time to complete procedure:** *5–10 minutes.*

PROCEDURE 58

SUCTIONING OROPHARYNGEAL OR NASOPHARYNGEAL AIRWAY

EQUIPMENT

Appropriately sized resuscitation equipment (mask, valve, bag)

Oxygen and humidity delivery source

Suction source, canister, and connecting tubing

Gloves, mask, goggles, gown (as appropriate)

Appropriately sized suction catheter pack

Age of child	Size of ETT (in millimeters)	Size of suction catheter (French)
Premature newborn–18 months	2.5–4.0	5½–6
6 months–3 years	3.5–4.5	8
5 years–12 years	5.0–6.5	10
16 years and older	7.0–10.0	12

Normal saline and container

Moisture-resistant disposable bag

NOTE: *Suction only after careful assessment indicates the need to do so. Coordinate suctioning with other pulmonary hygiene interventions (e.g., inhaled bronchodilators, chest physiotherapy). Provide adequate hydration to minimize mucosal drying and promote ciliary action.*

SAFETY

1. Use caution and care to avoid accidental dislodging of oropharyngeal or nasopharyngeal tube.
2. Be prepared to maintain airway and initiate resuscitation measures should the child exhibit progressive signs of respiratory or cardiac distress.
3. Initiate "Code Blue" and provide resuscitation if child experiences respiratory or cardiac failure.

PROCEDURE

1. Gather equipment. *Improves organization and effectiveness.*
2. Assemble suction canister and connecting tubing to suction source. Set suction levels as follows: 80–100 mm/Hg for infants and children under 10–12 years, 100–120 mm/Hg for older children. Ensure that appropriate resuscitation equipment (mask, valve, bag) is at bedside. *Improves organization and efficiency.*
3. Turn on oxygen source attached to the resuscitation bag *to inflate the reservoir bag.*
4. Wash hands. *Reduces transmission of microorganisms.*
5. Identify an assistant to help position, hold, and comfort child as necessary. *Improves organization and efficiency.*
6. Prepare child and family. Consider having someone support or comfort the child. *Enhances cooperation and parental participation; reduces anxiety and fear.*
7. Perform baseline respiratory assessment. *To determine if changes occur after procedure is completed; to determine child's respiratory status.*
8. Open and prepare suction pack and normal saline container, maintaining clean technique. *Improves organization and effectiveness.*
9. Don mask, gloves, goggles, and gown (as needed). Observe standard and droplet precautions according to policy. *To prevent transmission of microorganisms.*
10. Using dominant hand, remove protective covering, pick up suction catheter, and connect it to the suction tubing with nondominant hand. Check suction pressures once the suction catheter is connected. Place distal end of catheter in a cup of sterile saline *to test the suction. Improves organization and efficiency.*
11. If the child is being ventilated, have assistant disconnect the ventilator and hyperoxygenate with bag and mask three to five times. *Provides respirations for child before procedure is started.*
12. Remove the resuscitation bag. Using dominant hand, place the suction catheter into the orophraygeal or nasopharyngeal tube, making sure no suction is applied. Advance the catheter no farther than ¼ inch below the edge of the oropharyngeal or nasopharyngeal tube. *Further insertion may damage oropharynx or nasopharynx.*

NOTE: *To assist in judging how far to insert the catheter, place an appropriately sized catheter into an extra oropharyngeal or nasopharyngeal tube of the same size. Verify appropriate depth for suctioning; mark suction catheter to the appropriate depth with tape, or make a visual comparison of the tube length and the airway. If suction catheter is advanced more than necessary, it may cause injury to the child's trachea.*

13. Apply intermittent suctioning by covering the suction control hole with thumb. Gently rotate the catheter while withdrawing the catheter. Limit continuous

suction within the airway to no more than 5 seconds (infants) to 15 seconds (child). *Rotating catheter assures that hole in catheter tip has better access to secretions.*

14. Remove the catheter and flush with sterile saline. *Removes secretions that may be inside catheter.*

15. Repeat steps 13–16 as necessary, being sure to hyperoxygenate between suctioning. Allow 20–30-second intervals between each episode of suctioning. Limit suctioning to a total of 5 minutes. *Procedure may need to be repeated to remove sufficient secretions; suctioning longer than 5 minutes may cause hypoxia.*

16. Assess respiratory status, including respiratory rate, color, and effort. Auscultate breath sounds and observe chest expansion. *To determine if child's respiratory status has improved.*

17. Comfort child. *So child is less anxious and afraid.*

DOCUMENTATION

Assess and document the following prior to and following the procedure:

1. Child's general condition.
2. Client assessment prior to and immediately following suctioning. Include oxygen saturation, respiratory rate, effort, color, breath sounds, chest expansion, and heart rate. Note any hypoxia.
3. Note child's response to procedure, and whether there is increased anxiety or discomfort.
4. Color, consistency, and amount of secretions.
5. Note ventilator settings, oxygen requirements, type of oxygen delivery device, and flow rate immediately and every four hours (if using a hood, FiO_2, flow rate, and temperature every four hours) or more frequently as needed.
6. Any complications that occurred.

 Estimated time to complete procedure: *10 minutes.*

Endotracheal Tubes

OVERVIEW

Endotracheal tubes are sterile, disposable plastic airways used to maintain and secure an airway in an infant or child. The tapered distal end has an opening in the sidewall, and there are centimeter marks along the length of the tube that can be used when determining placement. The tubes are made with and without a cuff. Children under 8–9 years of age have a narrow airway and therefore do not need a tube with a cuff; older children, on the other hand, will need an endotracheal tube that has a cuff so that the airway can be sealed.

PROCEDURE 59

MONITORING ENDOTRACHEAL TUBES (ETT)

EQUIPMENT

Appropriately sized resuscitation equipment (mask, valve, bag)
Oxygen and humidity delivery source
Suction source, canister, and connecting tubing
Gloves, mask, goggles, gown (as appropriate)
Yankauer suction or closed port suction
Sterile suction kit (appropriately sized for ETT)

Age of child	Size of ETT (in millimeters)	Size of suction catheter (French)
Premature newborn–18 months	2.5–4.0	5½–6
6 months–3 years	3.5–4.5	8
5 years–12 years	5.0–6.5	10
16 years and older	7.0–10.0	12

Sterile unit dose normal saline and water
Sterile single-use water container
Benzoin
Tape, 2 × 2 gauze
Hypoactive dressing
Tape remover
3-way stopcock
Pressure manometer
5 ml syringe
Stethoscope
Pulse oximeter
Cardiorespiratory monitor
Moisture-resistant disposable bag

SAFETY

1. Infants and children unable to notify others of distress must be observed at all times.
2. The child, when transported outside of the client room, must be accompanied by trained personnel.
3. Initiate "Code Blue" and provide resuscitation if child experiences respiratory failure.
4. The following items must accompany the child when leaving the room: self-inflating resuscitation bag, mask, suction catheter, connecting tubing, normal saline, stethoscope, portable oxygen, and suction setup.
5. Be alert to complications, including obstruction, hemorrhage, subcutaneous emphysema, and tube dislodgement.

PROCEDURE

1. Wash hands. *Reduces transmission of microorganisms.*
2. Prepare child and family for procedure. Consider having someone support or comfort the child. *Enhances cooperation and parental participation; reduces anxiety and fear.*
3. Assess patency of airway, ETT placement (note the centimeter marking), size, security of ETT, proper humidification to airway, level of consciousness every two hours (more frequent as determined by physician's order or assessment). Include respiratory rate, work of breathing (retractions, flaring, grunting), breath sounds, chest symmetry, color, oxygen saturation. Monitor cardiorespiratory monitor and pulse oximeter. Identify ventilator settings and verify physician's orders regarding oxygen concentration, humidity, air temperature, pressure, tidal volume, and inspiratory/ expiratory ratio and rate. Support the ventilator tubing by securing to bed. *Determines child's condition; determines if ventilator is set according to physician orders; so ETT is not removed before ordered.*
4. Position child to prevent airway occlusion and promote secretion drainage. *So child's respiratory situation is not compromised and secretions are able to be removed easily.*
5. Monitor security of ETT. If tape loosens and ETT appears to not be secured, resecure (with assistance as needed). *To be sure ETT is still secure and able to function correctly.*
6. If it is necessary to completely retape ETT, gently remove hypoactive dressings while assistant secures ETT. Tear two pieces of tape long enough to reach from one cheek to the other. Split each piece of tape approximately two-thirds of its length. Paint each cheek and above the mouth over the nasal philtrum with benzoin. Affix the hypoactive dressing on each cheek after the benzoin is dry (tacky). Place the unsplit end of the tape to the square of hypoactive dressing. Carry the upper split portion of the tape over the nasal philtrum onto the opposite cheek. Bring the lower split end of the tape under the tube and wrap in a spiral. Fold the last 5 mm of the tail onto itself. Affix the second split tape in the same manner. *To be sure ETT is securely fastened and does not become unattached.*
7. Auscultate breath sounds and observe chest expansion. Record length of the ETT. Observe for air leaks. Ensure that ventilator is securely attached to ETT.

Suction as needed. *To determine if ETT is allowing air to enter respiratory track; to be sure ETT is patent and has no leaks which will decrease efficiency.*

8. Assist in obtaining chest x-ray if there is concern regarding displacement. *To check placement of ETT.*

9. Insert nasogastric tube if one is not already placed. (Follow procedures described earlier.) *To prevent aspiration of stomach contents, abdominal distention due to positive pressure ventilation, and air trapping.*

10. Measure arterial blood gases according to physician's orders. Assess hydration status in relation to viscosity of secretions. Note heated humidity, medications, skin turgor, mucous membranes, and intake and output. *To determine if ETT placed correctly and delivering adequate oxygen to child; if child is not adequately hydrated, secretions will be viscous.*

11. Provide oral care b.i.d. or more frequently as needed. *Oxygen is drying; if child is NPO, will need frequent oral care.*

12. Assess means and effectiveness of communicating daily needs (acutely and long term). Provide alternative methods as needed (e.g., eye blinks, tapping on bed, paper and pencil). *Child with ETT will have difficulty communicating normally.*

13. Promote ongoing nutritional needs. *For continued physical and psychological growth.*

14. Assess ongoing psychosocial needs of child and family coping with endotracheal tube. *ETT can be frightening to child and family; ETT may restrict child's movement and communication ability.*

15. Assess developmental needs. *Child with ETT may not be able to communicate normally, but will need to have developmental needs met.*

DOCUMENTATION

1. Child's general condition. Results of chest x-ray (CXR) and ABGs as applicable.

2. Client assessment, with a focus on respiratory status (e.g., respiratory rate, effort, color, breath sounds, chest movement, oxygen saturation, ventilator settings, presence of air leaks).

3. Note size, centimeter marking, and security of ETT.

4. Care child receives (e.g., oral care, repositioning).

5. Child's response to nursing cares.

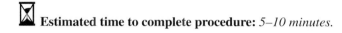 **Estimated time to complete procedure:** *5–10 minutes.*

PROCEDURE 60

ENDOTRACHEAL SUCTIONING

EQUIPMENT

Appropriately sized resuscitation equipment (mask, valve, bag)
Oxygen and humidity delivery source
Suction source, canister, and connecting tubing
Gloves, mask, goggles, gown (as appropriate)
Appropriately sized suction catheter pack

Age of child	Size of ETT (in millimeters)	Size of suction catheter (French)
Premature newborn–18 months	2.5–4.0	5½–6
6 months–3 years	3.5–4.5	8
5 years–12 years	5.0–6.5	10
16 years and older	7.0–10.0	12

Normal saline and container
Moisture-resistant disposable bag

NOTE: *Suction only after careful assessment indicates the need to do so. Coordinate suctioning with other pulmonary hygiene interventions (e.g., inhaled bronchodilators, chest physiotherapy). Provide adequate hydration to minimize mucosal drying and promote ciliary action.*

SAFETY

1. Use caution and care to avoid accidentally dislodging ETT.
2. Be prepared to maintain airway and initiate resuscitation measures should the child exhibit progressive signs of respiratory or cardiac distress.
3. Initiate "Code Blue" and provide resuscitation if child experiences respiratory or cardiac failure.

PROCEDURE

1. Gather equipment. *Improves organization and effectiveness.*
2. Assemble suction canister and connecting tubing to suction source. Set suction levels as follows: 80–100 mm Hg for infants and children under 10–12 years, 100–120 mm Hg for older children. Ensure that appropriate resuscitation equipment (mask, valve, bag) is at bedside. *Improves organization and efficiency. Set level appropriate for children of specific ages.*
3. Turn on oxygen source attached to the resuscitation bag *to inflate the reservoir bag.*
4. Wash hands. *Reduces transmission of microorganisms.*
5. Identify an assistant to help position, hold, and comfort child as necessary. *Improves organization and efficiency as well as cooperation.*
6. Prepare child and family. Consider having someone support or comfort the child. *Enhances cooperation and parental participation; reduces anxiety and fear.*
7. Perform baseline respiratory assessment. *Determines child's condition; used to determine if there are any changes after suctioning.*
8. Open and prepare suction pack and normal saline container, maintaining clean technique. *Improves organization and efficiency; procedure is a clean procedure.*
9. Put on mask, gloves, goggles, and gown (as needed). Observe standard and droplet precautions according to policy. *Reduces transmission of microorganisms; protects caregiver from microorganisms.*
10. Using dominant hand, remove protective covering, pick up suction catheter, and connect it to the suction tubing with nondominant hand. Check suction pressures once the suction catheter is connected. Place distal end of catheter in a cup of sterile saline to test the suction. *Promotes organization and efficiency; to be sure all tubing is connected correctly.*
11. If the child is being ventilated, have assistant disconnect the ventilator and hyperoxygenate with bag and mask three to five times. *Promotes organization and efficiency; reduces chance of hypoxia developing.*
12. Remove the resuscitation bag. Using dominant hand, place the suction catheter into the ETT, making sure no suction is applied. Advance the catheter no farther than ¼ inch below the edge of the ETT. *If suction catheter is advanced more than necessary or if suction is applied too soon, may cause injury to child's trachea/lungs.*

NOTE: *To assist in judging how far to insert the catheter, place an appropriately sized catheter into an extra ETT of the same size. Verify appropriate depth for suctioning; mark suction catheter to the appropriate depth with tape, or make a visual comparison of the ET tube length and the airway.*

13. Apply intermittent suctioning by covering the suction control hole with thumb. Gently rotate the catheter while withdrawing the catheter. Limit continuous suction within the airway to no more than 5 seconds (infants) to 15 seconds (child). *Rotating catheter*

assures that hole in catheter tip has better access to secretions; constant suction of more than 5–15 seconds may cause injury to child's trachea.

14. Remove the catheter and flush with sterile saline. *Removes secretions that may be on inside or outside of catheter.*

15. Repeat steps 13–16 as necessary, being sure to hyperoxygenate between suctioning. Allow 20–30-second intervals between each episode of suctioning. Limit suctioning to a total of 5 minutes. *Procedure may need to be repeated to remove sufficient secretions to improve child's respiratory status.*

16. Assess respiratory status, including respiratory rate, color, and effort. Auscultate breath sounds and observe chest expansion. *To determine if there are any changes from assessment prior to suctioning.*

17. Comfort child. *Procedure can be frightening to child and family; to obtain cooperation in the future if child needs to be suctioned again.*

DOCUMENTATION

Assess and document the following prior to and following the procedure:

1. Child's general condition.
2. Assessment prior to and immediately following suctioning. Include oxygen saturation, respiratory rate, effort, color, breath sounds, chest expansion, and heart rate. Note any hypoxia.
3. Note child's response to procedure and whether there is increased anxiety or discomfort.
4. Color, consistency, and amount of secretions.
5. Note ventilator settings, oxygen requirements, type of oxygen delivery device and flow rate immediately and every four hours (if using a hood, FiO_2, flow rate, and temperature every four hours) or more frequently as needed.
6. Any complications that occurred.

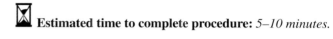 **Estimated time to complete procedure:** *5–10 minutes.*

Tracheostomies

OVERVIEW

A tracheostomy is an incision made into the trachea with insertion of a cannula for airway management. Tracheostomies are performed for the child who has a potential or present airway obstruction, for ventilatory assistance, to provide pulmonary hygiene, to decrease dead anatomic space in the child who has chronic obstructive pulmonary disease, and to avoid prolonged endotracheal intubation.

The tracheostomy is performed below the level of the vocal cords, allowing air to enter and exit the tracheostomy rather than entering and exiting through the upper airway.

The tracheostomy tube can be plugged to evaluate the child's ability to tolerate removal of the tracheostomy tube (decannulization) and to provide verbal speech for the child who has a tracheostomy. The plastic pediatric tracheostomy tube has an obturator, which is used for insertion and is held in place with twill tape that is tied around the child's neck.

Immediately after the tracheostomy has been performed, all care provided to the area must follow sterile technique. After the family learns to care for the tracheostomy, it becomes a clean procedure. Tracheostomies are monitored closely, and tracheostomy care is usually performed once per shift. Whenever performing tracheostomy care, a second person should always be available to help.

The tracheostomy is a surgical procedure. The nurse's role after the tracheostomy has been placed is to monitor and care for the child.

PROCEDURE 61

MONITORING A TRACHEOSTOMY

EQUIPMENT

Note: *Equipment is kept at bedside or in room when client has a tracheostomy.*

Appropriately sized resuscitation equipment (mask, valve, bag)

Oxygen and humidity delivery source

Suction source, canister, and connecting tubing

Gloves, mask, goggles, gown (as appropriate)

Spare tracheostomy tubes (see note below)

Spare tracheostomy tube holder

Appropriately sized suction catheter pack (#8 to #10 French for children, #5 to #8 French for infants)

Oxygen flow meter and blender

Pulse oximeter

Cardiorespiratory monitor

Bandage scissors and small hemostats

Preslit Sof-Wick dressing, cotton-tipped applicators

Unit dose normal saline

Half-strength (1.5%) peroxide, sterile water/normal saline

Antibiotic ointment if ordered

NOTE: *For a new tracheostomy, spare tracheostomy tubes should include same size and ½ size smaller. For an established tracheostomy, spare tracheostomy tubes should be same size.*

SAFETY

1. Infants and children unable to notify others of distress must be observed at all times.
2. The child, when transported outside of the client room, must be accompanied by trained personnel.
3. Initiate "Code Blue" and provide resuscitation if child experiences respiratory failure.
4. The following items must accompany the child leaving the room: spare tracheostomy tubes, self-inflating resuscitation bag, mask, suction catheter, suction connecting tubing, normal saline, stethoscope, Sof-Wicks, tracheostomy tube holder, water-soluble jelly, bandage scissors, gloves, portable suction (if needed).
5. Prevent potential aspiration by maintaining environment free of safety hazards.
6. Be alert to complications including obstruction, hemorrhage, subcutaneous emphysema, tube dislodgement, periostomal irritation, redness, or breakdown.

PROCEDURE

1. Assess patency of airway, tube placement, tube size, security of tracheostomy, proper humidification to airway, level of consciousness every two hours (more frequent as determined by physician's order or assessment). Include respiratory rate, work of breathing (retractions, flaring, grunting), breath sounds, chest symmetry, color, oxygen saturation. Monitor cardiorespiratory monitor and pulse oximeter. *To obtain information about child's condition over time.*
2. Position child to prevent airway occlusion and secretion drainage. *So tracheostomy is able to function appropriately.*
3. Maintain pulmonary toilet (e.g., cough, deep breath, incentive spirometer, activity). *To lessen chance of developing respiratory track infection.*
4. Assess viscosity, color, odor, and amount of secretions when suctioned. *To determine if secretions indicate development of respiratory infection.*
5. Assess hydration status in relation to viscosity of secretions. Note heated humidity, medications, skin turgor, mucous membranes, intake and output. *If child becomes dehydrated, secretions may become viscous and therefore harder to remove from respiratory track.*
6. Provide oral care b.i.d. or more frequently as needed. *If child is receiving oxygen, it is drying; if child is NPO, will need frequent oral care.*
7. Assess means and effectiveness of child's ability to communicate daily needs (both acutely and long term). Provide alternative methods as needed (e.g., tongue clicking, tapping on bed, paper and pencil). Involve speech therapist. *Child with tracheostomy will have difficulty communicating normally.*
8. Promote ongoing nutritional needs, calorie counts as needed, and plan intake with respect to possible changes in smell, taste, and swallowing ability. *For continued physical and psychological growth; child with tracheostomy may have difficulty eating normally.*
9. Assess ongoing psychosocial needs of child and family coping with tracheostomy placement (acute and long term). *Tracheostomy tube can be frightening to child and family; child may have difficulty communicating normally.*
10. Assess developmental needs. *Tracheostomy may restrict child's movement and normal development;*

may need referral to developmentalist or developmental interventionalist.

11. Discuss with family discharge needs regarding equipment procurement for long-term tracheostomy plan. *Family will need to have information about care child will need while at home.*

DOCUMENTATION

1. Assessment every two hours (more frequently if necessary), respiratory rate, work of breathing (retractions, flaring, grunting), breath sounds, chest symmetry, color, oxygen saturation, patency of airway, tube placement, tube size, security of tracheostomy, and level of consciousness.

2. Appearance of stoma and neck every shift and as needed (p.r.n.).

3. Frequency of suctioning, appearance and quantity of secretions, and tolerance of procedures as performed.

4. Date of last tracheostomy tube change.

5. Child and caregiver education.

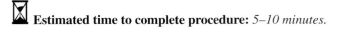 **Estimated time to complete procedure:** *5–10 minutes.*

PROCEDURE 62

CHANGING A TRACHEOSTOMY TUBE

EQUIPMENT

Appropriately sized resuscitation equipment (mask, valve, bag)

Oxygen and humidity delivery source

Suction source, canister, and connecting tubing

Gloves, mask, goggles, gown (as appropriate)

Spare tracheostomy tubes (see note below)

Spare tracheostomy tube holder

Appropriately sized suction catheter pack (#8 to #10 French for children, #5 to #8 French for infants)

Oxygen flow meter and blender

Pulse oximeter

Cardiorespiratory monitor

Bandage scissors and small hemostats

Preslit Sof-Wick dressing, cotton-tipped applicators

Tracheostomy tube with obturator

5 cc syringe if tube has cuff

Normal saline or sterile water

Water-soluble gel lubricant

Precut twill tape

Towel

NOTE: *For a new tracheostomy, spare tracheostomy tubes should include same size and half size smaller. For an established tracheostomy, spare tracheostomy tubes should be same size.*

SAFETY

1. The physician will be the first person to change the tracheostomy tube after surgery. After that, agency procedures regarding who changes the tracheostomy tube should be followed.
2. Do not use gauze dressing, as loose filaments may be inhaled into the tracheostomy.
3. All tracheostomy tube changes and replacements are a two-person procedure.
4. Be gentle in all aspects of care. *Clients should not feel any discomfort or unpleasant feelings at the site.*
5. Be alert to complications, including obstruction, hemorrhage, subcutaneous emphysema, tube dislodgement, periostomal irritation, redness, or breakdown.
6. Notify physician immediately if complications arise. Maintain patent airway via stoma or mouth/nose ventilation.
7. Initiate "Code Blue" and provide resuscitation if child experiences respiratory failure or does not have a patent airway.

PROCEDURE

1. Gather equipment. *Improves organization and effectiveness.*
2. Wash hands. *Reduces transmission of microorganisms.*
3. Identify an assistant to help position, assist in tube change, and hold and comfort child as necessary. *Improves organization and efficiency as well as child's cooperation.*
4. Prepare child and family. Provide child and family with age-appropriate explanation of procedure. Consider having someone support or comfort the child. *Enhances cooperation and parental participation; reduces anxiety and fear.*
5. Perform baseline respiratory assessment. *Determines child's condition; used to determine if there are any changes after suctioning.*
6. Don mask, gloves, goggles, and gown (as needed). Observe standard body substance precautions according to policy. *Reduces transmission of microorganisms; protects caregiver from microorganisms.*
7. Assemble supplies and equipment. Ensure that spare tracheostomy tube of appropriate size and type is at bedside. Open Sof-Wick dressing packets (as needed); pour normal saline/sterile water into containers. *Improves organization and efficiency.*
8. Prepare new tracheostomy tube. Attach tube holder. If a cuffed tube is being used, check cuff for leaks by injecting a small amount of air into the cuff. Deflate cuff completely. Insert obturator. Lubricate the tube with water-soluble gel or sterile water. *Improves organization and efficiency; lubrication will help place new tracheostomy tube easier.*
9. Position child by exposing the neck and straightening the airway (avoid hyperextension). If necessary, a rolled towel or diaper may be placed under the child's shoulders to extend the neck. The sniffing position is ideal. Use the least restrictive immobilizing methods when positioning the child (Figure VIII-5A). *So new tracheostomy tube can be placed without difficulty.*
10. Preoxygenate child as needed (and at any time during the procedure). Continually assess child for oxygenation and respiratory distress during the entire procedure. *Reduces chance of hypoxia developing.*
11. Remove the soiled dressing. *Reduces transmission of microorganisms.*
12. Deflate cuff (as appropriate); remove or cut tube holder while holding the tube to prevent accidental

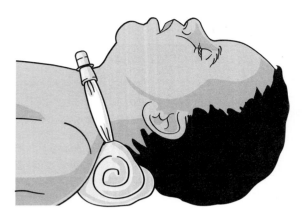

FIGURE VIII-5A Placement of towel under child's shoulders and neck to allow for straightening of the airway.

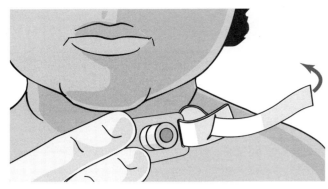

FIGURE VIII-5B Attach twill tape to the flange and tie securely.

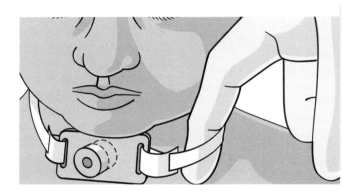

FIGURE VIII-5C Check that tape is tight enough to secure but loose enough to fit one finger between tie and child's neck.

dislodgment or displacement. *So old tube can be removed.*

13. Remove the old tube with a gentle steady motion, outward and downward following the natural curvature of the tracheostomy tube. *Decreases chance of injury to trachea.*

14. Insert the new tracheostomy tube. Use a gentle, arcing motion following the natural curvature of the tube. Do not force. If difficulty is encountered, pull the tube away from stoma, readjust entry angle, and reattempt tube placement. Use a gentle, steady upward or downward traction of the skin on the neck above or below the stoma to facilitate tube placement. *Decreases chance of injury to trachea.*

15. Immediately remove the obturator. Provide oxygen, ventilation, or suction as needed while holding the tube in place. *Reduces chance of hypoxia developing.*

16. Inflate the cuff as appropriate, using minimal leak technique. (Minimal leak technique: place stethoscope over the neck at cuff site. Slowly inject air into the cuff during positive inspiration until leak stops. Remove a small amount of air to allow a slight leak during peak inspiration. The leak is heard with the stethoscope.) *So tracheostomy tube remains in place.*

17. Observe for correct placement of the tube, chest movement, color, vital signs, and bilateral breath sounds. Note signs of respiratory distress or hypoxia. *To determine if tube is in correct place.*

18. Secure the tube with the tube holder. *So tracheostomy tube remains in place.*

19. Place new Sof-Wick dressing under the tracheostomy tube flanges (if used) using hemostats and fingers. While assistant holds the tube in place, remove soiled ties from flange. Attach twill tape to the flange and tie securely. This should be tight enough to prevent dislodgement but loose enough to fit one finger between tie and child's

neck (Figures VIII-5B and VIII-5C). *So tracheostomy tube remains in place; to protect neck skin from twill tape that may become moist or irritate neck.*

20. Clean old tube and obturator following procedure. *So it is ready to be used when tracheostomy is changed again.*

21. Monitor respiratory status and client response to procedure. *To determine if tracheostomy is in correct position.*

DOCUMENTATION

1. Procedure, child's preparation and response to procedure, including respiratory status and breath sounds.
2. Reason for tracheostomy tube change, tracheostomy tube size and type, condition of stoma.
3. Complications that might have occurred.
4. Quantity and viscosity of respiratory secretions.

 Estimated time to complete procedure: *10–15 minutes.*

PROCEDURE 63

CLEANING A TRACHEOSTOMY TUBE OR INNER CANNULA

EQUIPMENT

Appropriately sized resuscitation equipment (mask, valve, bag)

Oxygen and humidity delivery source

Suction source, canister, and connecting tubing

Gloves, mask, goggles, gown (as appropriate)

Spare tracheostomy tubes (see note below)

Spare tracheostomy tube holder

Appropriately sized suction catheter pack (#8 to #10 French for children, #5 to #8 French for infants)

Oxygen flow meter and blender

Pulse oximeter

Cardiorespiratory monitor

Bandage scissors and small hemostats

Half-strength peroxide

Normal saline or sterile water

Preslit Sof-Wick dressing

Cotton-tipped applicators

Precut twill tape

Clean, dry containers (2)

Towel

NOTE: *For a new tracheostomy, spare tracheostomy tubes should include same size and half size smaller. For an established tracheostomy, spare tracheostomy tubes should be same size. Equipment may be available in a prepackaged kit.*

SAFETY

1. Prevent potential aspiration by maintaining environment free of safety hazards.
2. Routine site care should not be done for the first 48 hours following the initial tracheostomy tube placement.
3. Routine tracheostomy site care and dressing change should be done at least once a shift or any time the site or dressing becomes wet or soiled. Do not use gauze dressing, as loose filaments may be inhaled into the tracheostomy.
4. All tracheostomy tube changes and replacements are a two-person procedure.
5. Be gentle in all aspects of care. *Clients should not feel any discomfort or unpleasant feelings at the site.*
6. Be alert to complications, including obstruction, hemorrhage, subcutaneous emphysema, tube dislodgement, periostomal irritation, redness, or breakdown.
7. Notify physician immediately of dislodged or displaced tube. Maintain patent airway via stoma or mouth/nose ventilation.

8. Initiate "Code Blue" and provide resuscitation if child experiences respiratory failure or does not have a patent airway.

PROCEDURE

1. Gather equipment. *Improves organization and effectiveness.*
2. Wash hands. *Reduces transmission of microorganisms.*
3. Identify an assistant to help position, assist in tube change, and hold and comfort child as necessary. *Improves organization and efficiency as well as child's cooperation.*
4. Prepare child and family. Provide child and family with age-appropriate explanation of procedure. Consider having someone support or comfort the child. *Enhances cooperation and parental participation and reduces anxiety and fear.*
5. Perform baseline respiratory assessment. *Determines child's condition; used to determine if there are any changes after suctioning.*
6. Don mask, gloves, goggles, and gown (as needed). Observe standard body substance precautions according to policy. *Reduces transmission of microorganisms; protects caregiver from microorganisms.*
7. Assemble supplies and equipment. Open Sof-Wick dressing packets and cotton-tipped applicators; pour normal saline/sterile water and hydrogen peroxide into containers. *Improves organization and efficiency.*
8. Position child by exposing the neck and straightening the airway (avoid hyperextension). If necessary, a rolled towel or diaper may be placed under the child's shoulders to extend the neck. The sniffing position is ideal. Use the least restrictive immobilizing methods when positioning the child. *So new tracheostomy tube can be placed without difficulty.*
9. Preoxygenate child as needed (and at any time during the procedure). *Reduces chance of hypoxia developing.*
10. Unlock the inner cannula; inspect for any damage, cracks, chips, rough areas, and so forth. Clean inside and outside of the tracheostomy tube or cannula with tap water using pipe cleaners and soft-tipped applicators. Rinse cannula. *Reduces transmission of microorganisms.*
11. Place cannula into the container with hydrogen peroxide. Agitate vigorously for one to two minutes. Allow cannula to air dry for as long as possible. Replace the inner cannula and lock into place. *Cleans cannula and removes thickened secretions.*

12. Gently lift the tracheostomy tube flange and remove the soiled dressing. *Reduces transmission of microorganisms; gentle movements lessen chance of dislodging cannula.*

13. Using the cotton-tipped applicators moistened with half-strength peroxide, begin cleaning around the stoma site, always moving outward from the stoma. Never clean toward the stoma. Use as many applicators as needed to remove secretions. Avoid dripping peroxide into stoma site (Figure VIII-6). *Reduces transmission of microorganisms; gentle movements lessen chance of dislodging cannula.*

14. Rinse the area using applicators soaked with normal saline or sterile water, always moving outward from

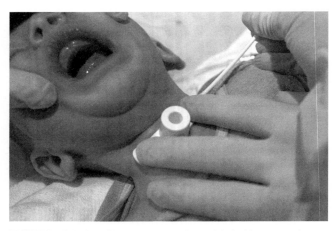

FIGURE VIII-6   Clean stoma site with half-strength peroxide, moving outward from stoma site in a circular fashion.

the stoma. Cleanse the area behind the flanges of the tracheostomy and around the neck with damp gauze, observing for redness or skin breakdown. *Reduces transmission of microorganisms; gentle movements lessen chance of dislodging cannula.*

15. Dry the skin around the stoma and neck thoroughly, using clean, dry applicators and gauze as appropriate. *To lessen the chance of moisture causing skin irritation and breakdown.*

16. Place new Sof-Wick dressing under the tracheostomy tube flanges (if used) using hemostats and fingers. While assistant holds the tube in place, remove soiled ties from flange. Attach twill tape to the flange and tie securely. This should be tight enough to prevent dislodgement but loose enough to fit one finger between tie and child's neck. *To protect neck skin from twill tape that may become moist or irritate neck.*

17. Monitor respiratory status and client response to procedure. *To determine if child's condition was impacted by procedure.*

DOCUMENTATION

1. Client preparation and response to procedure, including respiratory status.
2. Condition of skin around stoma and neck.
3. Complications that might have occurred (e.g., accidental tube dislodgement or displacement).
4. Quantity and viscosity of respiratory secretions.

Estimated time to complete procedure: *15–20 minutes.*

PROCEDURE 64

SUCTIONING A TRACHEOSTOMY

EQUIPMENT

Appropriately sized resuscitation equipment (mask, valve, bag)
Oxygen and humidity delivery source
Suction source, canister, and connecting tubing
Gloves, mask, goggles, gown (as appropriate)
Spare tracheostomy tubes (see note below)
Spare tracheostomy tube holder
Appropriately sized suction catheter pack (#8 to #10 French for children, #5 to #8 French for infants)
Normal saline and container
Moisture-resistant disposable bag

NOTE: *For a new tracheostomy, spare tracheostomy tubes should include same size and half size smaller. For an established tracheostomy, spare tracheostomy tubes should be same size.*

SAFETY

1. Be gentle in all aspects of care. *Clients should not feel any discomfort or unpleasant feelings at the site.*
2. Be prepared to maintain airway and initiate resuscitation measures should child exhibit progressive signs of respiratory or cardiac distress.
3. Initiate "Code Blue" and provide resuscitation if child experiences respiratory or cardiac failure.

NOTE: *Suction only after careful assessment indicates the need to do so. Coordinate suctioning with other pulmonary hygiene interventions (e.g., inhaled bronchodilators, chest physiotherapy). Provide adequate hydration to minimize mucosal drying and promote ciliary action.*

PROCEDURE

1. Gather equipment. *Improves organization and effectiveness.*
2. Assemble suction canister and connecting tubing to suction source. Set suction levels as follows: 80–100 mm Hg for infants and children under 10–12 years, 100–120 mm Hg for older children. Ensure that appropriate resuscitation equipment (mask, valve, bag) is at bedside. *Improves organization and efficiency. Choose suction level for child according to age so is at appropriate level.*
3. Turn on oxygen source attached to the resuscitation bag *to inflate the reservoir bag.*
4. Wash hands. *Reduces transmission of microorganisms.*

5. Identify an assistant to help position, hold, and comfort child as necessary. *Improves organization and efficiency as well as child's cooperation.*
6. Prepare child and family. Consider having someone support or comfort the child. *Enhances cooperation and parental participation; reduces anxiety and fear.*
7. Perform baseline respiratory assessment. *Determines child's condition; used to determine if there are any changes after suctioning.*
8. Open and prepare suction pack and normal saline container, maintaining clean technique. *Improves organization and efficiency.*
9. Place head of the bed at a 30° angle. Use least restrictive immobilizing techniques (use assistant as necessary). *Allows visualization of and access to tracheostomy; improves organization and efficiency as well as child's cooperation.*
10. Don mask, gloves, goggles, and gown (as needed). Observe standard and droplet precautions according to policy. *Reduces transmission of microorganisms; protects caregiver from microorganisms.*
11. Using dominant hand, remove protective covering, pick up suction catheter, and connect it to the suction tubing with nondominant hand. Check suction pressures once catheter is connected. Place distal end of catheter in a cup of sterile saline to test the suction. *Improves organization and efficiency; assesses whether or not suction is connected correctly.*
12. With nondominant hand, remove humidity source from the tracheostomy tube. Oxygenate the child before suctioning, using resuscitation bag in nondominant hand. Give several breaths (Figure VIII-7A). *Reduces chance of hypoxia developing.*
13. Remove the resuscitation bag. Using dominant hand, place the suction catheter into the tube, making sure no suction is applied. Advance the catheter no farther than ¼ to ½ inch below the edge of the tracheostomy tube (Figure VIII-7B). *Reduces chance of hypoxia developing; reduces chance of injuring trachea.*

NOTE: *To assist in judging how far to insert the catheter, place an appropriately sized catheter into an extra artificial airway of the same size. Verify appropriate depth for suctioning and mark suction catheter to the appropriate depth with tape.*

14. Apply intermittent suctioning by covering the suction control hole with thumb. Gently rotate the catheter while withdrawing the catheter. Limit continuous

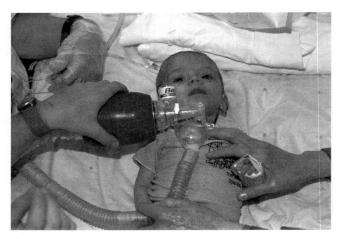

FIGURE VIII-7A   Oxygenating child prior to suctioning.

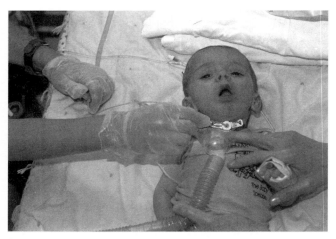

FIGURE VIII-7B   Using dominant hand, place the suction catheter into the tube.

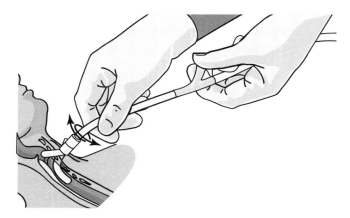

FIGURE VIII-7C   Gently rotate the catheter while withdrawing it.

suction within the airway to no more than 5 seconds (infants) to 15 seconds (child) (Figure VIII-7C). *Reduces chance of hypoxia developing; decreases chance of injury to trachea; rotating catheter assures that hole in catheter tip has better access to secretions; constant suction of more than 5–15 seconds may cause injury to child's trachea.*

15. Remove the catheter and flush with sterile saline. *Removes secretions that may be on inside or outside of catheter.*

NOTE: *The use of normal saline to irrigate the tracheostomy tube remains controversial. Follow policy, keeping the following guidelines in mind: 3–5 drops for an infant, 0.5 ml for a child, up to 1–3 ml for an adolescent.*

16. Oxygenate child. If necessary, repeat steps 13–15, being sure to oxygenate (or hyperoxygenate) between suctioning. Allow 20–30-second intervals between each episode of suctioning. Limit suctioning to a total of 5 minutes. *Procedure may need to be repeated to remove sufficient secretions to improve child's respiratory status.*

17. Assess respiratory status, including respiratory rate, color, and effort. Auscultate breath sounds. *To determine if there are any changes from assessment prior to suctioning.*

18. Comfort child. *Procedure can be frightening to child and family; to obtain cooperation in the future if child needs to be suctioned again.*

DOCUMENTATION

Assess and document the following prior to and following the procedure:

1. Child's general condition prior to and immediately after suctioning. Note how well the procedure was tolerated and if any difficulties occurred during the procedure.
2. Client assessment prior to and immediately following suctioning. Note oxygen requirements, oxygen saturation, respiratory rate, effort, color, breath sounds, and heart rate. Particularly note periods of desaturation.
3. Color, consistency, and amount of secretions.
4. Note any complications that occurred.
5. Note notification of physician regarding complications or unexpected responses that occurred.
6. Client cardiorespiratory assessment every four hours or more frequently if needed; type and flow rate of oxygen on follow-up visits.

 Estimated time to complete procedure: *5–10 minutes.*

Peak Expiratory Flow Rates (PEFRs)

OVERVIEW

A peak flow meter measures how well air moves out of the child's lungs. The peak expiratory flow rate (PEFR) is the fastest speed at which air is forced out of the lungs during expiration and is measured in liters per minute. The test, usually reserved for children over 3 years of age, is most helpful in determining the extent of a child's asthma. The PEFR is lower during acute episodes of asthma because of impaired expiration and air trapping that occur when there is an airway obstruction. Since there are a variety of peak flow meters on the market, it is important to become familiar with the equipment before having a child use it.

PROCEDURE 65

MEASURING PEFR

EQUIPMENT

Peak flow meter with mouthpiece (see figure VIII-8)
Peak flow record/chart
calculator

PROCEDURE

1. Set up equipment needed (peak flow meter with mouth-piece, record or chart, and calculator. *Improves organization and effectiveness.*
2. Wash hands. *Reduces transmission of microorganisms.*

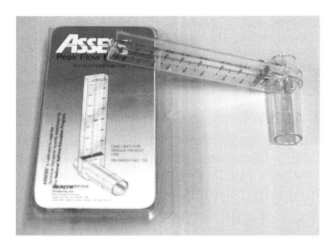

FIGURE VIII-8   One type of peak flow meter.

3. Prepare child and family. Consider having someone support or comfort the child. *Enhances cooperation and parental participation; reduces anxiety and fear.*
4. Ask child to sit up straight or stand up. *Expands lungs to maximum.*
5. Ask child to place the mouthpiece of the meter in his/her mouth, keeping tongue away from the opening; take a deep breath; close the lips around the mouthpiece; and then blow as fast and as hard as possible into the mouthpiece. *Ensures effective seal and accurate measurement.*
6. Read the number on the meter. *Ensures accurate documentation.*
7. Ask the child to repeat the process two or three more times; with a rest of 20–30 seconds between readings. *Ensures most accurate measurement of the PEFR.*
8. Record the highest of the readings, not the average. *The highest number will reflect the child's best expiratory flow rate.*

DOCUMENTATION

1. Time and date.
2. Reading.
3. How well child tolerated procedure.
4. Any interventions needed.

Estimated time to complete procedure: *2–5 minutes.*

Chest Physiotherapy and Postural Drainage

OVERVIEW

Chest pulmonary therapy and postural drainage (CPPD), also referred to as chest physiotherapy (CPT), is used to facilitate airway clearance by using proper positioning and chest wall percussion, coughing, and breathing. CPT is ordered most commonly in children who have difficulty coughing up bronchial secretions or have increased sputum production. Chest physiotherapy is often done in the morning before breakfast and in the evening before bedtime. It may be ordered more frequently if the child has a respiratory infection or copious, thick secretions. It is not uncommon for children to receive bronchodilators prior to the procedure to help loosen secretions.

PROCEDURE 66

POSITIONING FOR CPT

EQUIPMENT

Chest vibrator
Round oxygen mask or manufactured percussor
Stethoscope

NOTE: *Bronchodilators, via nebulizer or aerosol, are frequently administered prior to chest physiotherapy.*

SAFETY

1. Schedule CPT at least 1 hour prior to meals; should not be performed immediately before eating. *May cause loss of appetite or emesis, which could lead to aspiration.*
2. Children who receive nutritional support from continuous enteral feedings should have their feeding discontinued at least 30 minutes prior to CPT.
3. Closely monitor infants with a history of gastroesophageal reflux. *They are at higher risk of emesis, leading to possible aspiration.*
4. Assess the child for pain, and administer medications as ordered prior to CPT. *So child is comfortable (pain free) during CPT.*

PROCEDURE

1. Gather equipment *to assure organization and efficiency.*
2. Wash hands. *Reduces transmission of microorganisms.*
3. Prepare child and family. Consider having someone support or comfort the child. *Enhances cooperation and parental participation; reduces anxiety and fear.*
4. Perform baseline respiratory assessment, respiratory rate, rhythm, effort, color, and breath sounds. *Determines child's condition; used to determine if there are any changes after chest physical therapy.*
5. Place child in the recommended position and maintain that position for 10–15 minutes. Positions are determined based on the location of decreased breath sounds and mucus secretion. Generally, considering lobe anatomy, the lower lobes are drained first, then the middle lobes and lingua, followed by the upper lobes. See the Positions for CPT below. *So chest PT will effectively treat correct lobe of lung; lower lobes are treated first to improve drainage and prevent secretions loosened from upper lobes from pooling in lower lobes.*
6. Ensure that child has a T-shirt or gown covering the chest area. A towel may also be used. To produce chest vibrations (percussion) that dislodge secretions, cup

hands, holding fingers together, with wrist loose and relaxed (to conform with the configuration of the chest wall). Clap area with palm of hand, causing a hollow sound to be emitted, with a rhythmic pattern. Clap for approximately five minutes over identified chest area. (A round oxygen mask or manufactured percussor may be used instead.) *To prevent injury to skin; vibrations will loosen secretions.*
7. Encourage child to breathe deeply (inhaling through the nose and exhaling through the mouth), cough, and expectorate sputum following each percussion or vibration session. Allow child to assume normal position. *To encourage child to cough up secretions loosened by CPT.*
8. Vibration may also be done using manual pressure or with a chest vibrator. If using the manual technique, place one hand on top of the other over the desired area. Keep arms and shoulders in a straight position. Tense and relax arms for 10–15-second intervals. Repeat procedure for 10–15 minutes. *Vibrations will loosen secretions.*
9. Perform post treatment respiratory assessment. *To determine if there are any changes from assessment prior to CPT.*

DOCUMENTATION

1. Child's general condition.
2. Baseline assessment prior to chest physiotherapy (see step 4 above) and following procedures.
3. Child's response to chest physiotherapy (e.g., pain, respiratory difficulty).
4. If child is using oxygen, note flow rate and method of administration.

POSITIONS FOR CPT

Lower Lobes

1. Elevate foot of bed approximately 30°. Place child in prone position, putting a pillow or rolled towel under hips, with head down. Child may flex leg for comfort. Percuss posterior basal segment.
2. Elevate foot of bed approximately 30°. Place child in prone position, turned part way to one side. Place a pillow under leg for support. Child may flex leg for comfort. Percuss lateral basal segment.
3. Elevate foot of bed approximately 30°. Place child in a side-lying position, with head down. A pillow may be

placed between legs for comfort. Percuss anterior basal segment.

4. Position child prone with a pillow under hips. Keep bed flat. Percuss superior segment.

Right Middle Lobe

1. Elevate foot of bed approximately 15°. Place child in a left-side lying position, head down, knees flexed, turned part way toward the back. A pillow should be placed behind the child as support. Percuss lateral and medial segments.

Upper Lobes

1. Elevate foot of bed approximately 15°. Place child in a right-side lying position, head down, knees flexed, turned part way toward the back. Place pillow behind child for support. Percuss lingular, superior, and inferior segments (left upper lobe).

2. On a flat bed, place child in supine position, knees bent with a pillow under them for support. Percuss anterior segment (between clavicle and nipple each side of the chest).

3. On a flat bed, place child in supine position, with the child leaning back at a 30° angle onto pillow(s) for support. Percuss apical segment (area between clavicle and scapula each side of chest).

4. Position child in upright position leaning forward, at about a 30° angle, over back of a chair (padded with towels or a pillow). Percuss posterior segment (upper back and both sides of the chest).

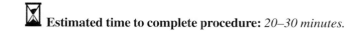 **Estimated time to complete procedure:** *20–30 minutes.*

Closed Chest Drainage and Chest Tubes

OVERVIEW

The chest drainage system is a closed system designed to drain air or fluid from the pleural cavity while restoring or maintaining the negative intrapleural pressure needed to keep the lung properly expanded. Large amounts of fluid or air in the pleural cavity impede lung expansion, causing respiratory distress. Excess fluid or air enters the pleural cavity due to chest trauma, chest surgery, or without any specific cause.

The drainage system uses a water seal to prevent air from returning into the pleural cavity. Once pleural air passes through the water seal and into the closed system, it cannot reenter the chest and is vented to the atmosphere. Occulsive dressings at the puncture site prevent air from entering the pleural space, and all connections between the tubing are usually taped to maintain an airtight system.

The chest drainage system can at times be attached to suction to increase the negative pressure between the pleural space and the drainage system, which improves drainage. The amount of suction is controlled by either a dial in some chest drainage setups or by the amount of saline added to the suction control container in other setups.

If a commercial drainage system is used, it is important to follow manufacturer's instructions.

PROCEDURE 67

ASSISTING WITH CHEST TUBE INSERTION

EQUIPMENT

Chest tube tray (generally includes):
    Chest tube (size designated by physician)
    Trocar
    Drainage system
    Suture scissors
    Hemostats
    Needle holder
    Syringes
    Needles of various sizes
    Stopcock
    4 × 4 gauze
    Medicine cup
    Y connector
    Forceps
    Drapes, towels
Sterile water or saline (1,000 cc bottle)
Local anesthetic
Gloves, sterile
Gown, mask
Stethoscope
Antiseptic (e.g., povidone-iodine)
Alcohol swabs
Petrolatum gauze
Clamp, padded
Adhesive tape
Rubber band and safety pin (optional)
Suture with needle (check if in tray)

PROCEDURE

1. Explain procedure and reason for procedure to child and family. *Enhances cooperation and participation; reduces anxiety and fear.*
2. Obtain signed consent. *An invasive procedure needs parent/guardian consent.*
3. Premedicate as ordered. *Decreases discomfort associated with chest tube insertion.*
4. Gather equipment. *Promotes organization and efficiency.*
5. Wash hands. *Reduces transmission of microorganisms.*
6. Assist physician in preparing child and necessary supplies. Set up drainage system according to instructions accompanying the system (see Preparing the Chest Tube Drainage System). *Enhances organization and efficiency.*
7. Assist physician as required. *Enhances organization and efficiency.*

8. Once the tube is in place and connected to the drainage system, ensure the integrity and functioning of the system.
    a. Ensure that the water in the suction control chamber/bottles is bubbling gently. *Bubbles indicate air is entering system.*
    b. Check the water seal for leaks. Potential sources of air include (1) a leak in the tubing, (2) a leak under the dressing, (3) a leak from the pleural cavity, (4) drainage of air from the pleural cavity, and (5) a crack in the unit. *If there is a leak in the system, it will not work efficiently.*
    c. Make sure all tubing connections are tight and wrapped with adhesive tape. *Loose connections will cause an air leak in the system and ineffective drainage of fluid and air.*
    d. Secure chest tube drainage tube to gown using the clamp that comes with the system or a rubber band and safety pin. *So tube cannot be pulled apart as child moves.*

NOTE: *Do not pin or secure tubing to the bedding. (Reduces the risk of accidentally dislodging the tube.)*

NOTE: *Policy at some agencies may prohibit the use of safety pins.*

9. Assist in obtaining a chest x-ray. *Confirms position of the tube and whether it has begun to evacuate fluid and air.*
10. Monitor vital signs, drainage, and insertion site every 15 minutes for 2 hours or according to agency policy. *To determine child's condition and condition of insertion site.*

DOCUMENTATION

1. Premedication given.
2. Insertion and how tolerated.
3. Size and location of tube.
4. Type of drainage system used.
5. X-ray results.
6. Functioning of drainage system, including if there is suction and at what pressure.
7. Amount, color, and consistency of drainage.
8. Respiratory status.

 Estimated time to complete procedure: *15–20 minutes.*

PROCEDURE 68

PREPARING THE CHEST TUBE DRAINAGE SYSTEM

PROCEDURE

1. If only water seal is ordered, fill the water seal chamber/bottle with sterile water or saline to the 2 cm level. *Provides a water seal and prevents air from entering the pleural cavity. The 2 cm level is sufficient to create a one-way valve to prevent air from entering the pleural cavity through the chest tube. Underfilling leaves water seal chamber/bottle tube exposed to air; overfilling inhibits air from exiting pleural space.*

2. If suction is ordered, fill suction control chamber/bottle to the ordered level of fluid, usually 10–20 cm of water. *Provides extra suction to increase drainage from the pleural cavity.*

3. If suction is ordered, attach suction tubing to the marked suction port and to the suction source. *Provides suction to the system.*

4. Turn on suction. Increase level of suction until there is gentle bubbling in the suction control chamber/bottle of the system. *Level of suction determined by air flow through the water in the suction chamber/bottle. Air flow indicated by water bubbling in the suction control chamber/bottle.*

5. Set up the system at the child's bedside, keeping drainage system below the level of the child. *Prevents backflow of fluid or air into the pleural cavity.*

DOCUMENTATION

1. Level of water seal.
2. Level of suction.

⊠ **Estimated time to complete procedure:** *5–10 minutes.*

PROCEDURE 69

CARING FOR A CHILD WITH A CHEST TUBE

PROCEDURE

1. Assessment
    a. Assess respiratory status every two hours or according to agency policy. *To determine change in child's condition.*
        1. Note rate, rhythm, depth, and ease of respirations. Also note anxiety and chest discomfort. *Indicates child's condition.*
        2. Auscultate lungs and percuss lung fields. Check for symmetry of chest movement. *Assesses for presence of air or fluid in pleural cavity, fluid in the lungs, and tension pneumothorax.*
        3. Assess for fluid fluctuation (with respiration) in the water seal chamber/bottle. *Fluctuations indicate changes in pressure in the pleural space, which occur when child breathes and the lung has not fully expanded.*
    b. Note amount and color of drainage from chest tube. Mark the level at the beginning of each collection and at the end of every shift. *To determine type and amount of fluid draining every shift.*

NOTE: *If the child is actively bleeding, assess drainage frequently, every 10–15 minutes.*

    c. Check dressing at least once a shift *to assure it is clean, dry, and intact.*

NOTE: *Dressing should be covered with adhesive tape. Change dressing in accordance with agency policy. Inspect entry site for drainage, inflammation, or subcutaneous emphysema.*

    d. Assess child's level of discomfort and medicate as ordered. *Manipulation of chest wall and insertion of chest tube are painful.*
    e. Assess functioning and integrity of drainage system every two hours or according to agency policy.
        1. Check for appropriate level of water in water seal and suction chambers/bottles, and refill with sterile water or saline as needed. *To be sure chest tube enters system below water level so vacuum is maintained.*
        2. Check for appropriate setting of wall suction. *So suction is maintained.*
        3. Assess for bubbling in water seal chamber/bottle. *Indicates air leak.*
        4. Check drainage tubing for kinks or obstructed flow. There should be no dependent loops of tubing or tubing laid horizontally on the bed. *Kinks, obstructions, and dependent loops interfere with chest tube drainage.*
        5. Check all connections between tubing to be sure they are tight and taped. *Loose connections cause air leaks and ineffective drainage.*
        6. Check that system is below level of child. *Facilitates drainage* (Figure VIII-9).
2. Do not strip or "milk" tubing unless specifically ordered by physician. *Stripping creates hazardously high pressure in the pleural cavity, which can damage lung tissue and pleura.*
3. Transporting the child with a chest tube.
    a. Disconnect from wall suction but keep connected to water seal. *Prevents air from entering the pleural space.*

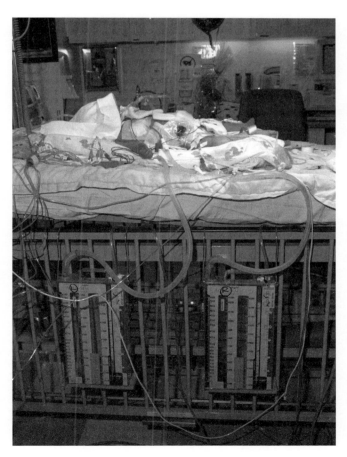

FIGURE VIII-9 Chest tube setup.

b. Do not clamp chest tube during transport. *No fluid or air can escape from pleural cavity when tube is clamped and potential for tension pneumothorax is decreased.*

c. Deep drainage system below level of chest and upright. *Facilitates drainage and maintains water seal.*

4. Have chest tube clamp at bedside to clamp off tube.

a. If bubbling occurs in water seal chamber/bottle while system is on suction. *Indicates leak in system.*

NOTE: *To check for air leak place clamp at various points, moving from the chest to the drainage system. Bubbling stops once clamp is placed between the air leak and the water seal.*

b. When changing the tube or replacing the drainage system. *Prevents air from entering the pleural cavity.*

c. When drainage system is cracked. *Prevents air from entering the pleural cavity.*

d. During chest tube removal. *Prevents air from entering the pleural cavity.*

DOCUMENTATION

1. Results of assessment of respiratory status.
2. Amount and color of chest tube drainage.
3. Condition of dressing.
4. Results of assessment of drainage system.

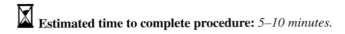 **Estimated time to complete procedure:** *5–10 minutes.*

PROCEDURE 70

ASSISTING WITH REMOVAL OF A CHEST TUBE

EQUIPMENT

Gloves, sterile (for physician and nurse)
Vaseline gauze
Dressings
Tape, foam
Chest tube clamp
Suture removal kit or sterile scissors
Sutures (if requested by physician)

PROCEDURE

1. Prepare child and family. *Enhances cooperation and participation; reduces anxiety and fear.*
2. Premedicate as ordered. *Decreases discomfort of chest tube removal.*
3. Gather equipment. *Promotes organization and efficiency.*
4. Assist child to appropriate position. *To better visualize area; remove tube more efficiently.*
5. Put on sterile gloves. *Reduces transmission of microorganisms.*
6. Assist physician as directed. *Enhances organization and efficiency.*

NOTE: *Removal consists of removing the dressing, clipping the sutures, clamping the chest tube, and removing the chest tube. A sterile occlusive dressing should be prepared and held ready to place as soon as the chest tube is removed.*

NOTE: *During the chest tube removal, instruct the child to take a deep breath and hold it, or to hum or yell loudly. Raises intrathoracic pressure and helps prevent recollection of air in the pleural cavity.*

7. Apply dressing (or assist physician as directed) and tape securely. *To prevent air from entering incision site.*

NOTE: *Dressing must be airtight. Dressing should not be removed for 24 hours. If drainage is soaking through, reinforce the dressing.*

8. Dispose of equipment properly. *Reduces transmission of microorganisms.*
9. Remove gloves. Wash hands. *Reduces transmission of microorganisms.*
10. Reevaluate the child's status regularly. Monitor vital signs, breath sounds, and respiratory distress, i.e., watch for signs of shortness of breath, decreased oxygen saturation, chest pain, or pain on inspiration. Monitor condition of dressing. *Identifies problems such as pneumothorax or mediastinal shift following chest tube removal.*
11. Assist in obtaining chest x-ray as ordered. *Promotes organization and efficiency.*

DOCUMENTATION

1. Time of chest tube removal and by whom.
2. Dressing site and its status.
3. How procedure tolerated.
4. Amount of drainage in system (since last recorded).
5. Assessment of child, especially respiratory status.
6. X-ray if ordered.
7. Premedication.

⧗ **Estimated time to complete procedure:** *10–15 minutes.*

UNIT IX

Gastrointestinal System and Nutritional Procedures

Gastrointestinal System

Nasogastric Tubes

Nasogastric (NG) tubes are used in infants and children for feeding when the child is comatose, semiconscious, or unable to consume sufficient food orally. The NG tube can also be used to empty or decompress the stomach after gastrointestinal surgery, clean and flush the stomach after the child has ingested a poisonous substance, document the presence of blood in the stomach, monitor the amount of bleeding from the stomach, or identify any recurrent bleeding. The size of the NG tube is determined by the age, weight, and size of the child. Since the gastrointestinal tract is considered to be a clean rather than a sterile, the procedure used to insert or care for the NG tube uses a clean technique.

Orogastric Tubes

The orogastric (OG) tube is most commonly used in place of the nasogastric tube for newborns and young infants who are obligate nose breathers. Occasionally, however, the OG tube is used in older children if they are intubated, unconscious, or unresponsive. The difference between the tubes is that the OG tube is passed through the mouth, whereas the NG tube is passed through the nose. The principles for insertion and care of both tubes are the same, except for using the oral rather than the nasal passage when initially inserting the tube.

Gastrostomy Tubes

Gastrostomy tubes (GT) are made of silicone or polyurethane. They are durable, compatible with formula, and used primarily for gavage feedings or to decompress the stomach. The gastrostomy tube is placed through an opening in the abdominal wall into the stomach and sutured in place. It is important to keep the tube as immobile as possible to avoid unintentional displacement or removal. Placement of the tube can be checked by aspirating small amounts of gastric contents prior to feeding. Whenever the tube is not being used for decompression or feeding, it should be clamped. It is important to observe the gastrostomy site for redness and abnormal drainage every shift and change the dressing around the site with a clean and dry dressing every shift. To change the dressing, a cut is made half way through a 2 × 2-inch or a 4 × 4-inch (depends on the size of the child) gauze pad, and then the pad is placed around the gastrostomy tube close to the site and taped in place. Nonsterile gloves are used to remove the old dressing, and then a clean pair of nonsterile gloves is used when placing the clean dressing.

PROCEDURE 71

INSERTING A NASOGASTRIC TUBE

PURPOSE

A nasogastric tube may be used to decompress the stomach, instill medications or feedings, or assess gastrointestinal function.

EQUIPMENT

Appropriate size nasogastric tube
Water-soluble lubricant
½-inch tape
1 transparent dressing
Syringe
1 hypoactive dressing
Blanket for restraint, if appropriate
Gloves, nonsterile (exam)
Pacifier, if appropriate
Emesis basis
Pin and rubber band
Towel
Stethoscope

Nasogastric Tube Selection

GUIDELINES

Type of tube	For gavage or lavage, use a single lumen tube.
	For intermittent gastric decompression, use a double lumen tube.
	For continuous long-term feeding, use a silicone tube.

	Weight of child	*Size*
Tube size	2 Kg	5 French
	3–9 Kg	8 French
	10–20 Kg	10 French
	20–30 Kg	12 French
	30–50 Kg	14 French
	> 50 Kg	16 French

PROCEDURE

1. Gather equipment. Select appropriate size and type of nasogastric tube. Some guidelines are presented above; however, the nurse must use his or her judgment or follow agency policies. *Promotes organization and efficiency.*
2. Wash hands. Put on nonsterile gloves. *Reduces transmission of microorganisms and protects from contact with body fluids.*

3. Prepare child and family. *Enhances cooperation and participation; reduces anxiety and fear.*
4. Position child supine at a 30°–45° angle if possible. *Allows efficient passing of tube.*
5. Assess patency of nares. *To determine if tube can be easily passed.*
6. Measure length of tube to be inserted and mark tube with a piece of tape. Several methods of measuring length of nasogastric tube to be inserted have been identified. *To determine how far to pass tube.*
   a. Measure from the tip of the nose to the earlobe and from the earlobe to the lower end of the xyphoid process. This is a commonly used method.
   b. Measure from the nose to the earlobe and from the earlobe to a point halfway between the xyphoid and the umbilicus (Figure XI-1A).
   c. Formulas based on height.
7. Place a towel over the child's chest *to protect clothing.*
8. Lubricate 1 to 3 inches of the tube with water or a water-soluble gel. *To enhance passing tube.*
9. Insert tube back and up into nostril; advance using gentle pressure. If resistance is met, withdraw the tube, relubricate, and try the other nostril (Figure IX-1B). *Follows anatomy of nose; gentle pressure will prevent tissue injury.*
10. If the child is able, ask child to swallow as the tube is advanced. A pacifier may be used for an infant over 3 months of age who does not need to mouth breathe. Continue to advance the tube until the tape mark is at the nostril. *Swallowing the tube will enhance passage.*
11. Check back of mouth for kinking of tube. *Occasionally tube will kink in back of throat; person passing tube is unaware of this unless back of throat is examined.*
12. Remove tube immediately if there is vomiting or signs of respiratory distress (e.g., cyanosis, tachypnea, nasal flaring, grunting, wheezing, prolonged coughing or choking) or if the child is unable to speak or cry. *These symptoms suggest that the tube is in the respiratory tract rather than the gastrointestinal tract.*
13. Remove guide wire if applicable. *Used only as a help in passing the tube; not needed after tube is passed.*

NOTE: *Some agencies have policies that limit insertion of nasogastric tubes with guide wires to physicians. Follow agency policy.*

14. Verify placement of nasogastric tube per agency protocol. The literature identifies several methods for

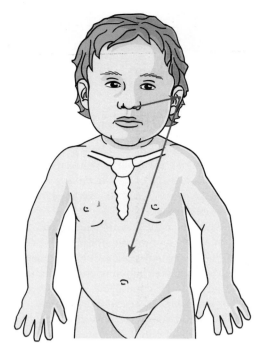

FIGURE IX-1A   Measuring NG tube distance.

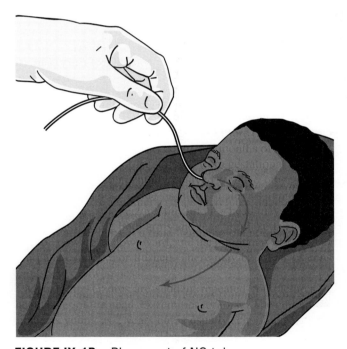

FIGURE IX-1B   Placement of NG tube.

determining appropriate placement of nasogastric tubes (Beckstrand et al., 1990; Gharib, Stern, Sherbin, & Rohrmann, 1996; Rakel et al., 1994). These include insufflation of air while listening for the sound of the air, withdrawal of gastric/intestinal contents, checking contents withdrawn for pH and other characteristics, and inserting end of tube in the water and watching for bubbles. Research has demonstrated that listening for air (a frequently identified method) is the least reliable method. The most reliable method for confirming placement is x-ray. *To be sure tube is in the stomach (GI track).*

15. Secure tube by placing hypoactive dressing on child's cheek and then securing the tube to the dressing with the transparent dressing or tape. The tube also may be taped to the upper lip or nose. Use a 4-inch length of tape, split about 2 inches of the tape lengthwise, place unsplit end on nose, wrap split ends around tube, and secure to nose (Figure IX-2). *To be sure tube does not come out of stomach.*

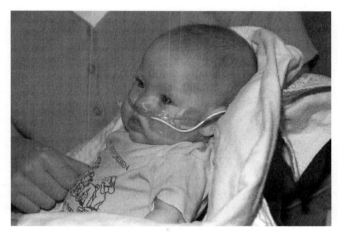

FIGURE IX-2   NG tube secured.

16. Attach tube to suction, feeding, or clamp as ordered. *So child can be fed or suctioned as ordered; tube is clamped if child is not being fed or suctioned.*
17. Remove gloves. Wash hands. *Reduces transmission of microorganisms.*

DOCUMENTATION

1. Insertion procedure with date and time.
2. How tolerated by child.
3. Type and size of tube.
4. Which nostril used.
5. Patency.
6. Amount, color, and consistency of returns.
7. Laboratory tests done on gastric contents, if applicable.

Estimated time to complete procedure: *5–10 minutes.*

PROCEDURE 72

MANAGING GASTROINTESTINAL SUCTION

EQUIPMENT

Source of suction with gauge
Suction tubing
Suction/collection cannister
Double lumen nasogastric tube
Tape
60 cc catheter tip syringe
Gloves, nonsterile

PROCEDURE

1. Check chart for order including type and level of suction. *Determines equipment needed; ensures appropriate application of gastric suction.*
2. Gather equipment. *Promotes organization and efficiency.*
3. Wash hands. *Reduces transmission of microorganisms.*
4. Explain procedure to child and family. *Enhances cooperation and participation; reduces anxiety and fear.*
5. Set up suction source. For wall suction, plug regulator into suction port. For portable suction, plug machine into power source. *Provides source of suction.*
6. Attach suction tubing and cannister to suction head. Turn on suction to test functioning of equipment. Turn suction off. *Evaluates functioning of equipment.*
7. Position child. *To visualize tube.*
8. Put on nonsterile gloves. *Protects nurse from contact with gastrointestinal fluids.*
9. If not already in place, insert nasogastric tube and check placement using procedure described previously. If nasogastric tube is already in place, remove syringe or plug from end of tube if present and check placement. *To be sure tube is correctly placed.*
10. Connect nasogastric tube to suction tubing. Tape connection site. *Protects integrity of suction.*
11. Ensure that vent of tubing is opened when suction is applied. *Prevents nasogastric tube from adhering to gastric wall.*
12. Turn on suction and set at appropriate level and type (i.e., intermittent or continuous). *To deliver needed suction.*

13. If air vent fills with fluid or is leaking, inject air vent with 5–10 cc air while suction is applied to the suction drainage. *To allow air vent to function appropriately.*
14. Position tubing to avoid dependent loops. *Prevents decrease in the efficacy of suction.*
15. Remove gloves. Wash hands. *Reduces transmission of microorganisms.*
16. Observe nasogastric tube for patency and proper function and pressure of suction every two hours or according to agency policy. When connected to suction there should be bubbling or fluid movement in the tube during the suction cycle. *To determine whether or not suctioning is functioning properly.*
17. Observe child for signs and symptoms of malfunctioning suction or complications. *To determine if suction is functioning properly.*
    a. Abdominal discomfort.
    b. Nausea or vomiting.
    c. Oral or nares discomfort.
    d. Leaking from the tubes.
    e. Gastric distention.
    f. Irritation or skin breakdown at site of entry (nares or mouth).
    g. Gastric distress/gastrointestinal (GI) bleeding.

NOTE: *In absence of documented GI bleed, notify physician if blood evident in gastric drainage.*

DOCUMENTATION

1. Type and pressure of suction.
2. Amount of drainage every shift or more often as needed.
3. Character of drainage every shift or more frequently if character changes.

 Estimated time to complete procedure: *5 minutes.*

PROCEDURE 73

IRRIGATING A NASOGASTRIC TUBE

EQUIPMENT

Warmed saline or water for irrigation
Catheter tip syringe
Chux pad and/or towel
Gloves, nonsterile
Stethoscope

PROCEDURE

1. Gather equipment. *Promotes organization and efficiency.*
2. Wash hands. *Reduces transmission of microorganisms.*
3. Prepare child and family. *Enhances cooperation and participation; reduces anxiety and fear.*
4. Put on nonsterile gloves. *Prevents nurse from contact with gastrointestinal fluids.*
5. Turn off suction or feeding as appropriate. Disconnect nasogastric tube from suction or feeding source or unclamp as appropriate. *Not needed during irrigation.*
6. Inject 5 cc of air while ascultating the abdomen. *To verify placement of NG tube.*
7. Fill the syringe with the prescribed amount of solution of 5–10 cc and inject it slowly into the tubing. Do not force. *Forcing may injure tissue and increase child's discomfort.*
   a. If solution does not flow easily,

1. Rotate the tubing or move it slightly. *Tube may be too close to stomach wall to allow solution to flow fully into stomach.*
2. Alternately push and pull the plunger of the syringe. *Alternating pressure helps work out the obstruction.*
   b. Notify physician if solution cannot be injected without considerable force. *May indicate a situation needing physician intervention.*
8. Aspirate the amount used in the irrigation from the tubing. *Prevents adding extra fluid volume to the stomach.*
9. Remove syringe and reconnect the nasogastric tube to the appropriate suction or type of feeding. *So bleeding or suctioning can continue.*
10. Remove gloves. Wash hands. *Reduces transmission of microorganisms.*

DOCUMENTATION

1. Verification of tube placement.
2. Time of procedure.
3. Type and amount of solution irrigated and amount of return.
4. Child's response to procedure and how tolerated.

Estimated time to complete procedure: *less than 5 minutes.*

PROCEDURE 74

PERFORMING NASOGASTRIC TUBE LAVAGE

EQUIPMENT

60 cc catheter tip syringe
Warmed NS for irrigation (body temperature)
Emesis basin
Towels
Gloves, nonsterile

PROCEDURE

1. Check for physician's order to obtain type and amount of irrigation solution and length of time of irrigation. *Physician order needed for NG tube lavage.*
2. Gather equipment. *Promotes organization and efficiency.*
3. Wash hands. *Reduces transmission of microorganisms.*
4. Prepare child and family for procedure. *Enhances cooperation and participation; reduces anxiety and fear.*
5. Position child in high Fowler's position or on left side with head elevated 15°. *To enhance organization and efficiency.*
6. Put on nonsterile gloves. *Protects nurse from contact with gastrointestinal fluids.*
7. Insert nasogastric tube and check placement per procedure as described under Inserting a Nasogastric Tube. *To be sure tube is placed correctly.*
8. Attach syringe to NG tube and pull back on the plunger to aspirate stomach contents. Aspirate contents until there is no more continual return. *Empties stomach before beginning lavage.*
9. Fill the syringe with the prescribed solution and slowly inject it into the stomach. The volume of each infusion should be about 20 cc. *Minimizes child's discomfort and reduces risk of vomiting.*

10. Pull back on plunger of syringe *to aspirate lavage solution via the nasogastric tube.* Discard in emesis basin. Not necessary to save aspirate.
11. Monitor amount of solution infused and amount removed. *Verifies good return of lavage solution, and permits monitoring of intake and output.*
12. Repeat process until results are clear or the prescribed amount of fluid has been delivered. *Clear fluid indicates tube has been inflated.*
13. During the procedure, monitor the child for airway patency, cramping, nausea and vomiting, comfort level, and obstructions in the tube. *Promotes the safety of the child.*
14. Remove nasogastric tube or attach to suction, or clamp as ordered. *Procedure is over; tube is clamped if child is not bag fed or suctioned. NG tube is removed according to MD order.*
15. Dispose of equipment and returned irrigation solution in appropriate containers. *Follows prescribed precautions.*
16. Remove gloves. Wash hands. *Reduces transmission of microorganisms.*

DOCUMENTATION

1. Time, type, and amount of solution used.
2. Character and amount of returned fluid.
3. Child's response to the procedure and how tolerated.

⧗ **Estimated time to complete procedure:** *5–30 minutes depending on reason for lavage or physician order.*

PROCEDURE 75

REMOVING THE NASOGASTRIC OR OROGASTRIC TUBE

OVERVIEW

When the nasogastric or orogastric tube is no longer needed, the physician or qualified practitioner will order its removal. If any problems are noted (poor gastric emptying, more gastric bleeding than expected, poor bowel sounds), the findings should be reported to the appropriate physician or qualified caregiver and the order to remove should be verified. After the tube is removed, the child's condition should be monitored for signs that the tube may need to be reinserted, such as vomiting and decreased bowel sounds.

EQUIPMENT

Nonsterile gloves
Emesis basin (depends on age of child)
Towel and tissue
Mouthwash or glass of water
10–20 ml syringe (smaller syringe if infant)

PROCEDURE

1. Check order for tube removal in chart. *Reduces risk of removing the tube prematurely.*
2. Gather equipment. *Improves organization and effectiveness.*
3. Wash hands. *Reduces transmission of microorganisms.*
4. Prepare child and family. *Enhances cooperation and parental participation; reduces anxiety and fear.*
5. Place child in a sitting position. *Helps removal of tube and prevents chance of aspiration if child vomits.*
6. Put on gloves. *Prevents exposure to bodily fluids.*
7. Place a clean paper towel on child's chest/lap. *Enhances cleanliness and comfort.*
8. Have child hold emesis basin if able. *In case child gags when tube is removed, it will be close by.*

NOTE: *If removing a NG or OG tube from an infant, step #8 is not necessary.*

9. Disconnect suction or feeding pump if any; remove tape and safety pin (if present). *Prevents spillage of gastric secretions or tube feeding solution. Protects esophageal tissue from suction pressure damage.*
10. Instill 10–20 ml of air into tube (amount may be less if an infant). *To remove any secretions or residual feeding that is in the tube.*
11. Pinch tube. *Prevents spillage of gastric contents or tube feeding solution while tube is being pulled.*
12. Ask child to take a deep breath and hold it while the tube is pulled out evenly and slowly over the course of 3–6 seconds. *Facilitates removal of tube.*

NOTE: *If removing the tube from an infant, pull tube evenly and gently while infant is exhaling if possible.*

13. Cover or wrap tube in paper towel and remove from child's bedside. *Seeing the tube may cause distress to the child.*
14. Provide oral hygiene (if appropriate). *Promotes child's comfort.*
15. Remove gloves, dispose of contaminated materials, wash hands. *Reduces transmission of microorganisms.*

DOCUMENTATION

1. Time and date.
2. Condition of nares (if an NG tube).
3. How child tolerated procedure.
4. Color and amount of any residual gastric contents in suction bottles (as appropriate).

⧖ **Estimated time to complete procedure:** *less than 5 minutes.*

PROCEDURE 76

ADMINISTERING A BOLUS FEEDING (NG, NJ, GASTROSTOMY)

EQUIPMENT

Formula
Water
Catheter tip syringe
Gloves, nonsterile

PROCEDURE

1. Check order for type, amount, and frequency of feeding. *Physician order needed for this procedure.*
2. Gather equipment. *Promotes organization and efficiency.*
3. Explain procedure to child and family. *Enhances cooperation and participation; reduces anxiety and fear.*
4. Wash hands. *Reduces transmission of microorganisms.*
5. Warm formula to room temperature. *Promotes comfort.*
6. Position child on right side or supine with head elevated. Have assistant hold or comfort child as necessary. *Reduces risk of reflux or vomiting.*
7. Put on nonsterile gloves. *Protects from contact with body fluids.*
8. Check placement of tube as appropriate for type of tube. *Tube could have moved since last feeding.*
   a. For nasogastric tube, check placement as described earlier.
   b. For a nasojejunal tube, check placement by measuring length of tube from nose to tube hub. This distance should have been recorded in the chart at the time of verification of placement and checked on a regular basis after verification.
   c. Placement check not needed for gastrostomy tubes.
9. Check for residual if indicated. Attach syringe and pull back on plunger. Note amount and character of residual. *Determines amount of feeding still in stomach.*
10. Return residual to child and flush tube. *Prevents electrolyte imbalance.*

NOTE: *If residual greater than half the amount of the previous feeding, notify the physician. For neonates, notify physician if residual exceeds 20% of previous feeding or more than 2 cc/Kg.* **This prevents distention of the stomach with possible reflux or vomiting.**

11. Attach empty syringe. Keep the tubing pinched. *Prevents air from entering the stomach.*
12. Flush tube. *Assesses patency and flow in the tube.*
    a. For neonates or fluid-restricted children, flush with 1–2 cc water or air.
    b. For other children, flush with 5–10 cc of water.
13. Add feeding to syringe and administer feeding. Control rate of feeding by raising or lowering the syringe. *Feeding too rapidly may cause vomiting.*

NOTE: **With a gastrostomy tube, hold straight up from insertion site,** *since this will put less stress on the tube.*

14. Following administration of feeding, flush tube with water. *Prevents tube from becoming clogged.*
    a. For neonate or fluid-restricted children, flush with 1–2 cc of water or air. If flushing with air and feeding gets sluggish, consider flushing with water.
    b. For other children, flush with 10–15 cc of water.
15. Remove syringe and rinse after each feeding. Syringe may be used for 12 hours before being discarded. *Reduces risk of contamination.*
16. Remove gloves. Wash hands. *Reduces transmission of microorganisms.*

DOCUMENTATION

1. Check for residual.
2. Amount of residual.
3. Time of feeding.
4. Type and amount of formula.
5. How procedure tolerated.

⧖ **Estimated time to complete procedure:** *The length of feeding should be similar to that of oral feeding, not less than 20 minutes. May take 30–60 minutes.*

PROCEDURE 77

ADMINISTERING NG, NJ, GASTROSTOMY, AND CONTINUOUS FEEDING

EQUIPMENT

Catheter tip syringe
Formula pump
Bag and tubing for pump
Formula
Water
Gloves, nonsterile

PROCEDURE

1. Check order for type, amount, and frequency of feeding. *Physician order needed for this procedure.*
2. Gather equipment. *Promotes organization and efficiency.*
3. Explain procedure to child and family. *Enhances cooperation and participation; reduces anxiety and fear.*
4. Wash hands. *Reduces transmission of microorganisms.*
5. Warm formula to room temperature. *Promotes comfort.*
6. Position child on right side or supine with head elevated. Have assistant hold or comfort child as necessary. *Reduces risk of reflux or vomiting; reduces fear/anxiety.*
7. Put on nonsterile gloves. *Protects from contact with body fluids.*
8. Check tube placement and residual as specified by agency policy. *To determine if tube remains in correct place; to determine if there is formula (feeding) present.*
9. Place up to four hours of formula in bag. Label with date and time. *Prevents accumulation of microorganisms.*

NOTE: *Do not add new formula to old formula already in bag.*

10. Hang feeding bag on IV pole. *Promotes organization and efficiency.*
11. Prime delivery tubing with formula and thread through formula pump according to manufacturer's instructions. *Promotes organization and efficiency.*
12. Attach tubing to end of NG/NJ/gastrostomy tube. *Promotes organization and efficiency.*
13. Turn on formula pump and set at prescribed rate. *So correct amount of formula delivered during alotted time.*
14. Remove gloves. Wash hands. *Reduces transmission of microorganisms.*
15. Flush tubing every 4–6 hours during feeding and at the completion of feeding. *Prevents tubing from becoming clogged.*
    a. For neonates and fluid-restricted children, flush with 1–2 cc of air or water.
    b. For other children, flush with 10–15 cc of water.
16. Replace disposable feeding bag and tubing every 24 hours. *Prevents accumulation of microorganisms.*

DOCUMENTATION

1. Type of formula.
2. Rate of administration.
3. Intake and output.
4. How feeding tolerated.

 Estimated time to complete procedure: *10–30 minutes.*

Ostomies

OVERVIEW

Ostomies are performed when the infant or child needs urinary or fecal diversion, such as with imperforate anus, prune belly syndrome, inflammatory bowel syndrome, Hirschprung's disease, necrotizing enterocolitis, spina bifida, trauma, or tumor. After surgery, the child will have either a dressing or an adhesive appliance. The appliance is a clear plastic bag with an opening at the end so that contents can be removed and measured. If the appliance is not used, the dressing used to cover the ostomy can be weighed before it is applied and then after it is removed to determine the amount of drainage. (Approximately 1 ml of fluid weighs 1 gm.) It is important to provide good skin care around the ostomy, because children's skin is more fragile than adults'.

PROCEDURE 78

CHANGING A FECAL OSTOMY APPLIANCE

EQUIPMENT

Appropriate drainable ostomy appliance (bag and skin barrier wafer)
Skin barriers (e.g., Stomahesive paste and powder)
Clean washcloth, 4 × 4 gauze, or cotton balls
Warm tap water
Ostomy soap (if prescribed by agency policy)
Scissors
Pen or pencil
Gloves, nonsterile

PROCEDURE

1. Gather equipment. *Promotes organization and efficiency.*
2. Explain procedure to child and family. *Enhances cooperation and participation; reduces anxiety and fear.*
3. Wash hands. *Reduces transmission of microorganisms.*
4. Assemble pouch according to instructions. *Promotes organization and efficiency.*
5. Put on nonsterile gloves. *Protects nurse from contact with body fluids.*
6. Empty current ostomy pouch of contents. *Prevents accidental contamination of surrounding environment if contents accidentally leak from appliance when removed.*
7. Remove current ostomy appliance. *No longer needed.*
8. Dispose of appliance in appropriate container. *Consistent with body fluid precautions.*
9. Remove gloves. Wash hands. *Prevents spread of microorganisms.*
10. Put on new nonsterile gloves. *Prevents spread of microorganisms.*
11. Cleanse stoma and surrounding skin with warm tap water or an ostomy soap as prescribed by agency policy. Rinse skin well. Pat dry. *Prevents injury to mucosa of stoma, which has no nerve endings and is very friable, and to surrounding skin.*
12. Assess stoma and surrounding skin. *To determine condition of skin.*
13. Measure stoma using measuring guide for appropriate width and length of stoma at base. *Ensures a good fit of the ostomy appliance without excess skin at the base of the stoma exposed to stool.*
14. Place gauze pad over stoma while preparing the skin barrier wafer and pouch for application. *Wicks stool away from skin and ensures a good seal of the wafer to the skin.*

15. Trace pattern of stoma opening onto paper backing of skin barrier wafer. *Ensures better fit and prevents laceration of the stoma or maceration of periostomal skin.*
16. Cut skin barrier wafer approximately ¹⁄₁₆ to ⅛ inch larger than stoma. *Ensures appropriate fit.*
17. Attach a clean pouch to the skin barrier wafer. Make sure the pouch is closed. *Prevents leaking of stool underneath the wafer during application process.*
18. Remove gauze pad from stoma. *Makes it easier to visualize the stoma.*
19. Remove paper backing from skin barrier wafer. If specified by agency policy, apply a thin ring of Stomahesive paste around the opening on the wafer and fan dry for 30–40 seconds or until dry to touch. *Promotes adhesion of bag to skin.*
20. Place the skin barrier wafer on the skin with the opening centered over the stoma. *So bag can attach to wafer and cover stoma.*
21. Place hand or warm washcloth over pouch for 3–5 minutes. *Helps seal the wafer to the skin.*
22. Remove gloves. Wash hands. *Reduces transmission of microorganisms* (Figure IX-3).

DOCUMENTATION

1. Pouch change.
2. Condition and color of stoma and skin.
3. How procedure tolerated.
4. Amount and character of stool.

⧗ **Estimated time to complete procedure:** *10–20 minutes.*

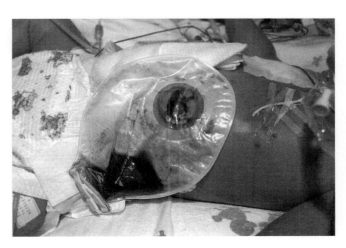

FIGURE IX-3   Infant with ostomy bag.

PROCEDURE 79

EMPTYING AN OSTOMY POUCH

EQUIPMENT

Receptacle for stool
Syringe (or bulb syringe) to aspirate contents of pouch of
  very small infants
Tissue
Water
Gloves, nonsterile

PROCEDURE

1. Gather equipment. *Promotes organization and efficiency.*
2. Explain procedure to child and family. *Enhances cooperation and participation; reduces anxiety and fear.*
3. Wash hands. Put on nonsterile gloves. *Reduces transmission of microorganisms and protects nurse from contact with body fluids.*
4. Open clamp or remove rubber band. *Allows contents to be removed.*

5. Empty contents into receptacle. Note amount, color, consistency, and the presence of any blood or mucus. *Determines amount and type of bag contents.*
6. Rinse inside of pouch using small amount of water. (May use a small paper cup, squirt bottle, or syringe.) Avoid stoma area. *Prevents premature loosening of skin seal. Cleans inside of pouch.*
7. Wipe end of pouch with tissue and replace clamp or rubber band. *So pouch will not leak contents.*
8. Dispose of stool in appropriate manner. *Consistent with body fluid precautions.*
9. Remove gloves. Wash hands. *Reduces transmission of microorganisms.*

DOCUMENTATION

1. Amount, color, and consistency of stool.

⧗ **Estimated time to complete procedure:** *less than 5 minutes.*

Enemas

OVERVIEW

An enema is a solution inserted into the rectum and sigmoid colon to remove feces or flatus or to instill medications. The cleansing enema, often used in preparation for lower bowel surgery or barium enema, stimulates peristalsis via irritation of the colon and rectum and by causing intestinal distention with the fluid. When giving an enema to infants or children, it is important to be aware of the type and amount of fluid administered as well as how far to insert the enema into the rectum. Most often, saline is used in pediatrics, although a Fleets enema or oil-retention enema may also be ordered. Enemas are contraindicated in clients with bowel obstruction, inflammation or infection of the abdomen, or if the child has had recent anal or rectal surgery. Table IX-1 offers guidelines on enema administration.

Table IX-1 Enema Administration Guidelines

Age	Volume (mL)	Distance to Insert Tube
Infant	40–100	2.5 cm (1 inch)
Toddler	100–200	5.0 cm (2 inches)
Preschooler	200–300	5.0 cm (2 inches)
School-Age	300–500	7.5 cm (3 inches)
Adolescent	500–700	10.0 cm (4 inches)

PROCEDURE 80

ADMINISTERING AN ENEMA

SAFETY

1. Never force catheter into anal canal. If a well-lubricated catheter does not advance easily, stop enema.
2. Use only isotonic solutions.
3. Give only the prescribed amount of solution. The smaller the child, the less the amount of fluid that can be safely given.
4. Give only the number of enemas prescribed.

EQUIPMENT

Prepackaged enema or container for enema solution, and rectal catheter
Towels
Lubricant
Bath thermometer
Waterproof pad
Bedpan, potty chair, diaper, and so forth
Gloves, nonsterile

PROCEDURE

1. Check physician's order. *Ensures that appropriate type of enema is given.*
2. Gather equipment. *Promotes organization and efficiency.*
3. Wash hands. *Reduces transmission of microorganisms.*
4. Explain procedure to child and family. *Enhances cooperation and participation; reduces anxiety and fear.*
5. Fill container with prescribed enema solution, unless it is a prepackaged enema. *Promotes organization and efficiency.*
6. Warm solution to body temperature or 37.7° C, 100° F. *Prevents cramping and discomfort. Cold fluid can cause hypothermia in a small child.*
7. Provide for child's privacy. *So child is not embarrassed; to enhance cooperation.*
8. Position waterproof pad under child. *Protects bed linens.*
9. Position child. *Promotes organization and efficiency; colon is on left side.*
   a. Left side, lateral recumbent position with knees up to chest.
   b. On back with legs lifted to expose anal orifice.
   c. Left side with right leg thigh flexed about 45° to body axis (Sims' position).

10. Put on nonsterile gloves. *Protects nurse from microorganisms in feces.*
11. Lubricate rectal catheter and enema tip. *Prevents irritation of mucosal lining of bowel and decreases discomfort.*
12. Prime rectal tube or nozzle of prepackaged enema. *Avoid introducing air into rectum.*
13. Have child take a deep breath. Introduce catheter past anal sphincter into anal canal and lower rectum. *Relaxes anal sphincter.*
14. Once tip of catheter is in place, elevate bag and instill fluid slowly or squeeze prepackaged enema. Do not elevate container more than 10 cm above rectum. *Fluid pressure increases with height of bag.*
15. If child shows signs of distress (e.g., abdominal pain, shortness of breath, or chest pain) flow should be stopped. *May indicate untoward effects.*
16. When solution is completely administered or child cannot hold any more, clamp tube and remove. *No longer needed.*
17. Clean lubricant and any feces from anus with toilet paper. *Promotes cleanliness; prevents irritation of skin.*
18. Have child try to retain enema for the prescribed amount of time. May hold buttocks together. *Allows enema to be more effective.*
19. After prescribed amount of time, place child on bedpan, potty chair, or toilet or apply clean diaper. *To expel enema, feces.*
20. After child expels the enema, cleanse the anal area as needed. *Prevents irritation of skin and mucous membranes of anus.*
21. Dispose of equipment in appropriate container. *Consistent with body fluid precautions.*
22. Remove gloves. Wash hands. *Reduces transmission of microorganisms.*

DOCUMENTATION

1. Procedure, including specific type of enema, and how child tolerated it.
2. Results of enema.

⧗ **Estimated time to complete procedure:** *10–15 minutes.*

UNIT X

Genitourinary System

Urinary Catheterization

— **Procedure 81: Performing Urinary Catheterization**

— **Procedure 82: Performing Routine Catheter Care**

Urinary Catheterization

OVERVIEW

Catheterization involves passing a rubber or plastic tube into the bladder via the urethra to drain urine from the bladder or to obtain a urine specimen. Intermittent catheterization is used to obtain a sample of urine or to relieve bladder distention. Indwelling catheters may be used short-term to keep the bladder empty, prevent urinary retention, or allow measurement of urine output. Long-term indwelling or retention catheters are used to control incontinence or prevent retention or leakage of urine. Catheterization in the hospital is a sterile procedure; however, when performed outside the hospital on children who need intermittent catheterization, it is a clean procedure.

PROCEDURE 81

PERFORMING URINARY CATHETERIZATION

EQUIPMENT

Catheter, straight or indwelling
Urethral catheterization tray:
   Gloves, sterile
   Cotton balls and povidone-iodine or Betadine swab sticks
      or cleansing solution specified by agency policy
Sterile, water-soluble lubricant
10 cc syringe, sterile
Sterile water
Light source
Blanket
Closed drainage system (for indwelling catheter)
Catheter plug (for children going to x-ray)
Tape or other tube-securing device

NOTE: *A second person is often helpful to assist with this procedure.*

RECOMMENDED SIZE AND TYPE OF CATHETER

< 3 Kg	5 French feeding tube or straight catheter
3–8 Kg	5–8 French straight or indwelling catheter
8–11 Kg	8–10 French straight or indwelling catheter
11–14 Kg	10 French straight or indwelling catheter
14–24 Kg	10–12 French straight or indwelling catheter
24–32 Kg	12 French straight or indwelling catheter

PROCEDURE

1. Check chart for order. *Physician order needed for this procedure.*
2. Gather equipment. *Promotes organization and efficiency.*
3. Wash hands. *Reduces transmission of microorganisms.*
4. Provide for privacy. *So child is not embarrassed; to enhance cooperation.*
5. Explain procedure to child and family. *Enhances cooperation and participation; reduces anxiety and fear.*
   a. Explanation should include that povidone-iodine or cleansing solution may feel cold, as catheter is passed may feel urge to urinate, and deep breathing or "panting" will help to pass catheter.
6. Place child on back in a recumbent position. Place a chux or other protection under the child's buttocks. *To visualize area; promotes organization and efficiency.*
7. Adjust light source to provide maximum lighting. *So area can be visualized.*

8. If needed, put on nonsterile gloves and cleanse perineum of stool. *Protects from contact with body fluids. Reduces risk of introducing fecal material into genitourinary tract.*
9. Remove gloves. Wash hands. *Reduces transmission of microorganisms.*
10. Prepare sterile field, maintaining strict aseptic technique. Open catheterization tray or sterile gloves, and drop sterile catheter and syringe onto sterile field. *To promote organization and efficiency. This is a sterile procedure.*
11. Put on sterile gloves. *Reduces transmission of microorganisms.*
12. If using catheterization tray, unfold waterproof underpad and place under child's buttocks. *Do not contaminate gloves while doing this. Prevents bed from getting wet.*
13. Prepare povidone-iodine or agency-prescribed cleansing solution and cotton balls or have assistant open povidone-iodine swabs. *Promotes organization and efficiency.*
14. Open sterile lubricant. If lubricant not part of catheterization tray, have assistant open and squeeze lubricant onto sterile field. *Promotes organization and efficiency.*
15. Maintaining sterile technique, fill syringe with sterile water. *Promotes organization and efficiency.*

NOTE: *Some catheterization trays come with prefilled syringe.*

16. Check catheter balloon prior to insertion by inflating and deflating it with sterile water. *Ensures functioning of catheter.*
17. Cleanse area and insert catheter. *To prevent transmission of microorganisms into collected urine.*
   a. Male
      1. Grasp shaft of penis gently but firmly with nondominant hand. This hand is now contaminated and stays in place throughout the procedure. *A firm pressure rather than a light pressure helps avoid an erection.*

NOTE: *Never catheterize a child with an erection.*

      2. Clean the meatus and then clean outward in a circular motion. Use each swab or cotton ball (generally held with forceps) only once. Be careful not to touch the penis with the sterile glove. *Prevents transmission of microorganisms.*

NOTE: *If child is uncircumcised, retract the foreskin. Do not leave the foreskin retracted following the procedure.*

    3. Pick up the catheter with free (sterile) hand and lubricate the tip. *Lubrication needed for easier insertion.*

    4. Hold the penis shaft perpendicular to the body and insert the catheter slowly and gently. *Prevents injury to urethra.*

    5. Insert the catheter to the hub. *Ensures that balloon will inflate in bladder, not in urethra.*

    6. Inflate the balloon with the recommended amount of water. *To prevent catheter from becoming dislodged.*

b. Female

    1. Separate labia using thumb and forefinger of nondominant hand. (This hand is now contaminated and stays in place during the procedure.) *Allows visualization of area.*

    2. Clean the labia and meatus from front to back using each swab or cotton ball (generally held with forceps) only once. Cleanse each side and then directly over the meatus. Be careful not to touch area with sterile glove. *Prevents microorganisms from contaminating urine.*

    3. Pick up the catheter with the free (sterile) hand and lubricate the tip. *Lubrication needed for easier insertion.*

    4. Align catheter opposite the meatus and insert gently downward. *Follows anatomy; prevents injury to urethra.*

    5. Insert to the hub. *Ensures that balloon will inflate in the bladder, not in urethra.*

    6. Inflate balloon with the recommended amount of water. *To prevent catheter from becoming dislodged.*

18. Connect catheter to closed drainage system *to collected urine.*

19. Attach drainage bag to bed below level of bladder and position catheter tubing in a loop on the bed. *Promotes drainage of urine.*

20. Secure catheter with tape or tube holder. *To prevent it from being pulled out accidently.*

    a. Male: On abdomen or outer thigh.

    b. Female: Inner thigh.

21. Clean the perineum to remove all Betadine. *Prevents skin/mucous membrane irritation.*

22. Make child comfortable. *To enhance cooperation and decrease anxiety.*

NOTE: *The procedure for a straight catheterization (not indwelling) is the same as described above. However, the catheter is inserted only long enough to obtain a urine specimen or to completely drain the bladder. The balloon is not inflated if a straight catheterization.*

DOCUMENTATION

1. Procedure and time done.
2. Size of catheter.
3. Amount of urine output.
4. Color and character of urine.
5. Child's response and how tolerated.

 Estimated time to complete procedure: *10–20 minutes.*

PROCEDURE 82

PERFORMING ROUTINE CATHETER CARE

OVERVIEW

Even though an indwelling catheter is used to drain urine from the bladder, it may provide a route for infection to enter the body. Therefore, care must be taken to ensure that the surrounding area is clean to decrease contamination by bacteria flora. It is important to repeat catheter care whenever it becomes soiled with stool or other drainage.

EQUIPMENT

Prepackaged kit
Antiseptic solution
Sterile swabs
Clean gloves
Sterile bowl
Washcloth, soap, water

PROCEDURE

1. Steps 1–7 of urinary catheterization procedure.
2. Put on clean gloves. *Reduces transmission of microorganisms.*

3. Cleanse perineal area with soap and water. *Soap has antibacterial qualities.*
4. Cleanse meatus in circular motion from the most inner surface to the outside. Use soap and water unless there is excessive purulent drainage. Then follow by using antiseptic solution on cotton balls. *Moving from the most clean area to the least clean decreases risk of recontamination.*
5. Cleanse catheter from meatus out to end of catheter, being careful not to pull on catheter. *Moving from the most clean area to the least clean decreases risk of recontamination. Pulling on catheter will traumatize bladder.*
6. Place cotton balls in proper receptacle and dispose. *Reduces transmission of microorganisms.*
7. Wash hands. *Reduces transmission of microorganisms.*

DOCUMENTATION

1. Time and date.
2. Condition of area around catheter.
3. Solution used.

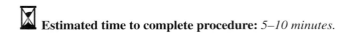 **Estimated time to complete procedure:** *5–10 minutes.*

UNIT XI

Neurological System

Neurological Status

Increased Intracranial Pressure

Seizures

Intraventricular Shunts

Extraventricular Drain (EVD)

— Procedure 83: Maintaining EVD System at Correct Level and Functioning

— Procedure 84: Assessing a Client with an EVD

— Procedure 85: Monitoring Cerebrospinal Fluid (CSF) in the Client with an EVD

— Procedure 86: Changing the EVD Drainage Bag

— Procedure 87: General Nursing Care and Safety with EVDs

Neurological Status

OVERVIEW

Infants and children with neurologic dysfunction display a wide variety of responses to neurologic injuries or illnesses. Changes in levels of consciousness are common, can be manifested in varying degrees, and need to be assessed. The youngster may demonstrate confusion and, although alert, may be disoriented to time, place, and person or unable to answer simple questions. The condition may deteriorate to delirium, where anxiety, fear, and agitation are seen. Level of consciousness may further diminish to stupor when the child is in an unresponsive state, reacts only to vigorous stimulation, and then returns to the original state once the insult is removed. Coma, the most severe form of depressed consciousness, is defined as no response to intense painful stimuli.

The child's level of consciousness may be evaluated several ways. AVPU is commonly utilized (refer to Box XI-1). However, it is necessary to state the exact stimulus and reaction elicited when used. For example, if assessing a painful response, the catalyst (pressure on a nailbed, a vigorous sternal rub) should be mentioned. The child's response should be specific—that is, whether the stimulus was removed by request or the child just moaned or did nothing at all.

BOX XI-1	AVPU
A	**Alert** and awake
V	Responsive to **Verbal** stimuli
P	Responsive to **Painful** stimuli
U	**Unresponsive**

A second way to determine level of consciousness is a neurological assessment that includes the Glasgow Coma Scale (Table XI-1). However, the child's chronological age must be taken into account when using this scale. For example, a toddler may keep the eyes closed so that what is happening in the environment will not be seen, whereas a five-year-old may not verbally respond to the nurse about opening his/her eyes because caregivers have told the child never to talk to strangers.

Table XI-1   Glasgow Coma Scale Adapted for Infants and Children

Criteria	Score	Infant and Child Response	Child Response
Eye Opening	4	Spontaneous	Spontaneous
	3	To loud noise	To verbal stimuli
	2	To pain	To pain
	1	No response	No response
Verbal Response	5	Smiles, coos, cries to appropriate stimuli	Oriented to time, place, person; speaks appropriately
	4	Irritable crying	Confused
	3	Inappropriate crying	Inappropriate words or phrases
	2	Grunts or moans	Incomprehensible words
	1	No response	No response
Motor Response	6	Spontaneous	Obeys commands
	5	Withdraws to touch	Localizes pain
	4	Withdraws to pain	Withdraws to pain
	3	Decorticate posturing	Decorticate posturing
	2	Decerebrate posturing	Decerebrate posturing
	1	No response	No response

Source: Teasdale & Jennett (1974).

Pediatric criteria have been developed for the Glasgow Coma Scale that consider age and developmental level in assessing the child's ability to open her/his eyes, provide verbal response, and provide motor response. Each category is scored and added together for a total score. The maximum score is 15, which indicates normal neurological functioning. The minimum score is 3, which indicates complete unresponsiveness.

The presence or absence of posturing is another important indicator of level of consciousness (Figure XI-1). Decorticate or flexor posturing is associated with bilateral cerebral hemisphere injury. Decerebrate or rigid extensor posturing is secondary to trauma to the midbrain or pons; it is associated with poor prognosis. Flaccid areflexia or the absence of response is indicative of severe brain stem injury and is evident most frequently in terminal coma.

The nurse caring for the child with alterations in neurologic function must be able to meet identified needs. This begins with making a basic assessment of the child's physical condition using the ABCs (Box XI-2).

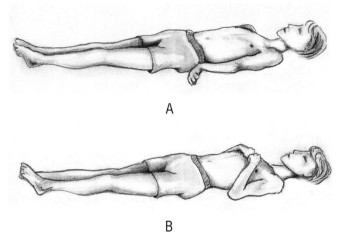

FIGURE XI-1   Motor system dysfunction. A. Decerebrate rigidity. B. Decorticate rigidity.

BOX XI-2   Assessment Using the ABCs

A = **A**irway
B = **B**reathing
C = **C**irculation
D = **D**isability or neurologic status
E = **E**xposure of body

Evaluation always follows the ABC progression, only moving to the next step once the area assessed is determined to be stable. If not, appropriate interventions are initiated before moving on. For example, if an airway cannot be determined as patent, intubation should occur immediately. Once the airway is secure, the remaining ABCs can be addressed.

Once the youngster's ABCs are stable, it is important to evaluate neurologic status, including:

- Level of consciousness that can be assessed using AVPU or the Glasgow Coma Scale
- Motor responses including strength, symmetry, spontaneity, and posturing
- Sensory evaluation including responses to temperature (hot versus cold), pressure (mild, moderate, or severe), pain (sharp versus dull), and proprioception
- Reflexes, noting presence, absence, symmetry, and strength of cranial nerves as well as the Babinski, biceps, triceps, patellar, and ankle reflexes (Table XI-2)
- Physical abilities compromised by the illness or injury
- Any sequelae associated with immobility such as contractures or skin breakdown

---

Table XI-2   Assessment of the Cranial Nerves in the Unconscious Child

Cranial Nerves	Reflex Evaluated	Evaluation
II and III	Pupillary	Shine light source directly into eye. *Intact response*: Pupils will immediately constrict.
II, IV, and VI	Oculocephalic	Hold eyes open and turn head from side to side only *after* cervical spine has been cleared of injury. *Intact response*: Eyes should be gazing upward.
III and VIII	Oculovestibular	*After* cervical spine has been cleared of injury and tympanic membrane has been determined to be intact, place child's head in midline with head elevated. Inject ice water into the ear canal. *Intact response*: Eyes will deviate toward irrigated ear.
V and VII	Corneal	Gently swab cornea with sterile cotton tipped applicator. *Intact response*: Blink.
IX and X	Gag	Irritate pharynx with tongue depressor or cotton swab. *Intact response*. Gag.

Increased Intracranial Pressure

OVERVIEW

Normal intracranial pressure is between 0 and 12 millimeters of mercury, although the body can adapt to 20 millimeters of mercury without detrimental effects. The infant is better able to accommodate the rising pressure than an older child because the skull is more elastic, the fontanelles are not yet closed, and there is room inside the cranium for brain growth.

The early and late signs and symptoms of increased intracranial pressure are presented in Table XI-3.

Table XI-3   Signs and symptoms of increased intracranial pressure

Early Signs
• Headache
• Vomiting
• Slight change in vital signs
• Slight alteration in level of consciousness
• Pupils which are not symmetrical or responsive
• Sunsetting eyes where sclera can be seen above the iris
• Cranial nerve palsies of VI and VII
• Generalized seizures

Late signs
• Significant deterioration in level of consciousness
• Respiratory distress including shallow breathing and Cheyne-Stokes respirations
• Cushing's triad —Bradycardia —Wide pulse pressure —Increased systolic blood pressure
• One pupil fixed and dilated with extremities on the contralateral side either flaccid or spastic

In addition, the infant will also display:
- High-pitched cry
- Bulging fontanelle
- Dilated scalp veins
- Wide sutures
- Irritability

Seizures

OVERVIEW

Seizures are episodic, stereotypic behavioral syndromes that have an abrupt onset, generally are not provoked by external stimuli, and result in loss of responsiveness.

The cause of seizures is often unknown or idiopathic, although there may be genetic factors present predisposing children to particular types of seizures. Febrile seizures are an example of a type of seizure that has an unknown cause. Seizures can also be acquired, resulting from traumatic brain injury, central nervous system infection, hypoglycemia or other endocrine dysfunction, toxic ingestion or exposure, intracranial lesion, or vascular malformation. Typically, infants develop seizures because of birth injury, anoxic episodes, infection, intraventricular hemorrhage, or a congenital brain anomaly. Seizures in older children occur most often as secondary to trauma or infection. In addition, changes in diet or hydration status, fatigue, or not taking prescribed medications may precipitate seizure activity.

Status epilepticus is a prolonged seizure or series of convulsions where loss of consciousness occurs for at least 30 minutes. Refractory seizures last more than 60 minutes. Epilepsy, on the other hand, refers to a chronic seizure disorder that is often associated with central nervous system pathology.

There are two broad categories of seizures: generalized and partial. Clinical manifestations depend on the specific type of seizure. Partial seizures are characterized by local motor, sensory, psychic, and somatic manifestations. There are two types of partial seizures: simple partial seizures and complex partial seizures.

Simple partial seizures, or focal seizures, can be manifested at any age. There is no aura associated with these episodes, and consciousness is generally not lost. Most often, the symptoms seen are motor or sensory in nature. Movements may involve one extremity, a part of that extremity, or ipsilateral extremities with the head and eyes twisting in the opposite direction. The arm toward which the head is turned is abducted and extended with the fingers clenched. There may be numbness, tingling, or painful sensations as well that begin in one area of the body and spread out to others. Alterations in sensory perception may also be present. The child may have visual hallucinations and report seeing images or light flashes. In addition, a buzzing sound may be heard, unusual odors identified, or an odd taste experienced. The child may also report feeling emotional or anxious.

There are several specific types of simple partial seizures. Jacksonian seizures are motor episodes beginning with tonic contractions of either the fingers of one hand, toes of one foot, or one side of the face. The spasms progress into tonic-clonic movements that "march" up adjacent muscles of the affected extremity or side of the body. Rolandic or sylvian seizures are manifested as tonic-clonic movements of the face with increased salivation and arrested speech that occur commonly during sleep (Huff, 2000).

Complex partial seizures are also known as partial psychomotor or temporal lobe episodes. They can be manifested from age 3 years through adolescence. Just before the event, the child may have an aura—a somatic, sensory, or psychic warning that the event will occur—often described as a strange sensation in the stomach that rises up to the throat. In addition, the youngster may have feelings of anxiety, fear, or déjà vu (the sense that an event has occurred before) or complain of abdominal pain, an unusual taste in his mouth, an odd odor, or visual or auditory hallucinations. Consciousness is not completely lost; rather, the child will appear confused or dazed, especially at the onset. When the seizure begins, the child stops the activity he or she is involved in and begins purposeless behaviors such as staring into space or assuming an unusual posture. The child may also perform automatisms, or repeated nonpurposeful actions, such as lip smacking, chewing, sucking, uttering the same word over and over, wandering aimlessly, or removing clothing. Violent acts or rages are rare. A postictal period follows this type of seizure when the child will be drowsy, confused, or aphasic or display sensory or motor impairments. Children usually do not remember the behaviors displayed.

Generalized seizures, arising from both cerebral hemispheres, can occur at any time and last from several seconds to hours. There is no aura, but there is always loss of consciousness. Generalized seizures appearing in children under 4 years of age are frequently associated with developmental delays, learning disabilities, and behavior disorders. There are four types of generalized seizures: tonic-clonic, absence, myoclonic, and akinetic.

Tonic-clonic seizures, often referred to as grand mal seizures, can occur at any age. Onset is usually abrupt and begins when the child loses consciousness and falls to the ground. The initial phase is tonic when there are intense muscle contractions. The jaw clenches shut, the abdomen and chest become rigid, and often the child emits a cry or grunt as exhaled air is forced through the taut diaphragm. Pallor or cyanosis may occur as oxygenation and ventilation are impaired. The airway is compromised because of increased salivation that the youngster cannot manage due to muscular contractions as well as the diminished mental status. The neck and legs are also extended, while the arms are flexed or contracted. The eyes roll upward or deviate to one side, the pupils dilate, and there may also be bladder or bowel incontinence. The tonic phase of the seizure usually persists for 10–30 seconds. During the clonic phase, jerking movements are produced as a result of contraction and relaxation of the muscles. These spasms dissipate as the seizure ends and can last from 30 seconds to 30 minutes after onset of the seizure. A postictal or postconvulsive state follows in which the child may be somnolent or, if awake, confused or combative; have no memory of the event; and have hypertension and diaphoresis. Headache, nausea, vomiting, poor coordination, slurred speech, or visual disturbances may follow.

Febrile seizures are a type of tonic-clonic seizure usually associated with rapid rise in temperature that reaches a minimum of 39° Centigrade. These episodes usually occur in children between 6 months and 5 years of age. There is often a positive family history of febrile seizures, and the seizures frequently accompany infectious processes such as upper respiratory infections, pneumonia, pharyngitis, shigella, urinary tract infections, otitis media, roseola, and meningitis. The seizures are often self-limiting and with a postictal period of less than 15 minutes.

Absence seizures (petit mal) appear around the fourth birthday and generally disappear near adolescence. They are characterized by a transient loss of consciousness that may appear as cessation of current activity. The child seems to stare into space or the eyes may roll upward with ptosis or fluttering of the lids. There also may be lip smacking or a loss of muscle tone, causing the head to droop or any objects in the hands to be dropped. These events usually last from 5 to 10 seconds and can occur as often as 20 or more times per day.

Infantile spasms (salaam) begin at 3 months of age. Many children with this disorder suffered from gestational difficulties and are developmentally delayed or have other neurologic abnormalities. Twice as many males as females are affected. During the seizure, this infant's head may suddenly drop forward while both arms and legs are flexed. The eyes may roll upward or downward, and the infant may cry out and turn pale, cyanotic, or flushed. There may be a loss of consciousness or awareness.

Myoclonic seizures are sudden, repeated contractures of the muscles of the head, extremities, or torso. The child, who can be as young as 2 years but is usually school-age or adolescent, recovers quickly. These seizures occur when the child is drowsy and just falling asleep or just waking up. There is usually no loss of consciousness, nor is there any postictal period.

Atonic or astatic-akinetic seizures (drop attacks) occur between ages 2 and 5 years and are manifested by sudden loss of muscle tone with the head dropping forward for a few seconds. More significant events occur when the youngster loses consciousness and falls to the ground, most often facedown.

In either case, amnesia follows. These seizures often cause repetitive head injuries if the child is not protected by wearing a football or hockey helmet. Many children who experience the seizures have underlying brain abnormalities and are mentally retarded.

Akinetic seizures are manifested as total lack of movement as the child appears frozen in a position. Mental status during the event is diminished.

Nursing Intervention for Seizures

Adopt seizure precautions (prior to a seizure):

1. Pad side rails of bed and ensure that no objects in the bed can cause harm if the child has a seizure. *The child having a tonic-clonic seizure must have a safe environment in which to move during the episode.*
2. Keep side rails in up and locked position when child in bed. *Prevents child from falling out of bed during a seizure.*
3. Have seizure precaution equipment at the bedside: suction setup, ventilation bag/mask. *Improves organization and effectiveness if child has seizure.*

During the seizure:

1. If the child begins to convulse when standing or sitting, gently ease the child to the ground and remove any furniture or objects nearby that may be hazardous. *Will prevent a fall and possible trauma. The floor is a safe place as long as there is nothing in the area to injure child.*
2. Place child on side. *Helps prevent aspiration of secretions and emesis if vomiting occurs.*
3. Perform jaw thrust as needed; administer oxygen either by face mask or assisted ventilation. *Helps maintain patent airway and needed oxygenation.*
4. Do not put anything in child's mouth. *Can cause injury or obstruct breathing.*
5. Suction as necessary. *Seizing children often have increased secretions that may pool in the hypopharynx and occlude the airway or pose a risk for aspiration.*
6. Remove eyeglasses; loosen clothing. *Prevents eyes from being cut if glasses break; prevents restriction of movement and breathing.*
7. Assist with intubation if prolonged seizure activity. *To facilitate breathing and prevent aspiration.*
8. Assist with medications as needed. *Antiseizure medications may be administered to stop seizure.*
9. Time the event. *Most seizures are self-limiting and last less than five minutes. If they are longer, interventions will need to be instituted to curtail the activity.*
10. Monitor child during postictal period. *Alerts staff should seizures return; informs physician or qualified*

practitioner about child's recovery; child may be confused during postictal period.

11. Document time, date, any precipitating event or aura, how long seizure lasted, and what treatment was administered and by whom. *Necessary to monitor child's condition.*

Upon discharge from acute care:

1. Provide information to family about how to handle seizures at home. *Decreases anxiety; allows family to ensure child's safety.*
2. Teach caregivers about importance of giving all medications as ordered by the physician and need for periodic drug serum-level testing. *Missing doses may precipitate a seizure; as child gets older or grows in size, medication dosage may need to be adjusted.*
3. Ensure caregivers are aware of medication side effects. *Prepares them to handle any reactions that may occur.*
4. Work with family on accepting diagnosis. *Giving the family control of the child's well-being will empower them and make them less angry and frustrated by their child's condition.*

5. Stress the actions and activities in which child can participate rather than dwelling on what cannot or should not be done. *It is important to be positive with the family and encourage them to treat this youngster as normally as possible. Also, encourage them not to make this child their "special" one in the family at the expense of the other siblings.*

If a seizure is suspected, obtain the following information:

1. Did child suffer a loss of consciousness or awareness?
2. Did child become pale, cyanotic, or flushed?
3. Did child display any unusual movements, especially tonic-clonic actions, repeated muscle spasms, or head drops?
4. Did child have dilated pupils and/or did eyes roll upward or deviate to one side?
5. Was child incontinent of urine or stool?
6. What happened after the episode? Was there a postictal period? If so, describe it.
7. How soon after the event did the child's behavior return to normal?

Intraventricular Shunts

OVERVIEW

Ventricular shunts are used to treat hydrocephalus. The shunt system, made of radiopaque plastic material, has a ventricular catheter, a unidirectional pressure valve and pumping chamber, and a distal catheter that work together to direct the flow of cerebrospinal fluid from the ventricles to other areas of the body for absorption. In pediatrics, shunts are placed to manage progressive ventricular enlargement and increased intracranial pressure in the presence of large ventricles. Most often, they are ventriculoperitoneal (from the ventricle to the peritoneum) or ventriculoatrial (from the ventricle to the left cardiac atrium). The first is more commonly used in infants and children, as the peritoneal cavity provides both an adequate blood supply to ensure cerebrospinal fluid reabsorption and a large space to accommodate the coiled catheter tubing. In clients with congenital hydrocephalus, shunts are typically placed as soon as the diagnosis is made, and modifications to handle physical growth are planned at regular intervals. However, unexpected revisions may occur at any time.

Postoperative Nursing Interventions

Children who have a shunt placed are cared for as any other postoperative patient, with the following interventions that are specific to the procedure:

1. Place child in a flat position on the unoperated side. *To prevent rapid cerebrospinal fluid drainage and pressure on the valves.*
2. Monitor every two hours.
   a. Level of consciousness
   b. Head circumference
   c. Vital signs
   d. Neurologic checks
   e. Surgical site

To be aware of changes in condition; to document that child is not developing complications (infection, bleeding).

3. Care for shunt as indicated by physician order. *Some shunts are pumped; others are not. Check order.*
4. Provide pain medication or interventions as indicated. *Allows child to be more comfortable.*
5. Before discharge, speak with family about caring for the child with a shunt. *So they will be able to care for child at home.*
   a. Teach signs and symptoms of shunt failure and shunt infection.
   b. Advise about safety issues such as avoiding contact sports.
   c. Encourage caregivers to treat child as normally as possible.

Extraventricular Drain (EVD)

OVERVIEW

The extraventricular drain (EVD) serves both as a monitor of intracranial pressure as well as a portal through which cerebrospinal fluid (CSF) can be removed and therapeutic agents introduced. The drain is a Silastic catheter, with the proximal end inserted into the ventricle and the distal end tunneled under the skin and sutured in place. The distal end is then connected to a tubing, which in turn is attached to a drainage device, an injection apparatus, and a manometer (Figure XI-2). EVDs are most commonly used in pediatrics to treat an infected intraventricular shunt. If the shunt becomes infected, it is removed, an EVD is placed, and the child is treated with intravenous antibiotics.

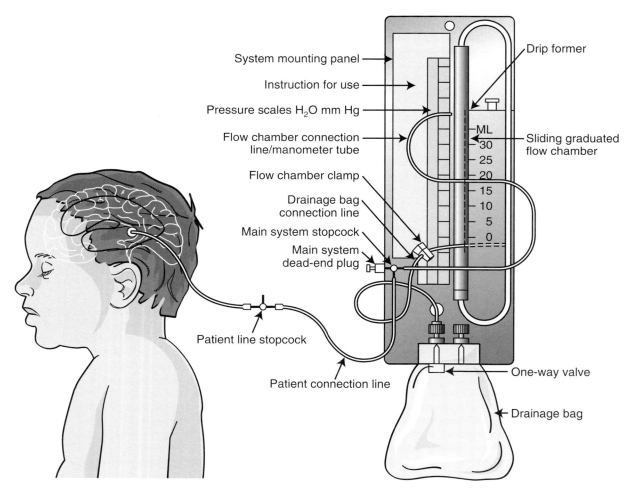

FIGURE XI-2   Placement of an external ventricular drain (EVD) shown with drainage collection setup.

PROCEDURE 83

MAINTAINING EVD SYSTEM AT CORRECT LEVEL AND FUNCTIONING

PROCEDURE

1. Check physician's order for pressure level at which the system is to be maintained. Most frequently, a positive pressure is ordered. Occasionally a negative pressure is ordered. *A physician order is required for the pressure level needed to be monitored.*
2. Ensure that "zero mm H_2O" on the scale monitoring level is at the anatomical reference point used to establish zero pressure. *Ensures that the pressure set will be accurate.*
   a. Supine at midear level.
   b. Side lying at nose.

NOTE: *These are the external anatomical reference points that correspond most closely with the foramen of Monro.*

3. Use a string held from the client to zero on the scale to determine that the two points are level. *More clearly demonstrates that the two points are level* (Figure XI-3).
4. Ensure that top of the flow chamber (marked with an arrow) is at the ordered level. If not, loosen the locking knob, slide the chamber up or down, and then tighten the knob. *Enables CSF to drain when it reaches the ordered pressure level while preventing excessive or too-rapid drainage.*
5. Check the patency of the system by movement of CSF with movement of the client, or slightly lower the drain system and observe for CSF drip and then return the drain to the ordered position. Make sure that all stopcocks are in the "on" position. *CSF will not drain when the tubing is occluded.*
6. Be sure that the clamp between drip chamber and collection bag is closed. *Allows for accurate monitoring of CSF output and ensures proper functioning of the system.*
7. Clamp the system off by turning the stopcock to the "off" position (off toward the client). Use the stopcock on the mounting board. *It is most clearly visible when the following situations occur:*
   a. Client or system will be moved out of alignment with each other (e.g., when repositioning the client). *When client and system are out of alignment, CSF can drain too rapidly or too slowly.*
   b. Crying or increased activity. *These increase CSF pressure and increase the flow of CSF into the system.*
8. After repositioning the client, realign the system and open clamp/turn stopcock to the "on" position. *Allows fluid to continue draining as ordered.*
9. Assess system every hour to ensure proper alignment. *So system is able to drain appropriately.*

NOTE: *Physician will determine how much activity the client can tolerate (e.g., whether client can get up and walk) and how long the system can be turned off. Generally, the system is not turned off for more than 30 minutes at a time.*

DOCUMENTATION

1. Pressure level of drain and level of drain itself (e.g., midear).
2. Patency of the system.
3. Times and duration when drain clamped and how client tolerated it.

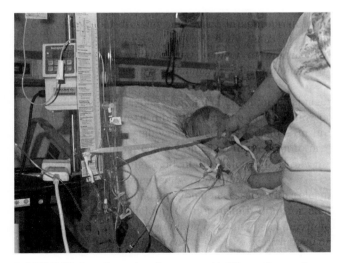

FIGURE XI-3 Ensuring "zero cm H_2O" on the scale, supine at midear level.

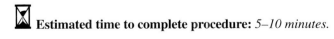 **Estimated time to complete procedure:** *5–10 minutes.*

PROCEDURE 84

ASSESSING A CLIENT WITH AN EVD

PROCEDURE

1. Monitor neurological status every four hours or as ordered. *To determine if condition has changed.*
2. Include the following in the assessment:
   a. Level of consciousness.
   b. Bilateral grip strength.
   c. Pupil size and response to light.
   d. Vital signs.
   e. Presence or absence of headache, nuchal rigidity, vomiting, double vision, slurred speech, dizziness, and ataxia.
   f. Blood or clear drainage from nose or ears.
   g. Presence or absence of seizures.
3. Assess insertion site and skin condition at least once a shift. Assess for redness and drainage. *To determine if inflammation/infection is present.*

DOCUMENTATION

1. Assessment findings.

 Estimated time to complete procedure: *10–15 minutes.*

PROCEDURE 85

MONITORING CEREBROSPINAL FLUID (CSF) IN THE CLIENT WITH AN EVD

PROCEDURE

1. Check CSF output every two hours or more frequently as needed. *If collection chamber fills completely, it will inhibit CSF drainage. If air filter at the top of the drip chamber becomes wet, the system will not function.*
2. Read volume of fluid using scale on drip chamber. *To determine amount of drainage.*
3. Note color and turbidity. *May indicate bleeding or infection.*
4. Drain drip chamber by: *(To allow more CSF to flow into chamber.)*
   a. Clamping system by turning stopcock to the off position. *If not clamped, there may be a momentary reduction in pressure resulting in temporary lack of drainage.*
   b. Carefully opening slide clamps at bottom of drip chamber and allow CSF to drain into collection bag.
   c. Leaving 5 cc of fluid in the bottom of the chamber.
   d. Closing both clamps. *Procedure to follow to drain chamber of fluid.*
5. Replace CSF (PO or IV) if/as ordered. *CSF contains sodium chloride, potassium, protein, and glucose. When large amounts are not replaced, this can result in fluid and electrolyte imbalance.*
6. Notify physician if CSF output is greater than 20 cc per hour. *Indicates child is losing more fluid than should over an hour; MD may readjust EVD system.*

DOCUMENTATION

1. Volume of CSF output.
2. Color and character of CSF.
3. Fluid replacement, if any.

Estimated time to complete procedure: *5 minutes.*

PROCEDURE 86

CHANGING THE EVD DRAINAGE BAG

EQUIPMENT

Gloves, sterile
Betadine stick swabs
New drainage bag, sterile

PROCEDURE

Change bag when three quarters full. *Prevents overfilling of drainage bag.*

1. Gather equipment. *Promotes organization and efficiency.*
2. Wash hands. *Reduces transmission of microorganisms.*
3. Prepare connection between tubing and bag by cleansing with Betadine swab sticks. *Reduces transmission of microorganisms.*
4. Allow to dry. *Betadine must dry to be effective.*
5. Ensure that clamps on tubing between drip chamber and bag are closed. *To prevent CSF from entering tubing.*

6. Open package containing new bag, maintaining sterile technique. *Promotes organization and efficiency.*
7. Put on sterile gloves. *Reduces transmission of microorganisms.*
8. Remove old bag from tubing and attach new bag. *Old bag no longer needed.*
9. Dispose of old bag containing CSF in biohazard container. *Consistent with guidelines for handling bodily fluids.*
10. Remove gloves. Wash hands. *Reduces transmission of microorganisms.*

DOCUMENTATION

1. Bag change.

 Estimated time to complete procedure: *10–15 minutes.*

PROCEDURE 87

GENERAL NURSING CARE AND SAFETY WITH EVDS

PROCEDURE

1. Keep free of kinks, constrictions, traction. *Allows system to drain properly and reduces chance of inadvertent dislodgement of needle or catheter.*
2. Take care to prevent dislodgement of catheter or needle when moving or caring for child. *So catheter/needle does not need to be replaced.*
3. Preserve closed system with as few interruptions as possible. *Minimizes introduction of microorganisms into CSF.*
4. Only physician enters the system to obtain samples or administer medications. *Usual agency procedure, to prevent chance of microorganisms entering system.*
5. Site care as prescribed by physician or agency policy.
   a. Strict aseptic technique for any care.
   b. If no dressing, site may be cleansed using prescribed solutions such as half-strength hydrogen peroxide followed by povidone-iodine.
   c. If dressing changes are ordered, use procedure for changing central line dressing.

DOCUMENTATION

1. Site care or dressing changes.
2. Laboratory specimens obtained.

⧗ **Estimated time to complete procedure:** *depends on physician order; 5–20 minutes.*

Musculoskeletal System

Casts

OVERVIEW

Casts are used to provide stabilization for fractured bones, to immobilize a surgical site, or to treat a musculoskeletal disorder (clubfoot, hip dysplasia). Casts are made of plaster of Paris or fiberglass. Casts covering forearms or lower legs are called short arm or leg casts; the spica or hip spica cast (commonly used to treat dysplasia of the hip) covers the hips and one or both legs. A cast should fit snugly and support the area needing immobilization. The cast may be changed several times if it becomes too loose or too tight. During the first 24 hours after the cast is applied, edema can create a tourniquet effect and inhibit circulation to the tissue. It is important to assess the cast site for edema or irritation to the skin. Nurses will often assist with the cast application and are responsible for cast care after it has been applied. Nurses also instruct the child and family on care of the cast at home.

PROCEDURE 88

PETALING A CAST

EQUIPMENT

Wet-proof adhesive tape: 1-inch, 2-inch, and ½-inch for very
small areas
Scissors
Moleskin (optional; not to be used around the perineum or an
area likely to get wet)

PROCEDURE

1. Prepare child and family. *Enhances cooperation and
participation; reduces anxiety and fear.*
2. Ensure that cast is dry. *Petaling is applied only after a
cast is dry.*
3. Gather equipment. *Promotes organization and efficiency.*
4. Wash hands. *Reduces transmission of microorganisms.*
5. Prepare petals by cutting strips of adhesive tape or
moleskin 1½ to 4 inches long, depending on thickness
of cast. Ends should be rounded. *Provides enough tape
to cover rough edges.*

NOTE: *Pointed petals wrinkle and come unattached more
easily than rounded petals.*

6. Pull stockinette lining taut over edge of cast and petal
the cast with adhesive tape or moleskin. *Assures that
stockinette padding stays in place.*
   a. Place one end of the tape on the inside of the cast,
   sticky side against cast.
   b. Bring other end of tape up over the cast and tape it
   down on the outside of the cast. Press firmly.
   c. Petals (tape strips) should overlap slightly and cover
   the entire exposed edge of the cast (Figure XII-1).
   *Provides smooth edge around cast opening. Over-
   lapping helps tape stick to itself/cast.*

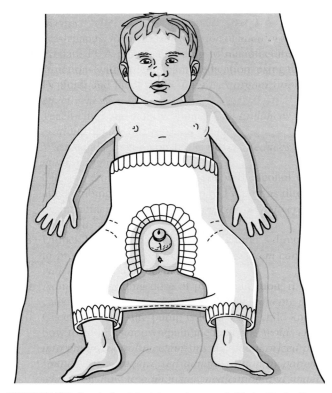

FIGURE XII-1   Infant in hip spica cast. Note that all
edges are petaled with adhesive strips, which overlap.

DOCUMENTATION

1. Time of procedure and material used.
2. Reaction of child to the procedure.
3. Teaching child and primary caregiver.

 Estimated time to complete procedure: *15–20 minutes.*

Braces

OVERVIEW

Children will wear braces temporarily (to treat scoliosis) or for long-term problems (cerebral palsy). Most children who need braces will be fitted by an expert and evaluated periodically to be sure the brace fits properly and is not causing skin breakdown.

Guidelines for family teaching related to braces include:

1. The brace should feel comfortable when worn.
2. The skin should be examined frequently (every one to two hours initially) and then less frequently (every four to six hours) once the skin has adapted. If the skin appears red where it contacts the brace, the child should not wear the brace until the redness disappears. If skin breakdown has occurred, the child should not wear the brace until the skin has healed.
3. A liner (sock, T-shirt) should be worn under the brace to help protect the skin.
4. The brace should be checked daily for rough edges or wear.

Skeletal Traction

OVERVIEW

Skeletal traction is applied directly to the bone using specialized equipment such as Steinmann pins, a Kirschner wire, Crutchfield tongs, nails, or screws, for the purpose of immobilizing a bone or to allow more precise alignment of fractured bone fragments. It provides a strong, steady pull and allows for longer periods of traction or can be used for short-term treatment of a fracture until it can be openly reduced and internally or externally fixated during surgery.

Skeletal traction uses pins implanted into the bone and held in place by an external metal frame. For example, halo traction provides support for cervical conditions and injuries by using pins placed in the skull, which are then attached to external metal bars fixed on a rigid chest vest.

Pins for skeletal traction are placed by an orthopedic surgeon. A potentially serious complication with pins inserted into the bone and exiting through the skin is osteomyelitis, which occurs when infection starting at the skin moves down the pin into the tissue and then into the bone. Another consideration with pins and nails is pain associated with pin placement or a fracture.

PROCEDURE 89

PERFORMING PIN SITE CARE

EQUIPMENT

Cotton-tipped applicators, sterile
Prescribed cleansing solution
Sterile normal saline
Sterile 2 × 2 gauzes
Povidone-iodine liquid or antimicrobial ointment
Sterile cotton-tipped applicators

PROCEDURE

1. Gather equipment. *Promotes organization and efficiency.*
2. Wash hands. *Reduces transmission of microorganisms.*
3. Explain procedure to child and family. *Enhances cooperation and participation; reduces anxiety and fear.*
4. Remove old dressing and inspect skin site. *To determine condition of skin at site.*

5. Dip applicators in prescribed solution and cleanse around pin sites. *To remove dried blood and secretions which may harbor microorganisms.*
6. Rinse pin sites with normal sterile saline using sterile cotton-tipped applicators. *To remove prescribed cleansing solution which may be irritating to skin.*
7. Apply povidone-iodine or antimicrobial ointment to the pin site as prescribed or per agency policy. *To reduce chance of pin site becoming infected.*
8. Place new 2 × 2 dressing on pin site. *To protect pin site from injury.*

DOCUMENTATION

1. Procedure and how tolerated.
2. Assessment of the pin site.

 Estimated time to complete procedure: *5–10 minutes.*

PROCEDURE 90

CARING FOR THE CHILD IN AN EXTERNAL FIXATION DEVICE

PROCEDURE

1. Assess pins, pin sites, and stability of frame every four hours. *Prevents complications and pin site infections.*
   a. Assess pins for breakage, bending, or shifting. Pins should be immobile.
   b. Assess pin sites for signs of infection (redness, edema, heat, tenderness, drainage). Pins sites should be clean and dry.
2. Assess neurovascular status of affected limb every four hours (capillary refill, color, temperature, movement, feeling). *Children with external fixation devices usually have extensive soft tissue, nerve, and vessel damage.*
3. Provide teaching to parent and child before discharge. *So parent and child are able to care for pin site after discharge.*
   a. Explain how to perform neurovascular checks, how to assess the pins sites, and when to call the physician. *To prevent complications.*
   b. Demonstrate pin care and have the provider give a return demonstration. *Ensures that caregivers use aseptic technique.*
   c. Reinforce instructions regarding activity level and weight bearing. *So fixation device is not damaged.*

   d. Explain that fixation device should not be used as a handle. *To prevent damage to fixation device.*
   e. Demonstrate range of motion exercises if appropriate and have child and caregiver return demonstration. *Ensures that appropriate exercises are being performed.*
   f. Instruct child and caregiver to elevate the extremity if edema occurs in the affected limb. *Improves venous return.*
   g. Teach appropriate use of assistive devices as necessary. *Prevents falls; inappropriate use of device could cause accidents.*

DOCUMENTATION

1. Neurovascular status and pin site condition.
2. Condition and status of fixation device.
3. Teaching done and parent and child comprehension. Return demonstrations given.

 Estimated time to complete procedure: *10–15 minutes.*

PROCEDURE 91

PERFORMING PIN CARE, EXTERNAL FIXATION DEVICE

EQUIPMENT

Cotton-tipped applicators, sterile
Prescribed cleansing solution
Gloves, sterile

PROCEDURE

1. Gather equipment. *Promotes organization and efficiency.*
2. Wash hands. *Reduces transmission of microorganisms.*
3. Explain procedure to child and family. *Enhances cooperation and participation; reduces anxiety and fear.*
4. Open applicators and cleansing solution. *Promotes organization and efficiency.*
5. Put on sterile gloves. *Reduces the transmission of microorganisms and protects the nurse from contact with body fluids.*
6. Cleanse the site. *To prevent infection at site.*
   a. Dip applicator in cleansing solution. *So applicator can cleanse site.*
   b. Cleanse each site using a circular motion. Cleanse from the pin site outward. *Cleanse from least contaminated to most contaminated area.*
   c. Use a new applicator for each pin site. *Reduces the transmission of microorganisms.*
7. Dispose of applicators in an appropriate container. *To reduce transmission of microorganisms.*
8. Remove and dispose of gloves. Wash hands. *Reduces transmission of microorganisms.*

DOCUMENTATION

1. Time procedure performed and cleansing solution used.
2. Condition of pin sites.

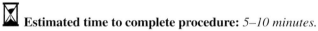 **Estimated time to complete procedure:** *5–10 minutes.*

UNIT XIII

Integumentary System

Rashes

OVERVIEW

Inflammatory skin conditions (rashes) can be acute or chronic in nature. Some accompany illnesses (e.g., measles), whereas others are an illness themselves (e.g., atopic dermatis). Whenever caring for a child with a rash, it is important to ascertain the type of rash (maculopapular, diffuse, urticarial, vesicular, petchial) as well as the area on the body where it occurs. Some rashes disappear with minimal or no treatment; others are challenging to care for, especially if they are chronic or become infected. The guidelines appearing below are more appropriate for a chronic rash such as atopic dermatis and can be taught to parents.

General Guidelines

1. Provide moist environment (dressing or occlusive ointment) for healing. *Provides moisture to the stratum corneum.*
2. Administer topical treatments and applications as ordered. *Topical medications and treatments prevent transdermal water loss.*
3. Administer systemic medication if prescribed. *Systemic medicines help reduce inflammation.*
4. Keep child away from irritant or allergen. *The best way to prevent reoccurrence.*
5. Avoid or reduce stimuli that exacerbate pruritis (clothing, bed linen, environmental allergens). *Reduces itching.*
6. Administer antipruritic medications. *Allergic reactions may be controlled by systemic medications.*
7. Administer soothing baths. Soaps may be drying; oils are hazardous with small children. Baking soda and oatmeal baths do not decrease moisture in the skin. *Cool water relieves itching; some additives may increase effectiveness of bath.*
8. Teach child and/or caregiver to pat skin dry rather than rub dry following a bath. *Rubbing further traumatizes skin and increases itching.*
9. Apply occlusive emollient reams immediately after bathing. *Helps retain moisture in skin and reduces itching.*
10. Keep child's fingernails short. *Contaminants under nails may harbor bacteria that can be introduced into open lesions by scratching.*
11. Cover child's hands with mittens or socks to prevent scratching. *Scratching can further damage skin, making it more susceptible to secondary infection.*
12. Dress child in clothing that is light, clean, and loose. *Tight clothing may cause more irritation and therefore more scratching; clean clothing will prevent further infection.*
13. Use hygienic methods, such as antibacterial soap pumps for hand washing, to prevent infection. *Keeps exposure to bacteria to a minimum.*

Wound Care

OVERVIEW

Wounds created surgically usually have minimal tissue reaction or destruction, minimal drainage, and minimal contamination. The wound edges are approximated, and rarely is dead space left to become infected after suturing. The dressing needed for this kind of wound is often a dry dressing. These wounds heal by primary intention. Wounds that heal by secondary and tertiary intention generally have tissue loss or delayed closure. Since the edges cannot be approximated, granulation tissue forms; the wound is left open, and healing occurs from the inside toward the outer surfaces.

There are four classifications of surgical wounds: clean, clean contaminated, contaminated, and infected. Clean wounds show no signs of infection, can be drained with a closed drainage system, and are able to be closed since the alimentary, respiratory, or genitourinary track were not entered. Clean contaminated wounds show no signs of infection or break in surgical technique and do involve the alimentary, respiratory, or genitourinary track. Contaminated wounds are open, fresh, or accidental wounds that show signs of infection or have experienced spillage of gastrointestinal contents. Infected wounds demonstrate an existing infection or perforated viscera and may be due to trauma with retained devitalized tissue.

Wounds are usually covered with a dressing in order to apply medications; maintain the moist environment; prevent cell dehydration; aid hemostasis; minimize edema; support, splint, or immobilize the area, protect the wound; protect and cushion against trauma and contamination; or absorb drainage.

Different types of wounds require different approaches to wound care. Wound care agents, including povidone-iodine, hydrogen peroxide, Dakin's solution, or other cleaning solutions, may need to be avoided, diluted, or used sparingly according to institutional policy or physician order since they can dry the wound and interfere with wound healing at the cellular level. Although they reduce the risk of infection, frequent application may not be necessary. Often, sterile water, sterile normal saline, or pH-neutral solutions are adequate to cleanse the wound.

The dry dressing and the wet-to-dry dressing are most commonly used in pediatrics.

PROCEDURE 92

APPLYING A DRY DRESSING

OVERVIEW

The dry dressing is most often used on a clean surgical wound with minimal drainage. Dry dressings cover and protect the wound as well as absorb drainage.

EQUIPMENT NEEDED

Gloves, nonsterile; 2 pairs
Montgomery straps or tape
Sterile forceps or sterile cotton swabs
Sterile 2 × 2s or 4 × 4s
Sterile ABD (abdominal dressing) pads
Moisture-proof or plastic bag
Washcloth

PROCEDURE

1. Review the physician's order and agency policy. *It is necessary to clearly understand the purpose of the prescribed procedure before proceeding.*
2. Gather equipment. *Promotes organization and efficiency.*
3. Wash hands. *Reduces transmission of microorganisms.*
4. Position child. Use bath blanket to drape so that only wound is exposed. *Provides privacy and prevents chilling.*
5. Place moisture-proof bag within easy reach. *Provides proper receptacle for disposal of contaminated dressing.*
6. Loosen Montgomery straps or remove tape from the dressing. Remove tape by pulling toward wound, small sections at a time, while holding down the skin in front of the tape. *Prevents skin breakdown and injury to newly formed tissue, and so old dressing can be removed.*
7. Put on nonsterile gloves. *Protects nurse from contact with body fluids.*
8. Remove old dressing and place old dressing and gloves in moisture-proof bag. *Dressings soiled with body fluids and exam gloves used to remove old dressing are considered contaminated and subject to biochemi-*

cal disposal in the correct manner per institutional protocol.
9. Assess wound. Note odor and color of any drainage. *Allows for evaluation of effectiveness of treatment; infected drainage has a dintinctive odor.*
10. Wash hands. *Reduces transmission of microorganisms.*
11. Put on second pair of clean gloves. *Reduces transmission of microorganisms and protects health care worker from contact with body fluids.*
12. Cleanse skin around incision if necessary with a clean, warm, wet washcloth. *Dried blood or drainage can irritate the skin.*
13. Apply new 4 × 4 or 2 × 4 dressing by grasping the edges of the dressing and placing it on the wound; cover with ABD pad if indicated; secure dressing with Montgomery straps or tape. If using tape, place at edges of dressing so that it cannot be lifted to expose wound. Use paper tape on thin, fragile, or sensitive skin. Write initials and date and time of the dressing change on a piece of tape and apply to dressing. *A light dressing of 2 × 2 or 4 × 4 may be all that is needed depending on the size of the wound; ABD pad helps protect the wound; Montgomery straps prevent skin breakdown from tape removal associated with frequent dressing changes; initials and date and time record help staff know when to change dressing again.*
14. Remove gloves. Wash hands. *Prevents transmission of microorganisms.*
15. Assist child to position of comfort and assess level of comfort. *To reduce anxiety and enhance well being.*

DOCUMENTATION

1. Wound appearance:
   a. Site,
   b. Type and amount of drainage,
   c. Condition of wound margin (the outside skin edge).
2. Dressing materials used.
3. Date and time of dressing change.
4. How child tolerated procedure.

 Estimated time to complete procedure: *5–10 minutes.*

PROCEDURE 93

APPLYING A WET-TO-DRY DRESSING

OVERVIEW

The purpose of a wet-to-dry dressing is to cover and protect the wound, collect exudates, promote healing, and promote light surface debridement. The decision to apply a wet-to-dry dressing depends on the wound bed, type of tissue, presence of eschar, amount of exudates, stage of wound healing, state of surrounding tissue, and the presence of infection.

Specifics of the wet-to-dry dressing vary according to the preferences of the surgeon and wound specialist, institutional policies, and outcome measurement standards used to evaluate the effectiveness of the dressing. Current evidence regarding dressing types and tracking wound outcomes should be reviewed periodically to help make the best dressing treatment choices in the clinical setting.

PURPOSE

Debridement of a wound; as it dries, the wet-to-dry dressing adheres to debris on the surface of the wound. When the dressing is removed, surface debris from the wound is removed along with the dressing.

EQUIPMENT

Gloves, sterile
Gloves, nonsterile
Sterile ABD (abdominal dressing) pads
Moisture-proof or plastic bag
Sterile gauze
Sterile container or bowl
Sterile drapes
Sterile normal saline or solution per physician's order
Montgomery straps or tape
Sterile forceps or sterile cotton swabs
Skin barrier
Bath blanket

PROCEDURE

1. Review the physician's order and agency policy. *The meaning/purpose of the term "wet-to-dry dressing" is variable. Any dressing that is moist at the wound surface and covered with a dry dressing may be referred to as a wet-to-dry dressing. Some moist dressings are designed to provide a moist healing environment, not to debride the wound. It is necessary to clearly under-stand the purpose of the prescribed procedure before proceeding.*

2. Gather equipment. *Promotes organization and efficiency.*

3. Wash hands. *Reduces transmission of microorganisms.*

4. Position child. Use bath blanket to drape so that only the wound is exposed. *Provides privacy and prevents chilling.*

5. Place moisture-proof bag within easy reach. *Provides proper receptacle for disposal of contaminated dressing.*

6. Loosen Montgomery straps or remove tape from the dressing. Remove tape by pulling toward wound small sections at a time while holding down the skin in front of the tape. *Prevents skin breakdown and injury to newly formed tissue. So dressing can be removed.*

7. Put on nonsterile gloves. *Protects nurse from contact with body fluids.*

8. Remove old dressing—outer protective dressing and inner layers of gauze packing. Remove packing by gently grasping gauze without touching the wound. Do not moisten to remove. *Moistening defeats the purpose of dressing, which is to remove necrotic tissue and exudate.*

9. Place old dressing and gloves in moisture-proof bag. *To reduce transmission of microorganisms.*

10. Assess wound. Note odor and color of any drainage. *To determine condition of wound.*

11. Wash hands. *Reduces transmission of microorganisms.*

12. Open supplies and set up sterile field. Using aseptic technique, place fine mesh gauze into sterile container. Pour enough solution into container to soak gauze. *Promotes organization and efficiency.*

13. Put on sterile gloves. *Reduces transmission of microorganisms and protects health care worker from contact with body fluids.*

14. Clean and/or irrigate wound as ordered by physician, from center of wound outward using a new swab for each stroke. *Prevents contamination of wound by going from least contaminated to most contaminated area.*

15. Take piece of mesh gauze from container and gently squeeze out solution until gauze is only slightly moist. *If gauze is too moist, wound bed gets too soupy and increases chance of bacterial growth.*

16. Open gauze and gently pack it into wound using either forceps or the tip of a cotton swab stick. *So gauze comes in contact with wound surface.*

  a. Continue until all wound surfaces are in contact with gauze. *So gauze comes in contact with all wound surfaces.*

b. Do not pack too tightly. *Prevents compression of capillaries.*

c. Do not overlap wound edges with wet packing. *Prevents maceration (softening and breakdown of tissues).*

17. Apply layer of dry gauze over wet gauze. Cover with ABD pad. *Protects the wound.*

18. Remove gloves and discard *to reduce transmission of microorganisms.*

19. Secure dressing with Montgomery straps or tape. If using tape, place at edges of dressing so that it cannot be lifted to expose wound. Use paper tape on thin, fragile, or sensitive skin. Montgomery straps prevent skin breakdown from tape removal associated with frequent dressing changes. *Paper tape is less traumatic when removed from fragile skin than adhesive tape.*

20. Wash hands. *Prevents transmission of microorganisms.*

21. Assist child to position of comfort and assess level of comfort. *To promote and maintain well being.*

DOCUMENTATION

1. Describe condition of wound:
   a. Color and type of tissue,
   b. Type and amount of drainage,
   c. Size of wound bed, including depth of wound (use tape measure to assess actual size of wound),
   d. Undermining of wound,
   e. Condition of wound margin (the outside skin edge).
2. Dressing materials/solution(s) used for irrigating wound and for moistening gauze.
3. Date and time of dressing change.
4. How child tolerated procedure.

 Estimated time to complete procedure: *15–20 minutes.*

Wounds with Drains

OVERVIEW

Wounds may have drains placed into them during surgery or during the healing process for the purpose of draining sanguineous, serosanguineous, purulent, gastrointestinal, biliary, or other body fluids from the surgical site or cavity. The drain may exit via a stab wound near the main incision or may exit via the incision line or open wound. Drains may be of the Jackson-Pratt or Hemo-Vac type, with a collection device that can be emptied, or the drain may be a hollow type drain such as a Penrose that is not connected to a collection device and simply drains into a dressing. Drain care varies according to the surgeon's preference and agency or institutional policy.

PROCEDURE 94

CLEANING AND DRESSING A WOUND WITH PENROSE DRAIN

EQUIPMENT

Clean exam gloves
Container for proper disposal of soiled dressing
Washcloths
Sterile gloves
Normal saline
Small sterile bowl
Sterile cotton-tip applicators
Sterile towel
Multiple sterile 4 × 4 gauze pads
ABD pads (optional)
Tape or Mongtomery straps
Precut drain sponges (or cut 4 × 4s halfway through with sterile scissors)

PROCEDURE

1. Gather supplies. *Promotes organization and efficiency.*
2. Provide privacy to child. *Maintains child's comfort and security while dressing is being changed.*
3. Explain procedure to child and parent. *Enhances cooperation and participation; reduces anxiety and fear.*
4. Wash hands. *Reduces transmission of microorganisms.*
5. Put on clean exam gloves. *Protects nurse from contact with body fluids.*
6. Remove old dressing and place in appropriate container. *Dressings soiled with body fluids are considered contaminated and subject to biochemical disposal in the correct manner per institutional protocol.*
7. Assess wound. Note odor and color of any drainage; the drain may exit directly from the incision line or from a separate stab wound near the incision. Ensure that the drain is securely attached to the skin to prevent it from being accidentally dislodged. *Allows for evaluation of effectiveness of treatment.*
8. Cleanse skin around incision if necessary with a clean, warm, wet washcloth; do not disturb drain or area under the drain. *Dried blood or drainage can irritate the skin; moving drain can cause it to be dislodged or shifted so that it does not drain.*
9. Remove exam gloves. *Exam gloves used to remove old dressing are considered contaminated and subject to biochemical disposal in the correct manner per institutional protocol.*
10. Wash hands. *Reduces transmission of microorganisms.*
11. Set up a sterile field, including pouring ordered solutions into appropriate containers if indicated for the dressing change. *To promote organization and efficiency.*
12. Put on sterile gloves. *To promote organization and efficiency and prevent transmission of microorganisms to wound.*
13. Cleanse suture line using sterile normal saline or other approved cleaning solution with sterile cotton-tip applicators using a rolling motion. Remove excess moisture after cleansing with dry cotton-tip applicators. *Normal saline will not interfere with healing of suture line; cleansing should be from the clean to contaminated area to avoid introducing microbes into the clean portion of the skin. Excess moisture causes excoriation of skin.*
14. Cleanse the wound under the drain. The open drain should be handled minimally. The drain may be elevated with a sterile finger or a cotton-tip applicator to facilitate cleansing as described above. *If the drainage is excessive or not adequately absorbed by the dressing, the skin beneath the drain will need to be cleaned. Drainage on the skin can be an irritant and medium for bacteria. The open drain is a portal of entry into the surgical site. It may or may not be sutured in place and requires care in handling to avoid spreading contaminants or dislodging.*
15. Apply needed layers of pre-cut drain sponges around Penrose drain. Top with one to two layers of uncut 4 x 4s. *Precut (or 4 x 4s cut with a sterile scissors) drain sponges allow a close fit of the dressing around the drain while allowing the drainage to exit onto an absorbent material.*
16. Apply new 4 × 4 or 2 × 4 dressing; cover with ABD if indicated; secure dressing with Montgomery straps or tape. If using tape, place at edges of dressing so that it cannot be lifted to expose wound. Use paper tape on thin, fragile, or sensitive skin. Write initials and date and time of the dressing change on a piece of tape and apply to dressing. *A light dressing of 2 × 2 or 4 × 4 may be all that is needed depending on size of wound. ABD helps protect wound. Montgomery straps prevent skin breakdown from tape removal associated with frequent dressing changes. Paper tape is easier to remove than adhesive tape. Initials and date and time record help staff know when to change dressing again.*
17. Remove gloves. Wash hands. *Prevents transmission of microorganisms.*

DOCUMENTATION

1. Wound appearance:
   a. Site,
   b. Type and amount of drainage,
   c. Condition of wound margin (the outside skin edge).
2. Site of Penrose drain.
3. Dressing materials used.
4. Date and time of dressing change.
5. How child tolerated procedure.

 Estimated time to complete procedure: *5–10 minutes.*

PROCEDURE 95

MONITORING JACKSON-PRATT AND HEMOVAC DRAINS

OVERVIEW

The Jackson-Pratt (JP) (Figure XIII-1) and Hemovac drains are placed surgically to allow for draining of body fluids postoperatively. The drain ends in a bulb that compresses to allow for creation of gentle suction, thereby enhancing the flow of the fluid from the operative site. The drain may be in place for 24 hours to several weeks. The nurse is responsible for monitoring the drainage device and observing and measuring the drainage.

EQUIPMENT

Gloves, nonsterile (exam)
Specimen cup
Absorbent pads

PROCEDURE

1. Gather equipment. *Promotes organization and efficiency.*
2. Explain procedure to child and family. *Enhances cooperation and participation; reduces anxiety and fear.*
3. Wash hands. Put on gloves. *Reduces transmission of microorganisms and protects nurse from contact with body fluids.*

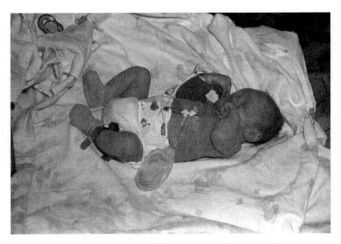

FIGURE XIII-1   Infant with Jackson-Pratt drain.

4. Expose drain site while keeping child draped. Place drainage system on absorbent pad. *Provides privacy, to prevent drainage from contaminating sheet.*
5. Examine system for patency, seal, and stability. *To determine condition of system.*
6. Remove cap from spout of drain. Do not touch tip of spout or cap to anything. *Reduces transmission of microorganisms.*

NOTE: *Policy at some agencies requires cleansing the drainage spout with povidone-iodine or alcohol before emptying.*

7. Pour drainage into specimen cup. *So can be removed from system and measured.*

NOTE: *Drain should be emptied at least once a shift or when half or two-thirds full.*

8. Compress Hemovac by pushing top and bottom together. Compress bulb on Jackson-Pratt. *Reestablishes suction and a closed drainage system.*
9. Keep Hemovac or Jackson-Pratt tightly compressed and reinsert plug. *Reestablishes suction and a closed drainage system.*
10. Position suction device on bed. *So there is no tension placed on system.*
11. Measure drainage. Note color, consistency, and odor. *So can document amount and description of drainage.*
12. Discard drainage and container appropriately. *Consistency with guidelines for handling body fluids; protects nurses and others.*
13. Remove gloves. Wash hands. *Reduces transmission of microorganisms.*
14. Send specimen to laboratory if ordered. *To determine if drainage has microorganisms; to determine contents of drainage.*

DOCUMENTATION

1. Amount, color, consistency, and odor of drainage.
2. Patency of drain.
3. Laboratory specimens sent, as appropriate.

Estimated time to complete procedure: *5 minutes.*

Care of the Pediatric Surgical Client

- Procedure 96: Assessing Pain
- Procedure 97: Monitoring Patient-Controlled Analgesia
- Procedure 98: Performing Preoperative Care
- Procedure 99: Performing Postoperative Care

PROCEDURE 96

ASSESSING PAIN

OVERVIEW

Pain, an important symptom seen in children, can be caused by pressure, overstretching, injury, or reduced oxygen supply to body tissues. It also can be a unique problem, a symptom of a specific disease or health problem, or the result of disease or treatment. Children of various ages perceive pain in the context of their development level and their perceptions. Their understanding of the world around them colors their behaviors and perceptions about pain (see Table XIV-1).

Table XIV-1   Developmental stage and pain responses

Phase	Developmental Task	Unique Pain Response
Infancy	Trust vs. mistrust Sensorimotor	Crying, withdrawal, furrowed brow, taut tongue
Toddlerhood	Autonomy vs. shame and doubt Sensorimotor Preoperational thought	Crying, screaming, protesting, withdrawal
Preschooler	Initiative vs. guilt Preoperational thought	Crying, able to point to or describe where pain is, anticipating painful procedures; body image concerns
School-age	Industry vs. inferiority Concrete operations	Body image concerns; may assume pain is punishment
Adolescent	Indentity vs. role confusion Formal operations	Assumption pain will be treated; can conceptualize pain relief

PAIN INTERVIEW AND HISTORY

The initial pain assessment should include comprehensive information about the child's pain experiences, treatments, and successes. The nurse should also query the child and parent(s) about interventions and coping strategies that have helped in the past. Questions should be asked about procedural and other types of painful experiences, and the PQRST format should be used to find out about pain. Following the PQRST system, the child is given the opportunity to describe and rate his or her pain using a self-rating scale (see Box XIV-1).

BOX XIV-1   The PQRST Pain Assessment

P (Presence of pain)	"Are you hurting today?"
Q (Quality)	"What words describe your pain?" (i.e., sharp, burning, tingling, etc.)
R (Radiation/location)	"Where is your pain? Does it shoot or radiate anywhere else?"
S (Severity)	"Give me a number between 0 and 10 for your pain."
T (Timing)	"How long have you had this pain? How long does the pain last when it comes?"

Parents should also be asked about the child's pain. For children developmentally or cognitively too young to rate or discuss their own pain, parent information should be valued as if the client had responded. Table XIV-2 lists questions the nurse can use in obtaining a pain history.

Table XIV-2   Pain history questions

Questions for Child	Questions for Parent
Tell me what pain is to you.	What words does your child use to describe pain?
Tell me about times you have hurt before today.	Describe the pain experiences your child has had.
Who do you tell if you hurt?	Who does your child tell when he/she hurts? How do you know when your child is in pain?
What do you do for yourself when you hurt?	How does your child usually react when he/she is in pain?
What do you want others to do for you when you hurt?	What do you do to help your child when he/she is hurting?
What don't you want others to do for you when you hurt?	What does your child do to help himself/herself when he/she hurts?
What helps the most to take your pain away?	What works best to decrease or relieve your child's pain?
Is there anything else you want to tell me about when you hurt? (If yes, describe.)	Is there anything special you would like me to know about your child's pain? (If yes, describe.)

Hester & Barcus (1986).

ASSESSMENT MEASURES

A number of assessment measures have been developed to quantify a child's pain. The measures are divided into two categories: objective measures used by the nurse or other health care professional to score patient behavior or vital sign changes, and self-reporting measures designed so that children can rate their own pain.

Objective Measures

Objective pain measures are ideal for the infant, preverbal child, or developmentally delayed child who is not able to actively participate in pain assessment. Most objective rating measures score behaviors and physiological changes to determine the intensity of pain experienced and are most useful for acute pain since reliability and validity are less well established for long-term pain. Objective pain assessment measures are most effective when combined with self-reporting tools for children and adolescents since they are able to report or score their own pain. The postoperative pain scale is valid for children over 12 years of age as a measure of acute pain and provides an objective means of assessing the pain. However, instruments such as this are best used for acute or short-term pain or when a child is unable to readily communicate pain. Objective measures are also a useful method of documenting improvements in pain intensity over time, such as postoperatively.

Subjective (Self-Rating) Measures

In all types of pain, the most information can be gained when children measure the pain themselves. Several methods assist children in rating their own pain, and the choice of a specific measure should be based on the child's developmental level and preferences, institutional policies, and instrument availability. A quantifiable measure of pain also adds to validity when discussing pain treatment with members of the health care team, because reporting a child's pain by numbers or measures is more credible than saying "she says she hurts." However, the limitation to all measures is their availability and consistency of use when accurately assessing pain. Figures XIV1–3 illustrate several pediatric pain assessment measures.

For the verbal child, a simple pain assessment scale of 0 to 10 or 0 to 5 may be the most helpful. Here, the nurse asks the child to rate pain on a scale where "0 is no pain at all" and "10 is the worst pain ever you can imagine." The scale points should be documented when recording the child's measure of pain (i.e., "rates pain 5 out of 10" rather than "rates pain a 5"). Drawing a 10 cm line and asking the child to point to the level of pain on the line may also be effective.

EQUIPMENT

Copy of appropriate pain scale depending on child's developmental level

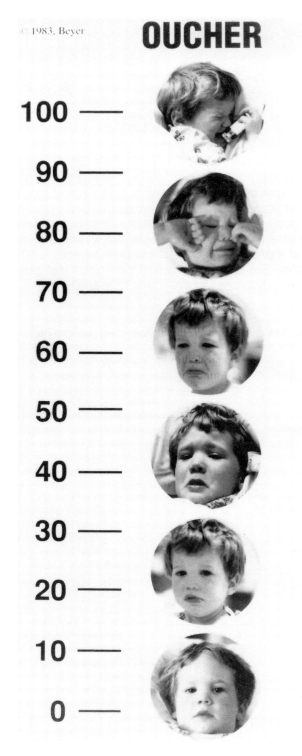

FIGURE XIV-1   The Oucher Pain Assessment Tool: For use with children 3–12 years of age. Child chooses photograph illustrating his/her pain. Caucasian, Hispanic, and African-American versions are available. The Caucasian version of the Oucher, developed and copyrighted by Judith E. Beyer, RN, PhD, 1983. Used with permission.

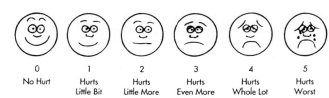

FIGURE XIV-2 Wong/Baker FACES Pain Rating Scale. Child chooses drawing illustrating how he/she feels. From Wong, Hockenberry-Eaton, Wilson, Winkelstein, & Schwartz (2001). *Wong's Essentials of Pediatric Nursing,* 6th ed., p. 1301, St. Louis: Mosby. Copyright Mosby. Reprinted with permission.

PROCEDURE

1. Gather equipment. *Improves organization and effectiveness.*
2. Teach child and family about pain scale chosen. *Enhances cooperation; reduces anxiety and fear.*

3. Ask child to point to picture or choose a number between 0 and 5 or 0 and 10 that reflects his/her current pain.
4. Document results.
5. Administer pain medication as ordered.
6. Reassess child's pain 30–45 minutes later.

DOCUMENTATION

1. Time and date.
2. Pain scale used.
3. Results of assessment.

⧖ **Estimated time to complete procedure:** *10 minutes.*

CODE _____

DATE _____

Adolescent and Pediatric Pain Tool (APPT)

INSTRUCTIONS:

1. **Color in the areas on these drawings to show where you have pain. Make the marks as big or small as the place where the pain is.**

Right Left   Left Right

2. Place a straight, up and down mark on this line to show how much pain you have.

| No pain | Little pain | Medium pain | Large pain | Worst possible pain |

3. Point to or circle as many of these words that describe your pain.

1	5	10	15
annoying	blistering	awful	off and on
bad	burning	deadly	once in a while
horrible	hot	dying	sneaks up
miserable	**6**	killing	sometimes
terrible	cramping	**11**	steady
uncomfortable	crushing	crying	
2	like a pinch	frightening	If you like,
aching	pinching	screaming	you may add
hurting	pressure	terrifying	other words:
like an ache	**7**	**12**	
like a hurt	itching	dizzy	_____
sore	like a scratch	sickening	
3	like a sting	suffocating	_____
beating	scratching	**13**	
hitting	stinging	never goes away	_____
pounding	**8**	uncontrollable	
punching	shocking	**14**	
throbbing	shooting	always	
4	splitting	comes and goes	
biting	**9**	comes on all of	
cutting	numb	a sudden	
like a pin	stiff	constant	
like a sharp knife	swollen	continuous	
pin like	tight	forever	
sharp			
stabbing			

For office use only.

BSA: _____
IS: _____

#S (2-9) _____ /37= _____ %
#A (10-12)_____ /11= _____ %
#E (1,13) _____ /8= _____ %
#T (14,15) _____ /11= _____ %

Total _____ /67= _____ %

FIGURE XIV-3 Adolescent and pediatric pain tool. Child fills out questionnaire. From Savedra, Tesler, Holzemer, & Ward. (1992). University of California, San Francisco, School of Nursing, San Francisco, CA 94143-0606. Copyright © 1989, 1992. Used with permission.

PROCEDURE 97

MONITORING PATIENT-CONTROLLED ANALGESIA

OVERVIEW

Patient-controlled analgesia (PCA) is a computer-operated pump that allows the client to self-administer pain medication. By pushing a button on the pump, children as young as five or six years old may self-administer intravenous opioids to relieve pain. The PCA dosing regimen allows for a steady drug state and more consistent analgesia while avoiding the undesired side effects associated with delivering relatively large doses of bolus analgesics. The delivery of small, frequent doses of opioids provides better pain relief without sedation. By maintaining a steady amount of the analgesic, the child receives better pain control at less risk.

PCA pumps offer several programming options. The pump may be programmed in "PCA only" mode, where doses of the medication are delivered only when the child demands a dose by pushing the button. In the "PCA plus (+) continuous" mode, the pump delivers a preprogrammed background infusion of the analgesic and administers additional medication according to patient request. The PCA (+) continuous mode is especially effective for young children who are often remiss or do not realize they need to push the button to administer their analgesic. The use of different modalities should be tailored to the child's ability to push the PCA button, considering developmental level and the anticipated pain management needs.

EQUIPMENT

Pump
Medication
Tubing
IV fluid
Alcohol wipes
Nonsterile gloves

PROCEDURE

1. Check physician's order. *Ensures that appropriate medication and dose are ordered for child.*

2. Gather equipment. *Improves organization and effectiveness.*
3. Wash hands. *Reduces transmission of microorganisms.*
4. Prepare PCA pump according to manufacturer's instructions with ordered pain medication, using tubing, IV fluid, and medication. *Improves organization and effectiveness.*
5. Teach child and family about PCA. *Enhances cooperation; reduces anxiety and fear.*
6. Wash hands; put on nonsterile gloves. *Reduces transmission of microorganisms.*
7. Clean one of the child's IV ports with alcohol wipe; attach tubing from PCA pump to IV port as directed by manufacturer. *So medication can be delivered to patient as needed.*
8. Unlock PCA pump; follow manufacturer's directions to program pump. *So PCA delivery system can provide medication as needed.*
9. Administer loading dose of pain medication, if indicated. *Allows pain medication to begin reducing pain.*
10. Check to make sure pump is locked and child knows how to administer own pain medication. *Avoids entry into pump control mechanisms by unauthorized personnel. PCAs require self-administration by patients who know how to administer medication and understand frequency of delivery.*

DOCUMENTATION

1. Time and date.
2. Amount and name of pain medication in PCA pump.
3. Child and family education on how to administer PCA.
4. Dose of pain medication delivered when PCA pump initially connected to child's IV.
5. Dose and interval of pain medication delivery.

 Estimated time to complete procedure: *10 minutes.*

PROCEDURE 98

PERFORMING PREOPERATIVE CARE

OVERVIEW

For most children, surgery is a frightening experience. To help allay this fright during the preoperative period, the nurse performs a baseline assessment and determines the child's and family's level of understanding regarding the surgery and what to expect during the postoperative period.

EQUIPMENT

Preoperative checklist
Stethoscope
Sphygmomanometer
Thermometer
Child's chart

PROCEDURE

1. Wash hands. *Reduces transmission of microorganisms.*
2. Verify admission orders regarding type of surgery, any risks, and child and family preparation. *Provides accurate and baseline information.*
3. Check to be sure child is wearing name band; if not, obtain another one and put it on child's wrist. *Provides for patient safety and protects physician legally.*
4. Check whether child or family has any questions regarding surgery and understands procedure; explain as indicated. *Decreases anxiety.*
5. Complete preoperative checklist, including history and physical assessment, especially vital signs and weight. *Provides baseline data.*
6. Ascertain any allergies or adverse reactions during previous surgeries or use of anesthesia. *Provides baseline data.*

7. Ascertain if parent or guardian has signed consent for surgery. *Provides legal basis for surgery.*
8. Complete any ordered preoperative procedures (enema, skin preparation, etc.) *Appropriate protocol.*
9. Dress child in appropriate attire according to surgical procedure; allow child to wear underwear or pajama bottoms. *Appropriate protocol; to protect privacy.*
10. Maintain child NPO as ordered. *To prevent aspiration.*
11. Remove valuables including eyeglasses from child's room; place in locked area or give to parent. *Provides security for items.*
12. Have child void. *To prevent incontinence or bladder distention.*
13. Administer preoperative medications as ordered. *Follow physician orders to promote rest and sleep or prevent against infection.*
14. Transport child to operative suite with a significant object (doll, stuffed animal, etc.). *Appropriate protocol. Helps decrease anxiety.*
15. Inform family of where surgical waiting area is and establish a way to contact them when surgery is completed. *Provides assurance to family.*

DOCUMENTATION

1. Time and date.
2. Preoperative checklist completed.
3. Unusual findings.
4. Any preoperative teaching done with parents and child.
5. Disposition of valuables.

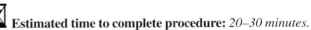 **Estimated time to complete procedure:** *20–30 minutes.*

PROCEDURE 99

PERFORMING POSTOPERATIVE CARE

OVERVIEW

The postoperative period extends from the completion of the surgical procedure through the time the child's condition is stabilized following surgery. Immediately after the surgical procedure, the child is sent to the postanesthesia care unit (PACU) for close monitoring while recuperating from the effects of anesthesia and the surgical procedure. When the child is received into the PACU, the admitting nurse assesses the child's baseline status, checking alertness, vital signs, cardiac rhythm, respiratory rate and efficiency, blood oxygen saturation, IV patency, and the condition of the surgical site. Once the child's condition is stabilized—indicated by stable vital signs for at least one hour, an intact surgical site, and an adequate respiratory status—the child is transferred to an area with less intensive monitoring, generally the surgical ward. Following this transfer, the nurse assuming care will repeat the thorough baseline assessment and continue to monitor the child's condition every 15 minutes for at least 1 hour, then every 30 minutes for the next hour, and then every hour for the next 4 hours.

EQUIPMENT

Stethoscope
Sphygmomanometer
Stethoscope
Oximeter
Sterile dressings as needed
Cardiac monitoring equipment
Incentive spirometer (may be optional)
Supplemental oxygen, if needed
Thermometer
Child's chart with postoperative orders
Nonsterile gloves
Lemon glycerine swab

PROCEDURE

1. Gather equipment. *Improves organization and effectiveness.*
2. Wash hands. *Reduces transmission of microorganisms.*
3. Move child from stretcher to bed. *Allows for easier care; bed is safer than stretcher.*
4. Teach child and family about postoperative monitoring; equipment needed; required position changes; need for frequent monitoring; importance of reporting any pain, nausea, shivering, or uncomfortableness; and reasons for deep breathing and coughing even though they may be painful. Reinforce preoperative teaching related to postoperative expectations and exercises. *Enhances cooperation; reduces anxiety and fear.*
5. Wash hands; put on nonsterile gloves. *Reduces transmission of microorganisms.*
6. Check child's vital signs (temperature, pulse, respiratory rate, blood pressure) upon arrival to unit. *Establishes baseline; indicates child's status.*
7. Check child's armband and verify child's identity with chart. *Protects from errors.*
8. Remind child that he/she has returned to the surgical unit. *Decreases anxiety; orients child.*
9. If ordered, attach leads for bedside electrocardiogram monitoring and run a baseline strip. *Establishes baseline data; provides constant monitoring.*
10. If ordered, attach oximeter to child and monitor oxygen saturation. *Establishes baseline data; provides constant monitoring.*
11. Check IV site using gloves; check IV solution and flow rate, and ensure that IV line is appropriately taped. *Prevents complications from infiltration of IV, allows appropriate rehydration, verifies appropriate solution, and prevents line from coming apart.*
12. Check surgical dressing and site if visible. Assess dressing for amount and type of drainage. Reinforce dressing as needed. Change dressing only if physician's orders say to. *Establishes condition of surgical site.*
13. Complete a brief head-to-toe assessment, being sure to check for patent airway, listen to breath sounds, check pulses distal to the surgical site, note temperature and color of extremities and capillary refill rate, check level of consciousness, listen for bowel sounds, evaluate urinary output (amount and color; make sure urinary catheter is draining), and presence and amount of pain. Pay attention to whether type of surgical procedure may require additional assessments (if NG tube present, etc.). *Provides baseline data; determines child's response to surgery.*
14. Encourage child to turn, cough, and deep breathe or use incentive spirometer (if ordered). *Improves lung expansion, prevents respiratory complications, and hastens clearance of anesthesia from lungs.*
15. Check and implement postoperative orders. Offer child fluids as ordered, or if NPO, moisten lips with lemon glycerine swab, etc. *Provides safe and appropriate postoperative care.*

16. Reposition child every two hours or more frequently as ordered and as indicated. *Prevents venous stasis, decreased circulation, disruption of skin integrity; reduces chance of pneumonia developing.*
17. Remove gloves and wash hands. *Reduces transmission of microorganisms.*

DOCUMENTATION

1. Time and date.
2. Vital signs.
3. IV information (solution, condition of site, rate).
4. Neuro checks, level of consciousness.
5. Oxygen saturation if obtained.
6. Condition of surgical site including any drains or appliances.
7. Any medications administered.
8. Unusual findings from assessment.
9. Position changes.
10. Presence or absence of pain.
11. Output.

 Estimated time to complete procedure: *20–30 minutes.*

Emergency Care

Fever and Hyperthermia Management

Definitions

Fever. Controlled elevation of body temperature above the normal range; results from an upward shift in the hypothalamic temperature set point; usually due to an infectious process in the body.

Hyperthermia. Elevation of core temperature above the hypothalamic temperature set point; results from a malfunction or an overload of the central thermoregulatory mechanisms (e.g., heat stroke, malignant hyperthermia).

In managing an elevated temperature, it is essential to determine whether the elevated body temperature is a fever or hyperthermia. Elevated body temperature may be treated with antipyretic medications (e.g., acetaminophen, ibuprofen) or by physical means such as sponging, cooling blankets, ice packs, air-conditioning, and fans.

Benefits of Fever

The literature identifies a number of benefits associated with fever (Klein & Cunha, 1996; Rowsey, 1997a; Rowsey, 1997b; Sharber, 1997; Thomas, 1995; Thomas et al., 1994). These benefits include increased host defenses and the enhanced effect of some antibiotics. The routine use of antipyretics to reduce mild to moderate fever is not recommended by some authorities. The primary purpose for treating fever is to promote comfort.

Management

- Administer antipyretic drug in appropriate dose based on child's weight.
- Give tepid water bath of 20–30 minutes' duration.
- Apply cool, moist towels or washcloths to skin. Expose only one area at a time; change towel or washcloth as needed and continue for approximately 30 minutes.
- Apply cooling blanket as ordered by clinician. Refer to agency policy.

Safety

1. Antipyretics work to reduce fever by lowering the thermoregulatory set point. Although salicylates (e.g., aspirin) are effective in reducing an elevated temperature, they have been associated with Reye's syndrome when given to children with influenza or varicella (chickenpox). Acetaminophen or ibuprofen are safer choices for fever management in children.
2. Physical modalities should not be used until 30 minutes to 1 hour after administering antipyretics. Use of physical modalities may activate heat-conserving and -producing mechanisms. Using physical modalities for treating fever provides no additional benefit over antipyretics alone and frequently are associated with increased client discomfort. Physical modalities, however, are appropriate measures for treating hyperthermia.
3. Never use cold water or alcohol for a sponge bath to reduce fever.
   a. Cold water can cause vasoconstriction and shivering, which raises the central body temperature.
   b. Alcohol reduces fever too rapidly and may lead to convulsions, especially in a small child.
   c. Alcohol fumes are toxic.
   d. Both can make the child uncomfortable.

PROCEDURE 100

ADMINISTERING A SPONGE BATH

USES

1. Children whose fever does not respond to antipyretics or who are very uncomfortable, e.g., fever > 104° F (40° C).
2. Children whose temperature elevation is caused by heatstroke or malignant hyperthermia.

NOTE: *The procedure is controversial and may not be used in all agencies.*

EQUIPMENT

Washbasin or bathtub
Tepid water (body temperature; should not feel warm or cold to touch)
Washcloths, small towels, or gauze squares
Dry towels and/or bath blanket
Plastic sheet to protect bed (optional)

SAFETY

1. Physical modalities should not be used until 30 minutes to 1 hour after administering antipyretics. Use of physical modalities may activate heat-conserving and -producing mechanisms. Using physical modalities for treating fever provides no additional benefit over antipyretics alone and frequently are associated with increased client discomfort. Physical modalities, however, are appropriate measures for treating hyperthermia.
2. Never use cold water or alcohol for a sponge bath to reduce fever.
   a. Cold water can cause vasoconstriction and shivering, which raises the central body temperature.
   b. Alcohol reduces fever too rapidly and may lead to convulsions, especially in a small child.
   c. Alcohol fumes are toxic.
   d. Both can make the child uncomfortable.

PROCEDURE

1. Gather equipment. *Promotes organization and efficiency.*
2. Explain procedure to child and family. *Enhances cooperation and participation; reduces anxiety and fear.*
3. Wash hands. *Reduces transmission of microorganisms.*
4. Take temperature, pulse, and respirations before proceeding. *Provides a baseline for determining effectiveness of treatment.*
5. Undress child or expose areas where there are large superficial blood vessels such as the axillary and inguinal regions. *Facilitates heat loss.*
6. Sponge with tepid water. Avoid chilling. *Shivering will increase heat production and decrease heat loss.*
   a. Child may be placed in tub for sponge bath or in bed using a basin of water. Protect the bed with a plastic sheet covered with a bath blanket. *So sheets do not get wet.*
   b. Use gentle friction and slowly stroke the wet washcloth over body. *Brings blood to surface to help dissipate heat.*
7. Sponge for 12–30 minutes unless child becomes chilled. *Amount of time needed to effectively sponge child.*
8. Pat child dry with a towel and redress in lightweight clothing. *So child does not become chilled.*
9. Take child's temperature immediately after discontinuing sponging and again 30 minutes later. *To determine if temperature decreased and stayed down.*

DOCUMENTATION

1. Time and duration of sponging.
2. Temperature and other vital signs.
3. How procedure tolerated, including child's response.

⧖ **Estimated time to complete procedure:** *15–30 minutes.*

Respiratory and Cardiac Emergencies

OVERVIEW

Respiratory or cardiac emergencies can occur at any time or place and be the result of a disease process (epiglottitis) or accident (foreign body aspiration, drowning). It is important during any respiratory or cardiac emergency to maintain tissue oxygenation by providing external cardiac compressions and/or artificial respirations if one or the other is needed.

PROCEDURE 101

TREATING AN INHALATION INJURY

OVERVIEW

Inhalation injuries are the result of inhaling noxious gases or smoke from a fire. The injury is suspected when there is a history of being exposed to a toxic gas or flames in an enclosed space, whether or not there are obvious burns to the skin. Other signs of a possible inhalation injury include a cough; hoarse voice; inspiratory or expiratory stridor; singed nasal hairs; sooty residue on the face or nose or in the sputum; burns of the lips, mouth, throat, or nose; or signs of respiratory distress.

EQUIPMENT

Stethoscope
Thermometer
Oxygen and necessary tubing
Pulse oximetry machine

PROCEDURE

1. Explain procedure to child and parent. *Enhances cooperation and participation; reduces anxiety and fear.*
2. Wash hands. *Reduces transmission of microorganisms.*
3. Position for best ventilation and comfort. *To allow for more effective breathing patterns.*

4. Take vital signs. *To determine child's baseline condition.*
5. Obtain a history of inhalation injury. *To determine appropriate treatment.*
6. Remove constricting clothing. *To allow for more effective breathing patterns.*
7. Administer oxygen or humidity (if ordered). *Facilitates oxygenation.*
8. Monitor oxygen saturation with pulse oximetry. *Determines need for oxygen and if child is receiving adequate oxygenation.*
9. Have emergency equipment available. *To avoid delay in treatment if needed.*

DOCUMENTATION

1. Time and date.
2. Child's initial condition.
3. Vital signs.
4. Pertinent information from history relative to cause of inhalation injury.
5. Treatment provided.
6. Child's response to treatment.

⧖ **Estimated time to complete procedure:** *5–10 minutes, depending on the seriousness of the injury.*

PROCEDURE 102

PERFORMING EMERGENCY AIRWAY MANAGEMENT
OVERVIEW

An open airway is essential for oxygenation. In an emergency, providing a patent airway is a priority. There are several causes of airway obstruction: the tongue may fall back into the pharyngeal cavity, obstructing the airway in an unconscious child (e.g., following grand mal seizures); thickened secretions may obstruct or narrow the airway; soft tissue edema may narrow or obstruct the airway; or the child may have aspirated a foreign body.

Use the acronym ABC when performing an initial assessment on a patient needing emergency airway management. A stands for airway, B for breathing, and C for circulation. If the airway is not patent, assisted ventilation will be needed until the child is able to breathe spontaneously or until a ventilator is provided.

EQUIPMENT

Although none of the listed items are required, they may be helpful:

Gloves
Supplemental oxygen
Oropharyngeal airway
Ambu bag and mask

PROCEDURE

1. Wash hands and put on gloves. *Reduces transmission of microorganisms.*
2. Assess airway; call for help if needed. *If airway is not open, child is at risk for injury or death.*
3. If mouth is not open, gently tilt head backward. Place one hand on the forehead and two fingers of the other hand under the mandible, tilting the jaw forward and the forehead back (Figure XV-1). *If tongue is blocking the airway, this will reposition the tongue, allowing air to go to the lungs.*
4. Assess for spontaneous respirations. *If spontaneous respirations are present, no other interventions may be required. If child is still not breathing, continue with interventions.*
5. Turn child on side and clear the mouth of secretions or obstructions, using the finger to sweep any secre-

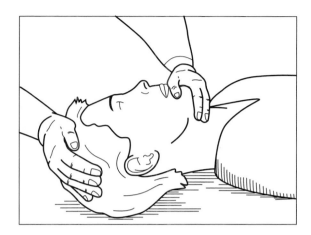

FIGURE XV-1 Tilt the jaw forward and the forehead back.

tions to the side (Figure XV-2). *Clearing the airway may cause spontaneous respirations to resume.*
6. Insert the oropharyngeal airway if available. *Helps keep the tongue from slipping into the phayrngeal area and blocking the airway.*
7. If spontaneous respirations occur, maintain the head in proper position. *Head must be positioned correctly once respirations resume to maintain patent airway.*
8. If respirations do not resume, initiate artificial respiration. *Hypoxia is not compatible with life.*
   a. Apply ambu mask to face; be sure there is a tight seal. Do not push the mask into the face. Rather, pull the jaw into the mask (Figure XV-3). *Failure to*

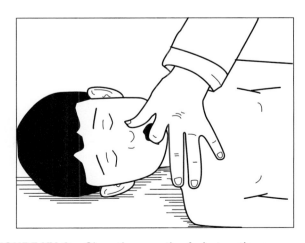

FIGURE XV-2 Clear the mouth of obstructions.

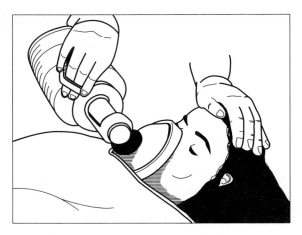

FIGURE XV-3   Bag-valve-mask ventilation.

achieve seal will not provide adequate air volume for resuscitation.

b. Begin ventilation by squeezing the ambu bag and then watching for the child's chest to rise. When chest rises, release bag. *Pushing too much air into the airway will cause air to be pushed into the stomach.*

c. Rate of ventilation should be 20 per minute in children and 30 per minute in infants. *Approximates normal respiratory rate.*

9. Continue efforts until assistance arrives or when child is stable. *Assures that every effort has been made to provide a patent airway.*

10. Remove gloves and wash hands. *Reduces transmission of microorganisms.*

11. When child is stabilized, talk to parents about situation; explain interventions. *Allays parental anxiety.*

DOCUMENTATION

1. Time and date.
2. Vital signs.
3. Measures taken for airway management.
4. Child's response.
5. Child's current condition.

⧗ **Estimated time to complete procedure:** *2–3 minutes or less.*

PROCEDURE 103

TREATING AN AIRWAY OBSTRUCTION

OVERVIEW

Airway obstruction in children may be caused by food (e.g., grapes, hot dogs, raisins, peanuts) or a foreign body (e.g., coins, beads, marbles, paper clips, thumbtacks) that becomes lodged in the airway or because of a respiratory disorder (e.g., croup, epiglottitis). Attempts to clear the airway should occur only when there is a witness to or a strong suspicion of aspiration of a foreign body or when the airway remains obstructed after attempting to provide artificial ventilation.

EQUIPMENT

Gloves (if available)

PROCEDURE

1. Determine if the obstruction is due to an infection or aspiration of a foreign body. *So treatment chosen is appropriate.*
2. Infants:
   a. Straddle infant over forearm in the prone position with the head lower than the trunk. Support the head by positioning a hand around the jaws and thigh. *Proper positioning is essential for success of the maneuver and prevention of other organ damage.*
   b. Deliver four back blows with the heel of your hand between the infant's shoulder blades (Figure XV-4). *Technique for dislodging the obstruction.*

   c. Keeping the head down, place the free hand on the infant's back and turn the infant over, supporting the back with your hand and thigh. *Safely rotates the infant's position to continue life-saving procedures.*
   d. With your free hand, place fingers in same position used for CPR; deliver four thrusts to the chest in the same manner as infant external cardiac compressions (Figure XV-5). *Technique for dislodging the obstruction.*
   e. Assess for a foreign body in the mouth of an unconscious infant, and utilize the finger sweep only if a foreign body is visualized. *The finger sweep may push a foreign object back down the throat unless the object is seen before the sweep is attempted.*
   f. Open the airway and assess for respiration. If respirations are absent, ventilate the infant. Assess for the rise and fall of the chest; if not seen, reposition the infant and attempt ventilation again. *Sometimes air can get around the foreign body; this allows for some oxygenation. If infant does not receive oxygen within 4–6 minutes, irreversible brain damage may occur.*
   g. Repeat the entire sequence again: four back blows, four chest thrusts, assessment for foreign body in oral cavity, and ventilation as long as possible. *Life-saving efforts must continue until they are successful or until the rescuer becomes exhausted and cannot continue.*
   h. If infant loses consciousness, begin CPR. *To provide ventilation and respirations.*
3. Small child—conscious, standing, or sitting:

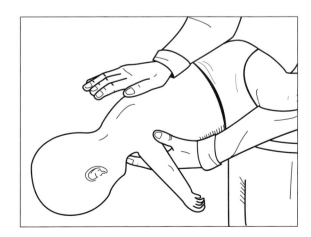

FIGURE XV-4   Back blows. (Infant)

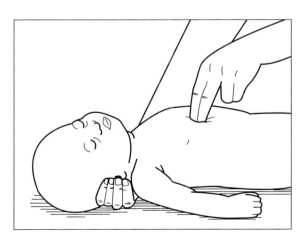

FIGURE XV-5   Chest thrusts. (Infant)

a. Assess air exchange and encourage coughing and breathing. Provide reassurance to child that you are there to help. *Inability to breathe is a distressing event for anyone, especially a small child who may not fully understand what is happening. Reassurance is important so that child will trust and cooperate with maneuvers needed to help. Coughing may dislodge the object.*

b. Ask child if he/she is choking. If is, follow instructions below. *Many small children are able to answer simple questions.*

1. Stand behind child. Wrap arms around waist and administer 6 to 10 subdiaphragmatic abdominal thrusts (Heimlich maneuver). Stand behind child. With arms under child's axilla and around the chest, place the thumb of one fist against the abdomen in the midline below the xiphoid and above the navel. Grasp your fist with your other hand. Deliver up to 5 quick upward thrusts. Each thrust should be a separate maneuver to try to dislodge the obstruction (Figure XV-6). *Proper positioning is essential for success of maneuver and prevention of other organ damage.*

2. Continue series of 5 thrusts until foreign object is expelled or child becomes unconscious. *Life-saving efforts must continue until they are successful or until the rescuer becomes exhausted and cannot continue.*

4. Small child—conscious or unconscious, laying down:

a. Position child supine and kneel at the child's feet. Gently deliver 6–10 subdiaphragmatic abdominal

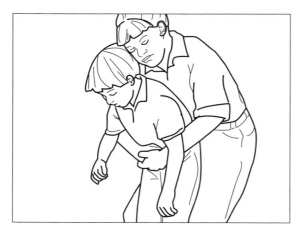

FIGURE XV-6   Abdominal thrusts (Heimlich maneuver) on conscious child.

thrusts (Heimlich maneuver). Place the heel of your hand on the child's abdomen in the midline between the xiphoid and navel. Place your other hand over your wrist. Press into the abdomen using both hands in quick, upward strokes. Deliver up to 5 quick upward thrusts. Each thrust should be a separate maneuver to try to dislodge the obstruction (Figure XV-7). *This is the recommended position for small children. Proper positioning is essential for success of the maneuver and prevention of other organ damage.*

b. Open the airway by lifting the lower jaw and tongue forward. Perform a finger sweep only if a foreign body is visualized. *Opening the airway allows for visualization of the oral cavity. The finger sweep may push a foreign object back down the throat unless the object is seen before the sweep is attempted.*

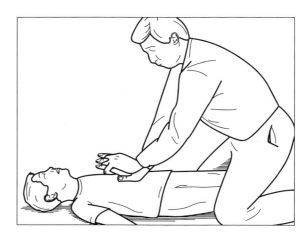

FIGURE XV-7   Performing abdominal thrusts on an unconscious child.

c. If breathing is absent, ventilate child. If the chest does not rise, reposition child and attempt ventilation again. *Sometimes air can get around the foreign body; this allows for some oxygenation. If child does not receive oxygen within 4–6 minutes, irreversible brain damage may occur.*

d. Repeat sequence a–c above as long as necessary. *Life-saving efforts must continue until they are successful or until the rescuer becomes exhausted and cannot continue.*

 Estimated time to complete procedure: *2–5 minutes.*

PROCEDURE 104

PERFORMING CARDIOPULMONARY RESUSCITATION

OVERVIEW

Cardiopulmonory resuscitation (CPR) is the basic life-saving skill used in the event of cardiac, respiratory, or cardiopulmonary arrest to maintain tissue oxygenation by providing external cardiac compression and/or artificial respiration. CPR is initiated when an infant, child, or adolescent is found without or develops the absence of a pulse or respiration or both. The goals of CPR, often referred to as the ABCs of emergency resuscitation, are:

a. Establish **A**irway
b. Initiate **B**reathing
c. Maintain **C**irculation

CPR should be initiated immediately once it has been determined that a cardiac or pulmonary arrest has occurred, since a lack of oxygen to the tissues can result in permanent cardiac and brain damage within four to six minutes.

CPR is a basic life-saving skill that nurses are expected to be able to perform not only in the hospital and other clinical settings but in the outside environment as well.

EQUIPMENT

Hard surface
Body substance precaution equipment
  Gloves
  Face shield
  Mask/CPR barrier device
Ambu bag
Oral airway
Emergency resuscitation cart
Documentation forms

PROCEDURE

I. One rescuer—adolescent.
  A. Assess responsiveness by tapping or gently shaking adolescent and asking if he/she is okay. If adolescent does not respond, call for help and begin basic life support. *Prevents injury to adolescent who is not experiencing a cardiac or respiratory arrest; assists in assessing level of consciousness and possible etiology of crisis.*
  B. Position adolescent in supine position on a hard surface. Be careful if a head or neck injury is suspected.

Proper positioning facilitates assessment of cardiac and respiratory status and successful external cardiac massage. Care must be taken if there is the chance of a head or neck injury so that further damage is prevented.

  C. Apply appropriate body substance isolation items (gloves, face shield, tissue) if available. *Prevents transmission of disease.*
  D. Position self. On knees, face adolescent parallel to his/her head. Begin assessing airway and breathing status. *Proper positioning prevents rescuer fatigue and facilitates CPR by allowing the rescuer to move from chest compressions to artificial breathing with minimal movement.*
  E. Open airway. Place one hand on the adolescent's forehead; apply a steady backward pressure to tilt the head back while placing the fingers of the other hand below the jaw at the location of the chin and lifting the chin. If a head or neck injury is suspected, the lift is modified and the jaw thrust is used. To perform the jaw thrust, place hands at the angles of the lower jaw and lift, displacing the mandible forward while tilting the head backward. Insert oral airway if available. *A patent airway is essential for successful artificial respiration. The head tilt and chin lift assist in preventing the tongue from obstructing the airway. The jaw thrust is used when a head or neck injury is suspected, because it prevents extension of the neck and decreases the potential of further injury.*
  F. Assess for respirations (Figure XV-8). Look, listen, and feel for air movement. *Due to the potential risk*

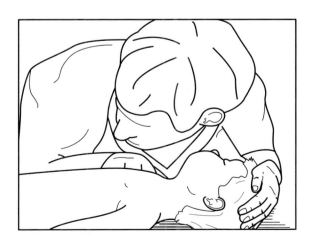

FIGURE XV-8   Assessing breathing.

of injury, CPR should not be administered to an ado-lescent with spontaneous respirations or pulse.

G. If respirations are absent, begin rescue breathing. *Hypoxia can cause irreversible brain and tissue damage after 4–6 minutes.*

   1. Occlude nostrils with the thumb and index finger of the hand on the forehead that is tilting the head back. *Occluding the nostrils and forming a seal over the mouth will prevent air leakage and provide full inflation of the lungs. Excessive air volume and rapid inspiratory flow rates can create pharyngeal pressures that are greater than esophageal opening pressures. This will allow air into the stomach, resulting in gastric distention and increased risk of vomiting.*

   2. Form a seal over the adolescent's mouth, using either your mouth or the appropriate respiratory assist device (Ambu bag and mask) and give two full breaths (½–2 seconds), allowing time for both inspiration and expiration (Figure XV-9). *Prevents air leakage; provides air for lungs.*

   3. Assess for the rise and fall of the chest. If the chest rises and falls, continue. If the chest does not move, assess for excessive oral secretions, vomit, airway obstruction, or improper positioning. *Visual assessment of chest movement helps confirm an open airway. A volume of 800–1,200 ml is usually sufficient to make the chest rise in most adolescents.*

H. Palpate the carotid pulse for 5–10 seconds (Figure XV-10). If present, ventilate at a rate of 12 times/minute. If absent, begin cardiac compressions. *Performing chest compressions on an adolescent with a pulse could result in injury. The carotid pulse may persist when peripheral pulses are no longer palpable. Hyperventilation assists in maintaining blood oxygen levels.*

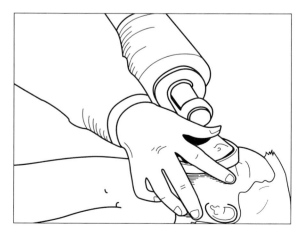

FIGURE XV-9   Bag and mask resuscitation.

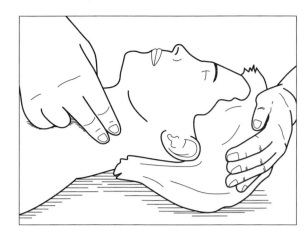

FIGURE XV-10   Checking for the carotid pulse.

I. Cardiac compressions. *Hypoxia can cause irreversible brain and tissue damage after 4–6 minutes. Proper positioning is essential so that damage to organs does not occur and there is maximum compression of the heart between the sternum and the vertebrae.*

   1. Maintain a position on knees parallel to adolescent's sternum. *So person performing cardiac massage can easily and more comfortably perform cardiac massage.*

   2. Position hands for compressions:

     a. Using the hand nearest to the legs, use the index finger to locate the lower rib margin and quickly move the fingers up to the location where the ribs connect to the sternum. *If compression performed over ribs, ribs may be fractured.*

     b. Place the middle finger of this hand on the notch where the ribs meet the sternum and the index finger next to it. *Determines correct placement on chest for cardiac massage.*

     c. Place the heel of the other hand next to the index finger on the sternum (Figure XV-11). *Determines correct site on chest for cardiac massage.*

     d. Remove the first hand from the notch and place it on top of the hand that is on the sternum so that they are on top of each other. *To enhance efficiency of cardiac massage.*

     e. Extend or interlace fingers, and do not allow them to touch the chest (Figure XV-12). *So fingers do not touch chest during massage.*

     f. Keep arms straight, with shoulders directly over hands on sternum, and lock elbows (Figure XV-13). *So cardiac massage can be performed more efficiently; so arms of person*

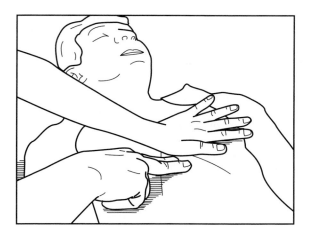

FIGURE XV-11 Place the heel of one hand next to the index finger on the client's sternum.

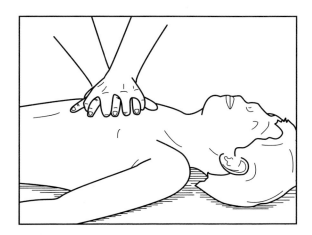

FIGURE XV-12 Extend or interface the fingers.

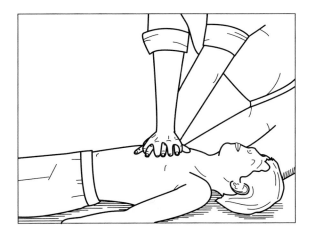

FIGURE XV-13 Keep arms straight and lock elbows.

performing cardiac massage do not tire prematurely.

3. Compress the sternum 3.8–5.0 cm (1½–2 inches) at the rate of 80–100 times/minute. *Provides enough pressure to circulate blood, provides sufficient rate to circulate blood.*

    a. The heel of the hand must completely release the pressure between compressions, but it should remain in constant contact with the adolescent's skin. *So heart is allowed to fill with blood during asystole.*

    b. Use the mnemonic "one and, two and, three and. . ." to keep rhythm and timing. *So rate of massage is maintained and constant.*

4. Ventilate adolescent as described above. *Helps maintain the open airway.*

5. Maintain the compression rate for 80–100 times/minute, interjecting ventilation after every 15 compressions. *Hypoxia can cause irreversible brain and tissue damage after 4–6 minutes. 80–100 is adequate rate for cardiac compression.*

6. Reevaluate the adolescent after 4 cycles. *Determines return of spontaneous pulse and respirations and need to continue CPR.*

    a. Palpate carotid pulse for 5 seconds. If absent, continue cycle for another 3–5 minutes before reassessing. *Determines if heart is beating spontaneously.*

7. Repeat cycle of 5 compressions and 1 breath until circulation returns or help arrives. *To deliver adequate amount of oxygenated blood to tissues.*

8. If adolescent does not have trauma and both pulse and respiration return, place in a side-lying position. *Protects the airway.*

II. One rescuer—child 1–7 years of age.

  A. Assess responsiveness by tapping or gently shaking child and asking, "Are you OK?" If child does not respond, call for help and begin basic life support. *Prevents injury to child who is not experiencing a cardiac or respiratory arrest; assists in assessing level of consciousness and possible etiology of crisis.*

  B. Position child in supine position on a hard surface. Be careful if a head or neck injury is suspected. *Proper positioning facilitates assessment of cardiac and respiratory status and successful external cardiac massage. Care must be taken if there is a chance of a head or neck injury so that further damage is prevented.*

  C. Apply appropriate body substance isolation items (gloves, face shield, tissue) if available. *Prevents transmission of disease.*

  D. Position self. On knees, face child parallel to child's head. Begin assessing airway and breathing status. *Proper positioning prevents rescuer fatigue and facilitates CPR by allowing the rescuer to move from chest compressions to artificial breathing with minimal movement.*

E. Open airway. Place one hand on the child's forehead; apply a steady backward pressure to tilt the head back while placing the fingers on the other hand below the jaw at the location of the chin and lifting the chin. If a head or neck injury is suspected, the lift is modified and the jaw thrust is used. To perform the jaw thrust, place hands at the angles of the lower jaw and lift, displacing the mandible forward while tilting the head backward. Insert oral airway if available. *A patent airway is essential for successful artificial respiration. The head tilt/chin lift assists in preventing the tongue from obstructing the airway. The jaw thrust is used when a head or neck injury is suspected because it prevents extension of the neck and decreases the potential of further injury.*

F. Assess for respirations. Look, listen, and feel for air movement. *CPR should not be administered to a child with spontaneous respirations or pulse due to the potential risk of injury.*

G. If respirations are absent, begin rescue breathing. *Hypoxia can cause irreversible brain and tissue damage after 4–6 minutes.*

1. Occlude nostrils with the thumb and index finger of the hand on the forehead that is tilting the head back. *Occluding the nostrils and forming a seal over the child's mouth will prevent air leakage and provide full inflation of the lungs. Excessive air volume and rapid inspiratory flow rates can create pharyngeal pressures that are greater than esophageal opening pressures. This will allow air into the stomach, resulting in gastric distention and increased risk of vomiting.*

2. Form a seal over the child's mouth using either your mouth or the appropriate respiratory assist device (Ambu bag and mask) and give 2 slow breaths (1–1½ seconds/breath), pausing to take a breath in between. *The volume of air in a small child's lungs is less than an adult's.*

3. Use only the amount of air needed to make the chest rise. When you see the chest rise and fall, you are using the right volume of air. *Excessive air volume and rapid inspiratory rates can increase pharyngeal pressures that exceed esophageal opening pressures, allowing air to enter the stomach and causing gastric distention, increasing the risk of vomiting, and further compromising the child's respiratory status.*

H. Palpate the carotid pulse for 5–10 seconds. If present, ventilate at a rate of once every 4 seconds or 15 times/minute. If absent, begin cardiac compressions. *Performing chest compressions on a child with a pulse could result in injury. The carotid pulse*

may persist when peripheral pulses are no longer palpable. Hyperventilation assists in maintaining blood oxygen levels.

I. Cardiac compressions. *Hypoxia can cause irreversible brain and tissue damage after 4–6 minutes; proper positioning is essential so that damage to organs does not occur and there is maximum compression of the heart between the sternum and the vertebrae.*

1. Maintain a position on knees parallel to child's sternum.

2. Place a small towel or other support under the child's shoulders. *The backward tilt of the head lifts the back of small children, and a small towel or some other type of support is necessary for effective cardiac compressions.*

3. Position hands for compressions.
   a. Locate the lower margin of the rib cage using the hand closest to the feet and find the notch where the ribs and sternum meet. *If compression performed over ribs, ribs may be fractured.*
   b. Place the middle finger on this hand on the notch, and then place the index finger next to the middle finger. *Determines correct placement on chest for cardiac massage.*
   c. Place the heel of the other hand in the sternum with the heel parallel to the sternum (1 cm above the xiphoid process). Make sure the hand is not over the xiphoid process. *Compressions over the xiphoid process can lacerate the liver; keeping the fingers off the chest during compressions reduces the risk of rib fracture.*
   d. Keeping the elbows locked and the shoulders over the child, compress the sternum 2.5–3.8 cm (1–1½ inches) at the rate of 80–100 times/minute. At the end of each compression, allow the chest to return to the normal position before beginning the next compression. *Provides enough compression to circulate blood at appropriate rate.*

4. Keep the other hand on the child's forehead. *Helps maintain the open airway.*

5. At the end of every fifth compression, administer a ventilation (1–1½ seconds). *Hypoxia can cause irreversible brain and tissue damage after 4–6 minutes.*

6. Reevaluate the child after 10 cycles. *Determines return of spontaneous pulse and respirations and need to continue CPR.*
   a. Palpate carotid pulse for 5 seconds. If absent, continue cycle for another 3–5 minutes before reassessing. *Determines if heart is beating spontaneously.*

    b. Repeat cycle of 5 compressions and 1 breath until circulation returns or help arrives. *To deliver adequate amount of oxygenated blood to tissues.*

    c. If child does not have trauma and both pulse and respiration return, place child in a side-lying position. *Protects the airway.*

III. One rescuer—infant 1–12 months old.

  A. Assess responsiveness by tapping or gently shaking infant. If infant does not respond, begin basic life support and call for help. *Prevents injury to infant who is not experiencing a cardiac or respiratory arrest; assists in assessing level of consciousness and possible etiology of crisis.*

  B. Position infant in supine position on a hard surface. Be careful if a head or neck injury is suspected. *Proper positioning facilitates assessment of cardiac and respiratory status and successful external cardiac massage. Care must be taken if there is a chance of a head or neck injury so that further damage is prevented.*

  C. Apply appropriate body substance isolation items (gloves, face shield, tissue) if available. *Prevents transmission of disease.*

  D. Position self. On knees, face infant parallel to infant and next to head. Begin assessing airway and breathing status. *Proper positioning prevents rescuer fatigue and facilitates CPR by allowing the rescuer to move from chest compressions to artificial breathing with minimal movement.*

  E. Open airway. Place one hand on the infant's forehead; apply a steady backward pressure to tilt the head back while placing the fingers on the other hand below the jaw at the location of the chin and lifting the chin. Be careful not to overextend the infant's neck (Figure XV-14). Place a towel or diaper under the infant's shoulders or use a hand to support the neck. If a head or neck injury is suspected, the lift is modified and the jaw thrust is used. To perform the jaw thrust, place hands at the angles of the lower jaw and lift, displacing the mandible forward while tilting the head backward (Figure XV-15). Insert oral airway if available. *A patent airway is essential for successful artificial respiration. The head tilt/chin lift assists in preventing the tongue from obstructing the airway. Overextension of the infant's head can cause a closing or narrowing of the airway. The jaw thrust is used when a head or neck injury is suspected, because it prevents extension of the neck and decreases the potential of further injury.*

  F. Assess for respirations. Look, listen, and feel for air movement. *CPR should not be administered to an infant with spontaneous respirations or pulse due to the potential risk of injury.*

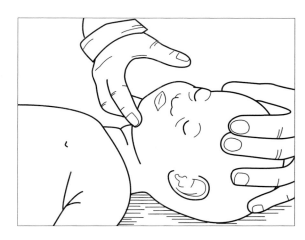

FIGURE XV-14   Head tilt—chin life maneuver.

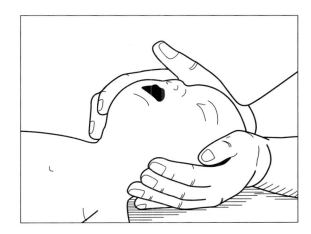

FIGURE XV-15   Jaw thrust maneuver.

  G. If respirations are absent, begin rescue breathing. *Hypoxia can cause irreversible brain and tissue damage after 4–6 minutes.*

    1. Make a tight seal over both the infant's nose and mouth and gently administer artificial respirations. Maintain patent airway with chin lift or jaw thrust (Figure XV-16). *Making a complete seal over the infant's mouth and nose prevents air leakage.*

    2. Give 2 slow breaths (1–1½ sec/breath), pausing to take a breath in between. *The volume of air in an infant's lungs is less than an adult's or child's.*

    3. Use only the amount of air needed to make the chest rise. When you see the chest rise and fall, you are using the right volume of air. *Excessive air volume and rapid inspiratory rates can increase pharyngeal pressures that exceed esophageal opening pressures, allowing air to enter the stomach and causing gastric distention, increasing the risk of*

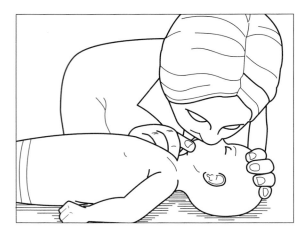

FIGURE XV-16   Mouth-to-mouth-and-nose resuscitation.

vomiting, and further compromising the child's respiratory status.

H. Palpate the brachial pulse for 5–10 seconds (Figure XV-17). (The brachial pulse is located on the inside of the upper arm between the elbow and shoulder. Place your thumb on the outside of the arm and palpate the proximal side of the arm with the index finger and middle fingers.) If present, ventilate at a rate of once every 3 seconds or 20 times/minute. If absent, begin cardiac compressions. *Performing chest compressions on an infant with a pulse could result in injury. The carotid pulse is difficult to locate in infants; therefore, the brachial artery is the recommended site. Hyperventilation assists in maintaining blood oxygen levels.*

I. Cardiac compressions. *Hypoxia can cause irreversible brain and tissue damage after 4–6 minutes; proper positioning is essential so that damage to organs does not occur and there is maximum compression of the heart between the sternum and the vertebrae.*

1. Maintain a position parallel to the infant. Infants can easily be placed on a table or other hard surface. *Enhances efficiency of cardiac compressions.*

2. Place a small towel or other support under the infant's shoulders. *A small towel or some other type of support is necessary for effective cardiac compressions.*

3. Position hands for compressions.
   a. Using the hand closest to the infant's feet, locate the intermammary line where it intersects the sternum. *Compressions over the xiphoid process can lacerate the liver.*
   b. Place the index finger 1 cm below this location on the sternum, and place the middle finger next to the index finger. Be sure fingers are not over the xiphoid process. *Keeping other fingers and hands off the chest during compressions reduces risk of rib fracture.*
   c. Using these two fingers, compress in a downward motion 1.3–2.5 cm (½–1 inch) at the rate of 100 times/minute. *Provides enough pressure to circulate blood, provides sufficient rate to circulate blood.*

4. Keep the other hand on the infant's forehead. *Helps maintain the open airway.*

5. At the end of every fifth compression, administer ventilation for 1–1½ seconds (Figure XV-18). *Hypoxia can cause irreversible brain and tissue damage after 4–6 minutes.*

6. Reevaluate the infant after 10 cycles. *Determines the return of spontaneous pulse and respirations and the need to continue CPR.*

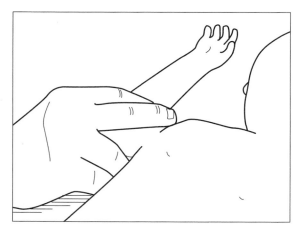

FIGURE XV-17   Checking for the brachial pulse.

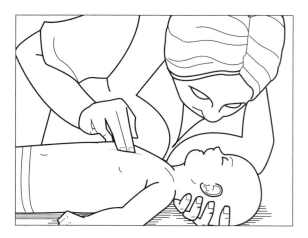

FIGURE XV-18   Alternating breathing and chest compressions.

a. Palpate brachial pulse for 5 seconds. If absent, continue cycle for 3–35 minutes before reassessing. *Determines if heart is beating spontaneously.*

7. Repeat cycle of 5 compressions and 1 breath until signs of circulation return or help arrives. *To deliver adequate amount of oxygenated blood to tissues.*

8. If infant does not have trauma and both pulse and respiration return, place infant on side. *Protects airway.*

IV. Two rescuers.

A. Follow the steps outlined above for either the adolescent, child, or infant CPR with the following changes:

1. One rescuer is positioned facing the infant/child parallel to the head while the other rescuer is positioned on the opposite side facing the infant/child parallel to the sternum and next to the trunk (Figure XV-19). *Proper positioning allows one rescuer to perform artificial respirations while the other administers chest compressions without getting in each other's way. In addition, this facilitates ease in changing positions when one of the rescuers becomes fatigued.*

2. The rescuer positioned at the trunk is responsible for performing cardiac compressions and maintaining the verbal mnemonic count. This is rescuer #1. *Promotes efficiency of CPR.*

3. The rescuer positioned at the infant/child's head is responsible for monitoring respirations, assessing pulses, establishing an open airway, and performing rescue breathing. This is rescuer #2. *Promotes efficiency of CPR.*

4. The compression to ventilation rate changes to 3:1, delivering the ventilation on the upstroke of the third compression. *Delivering compressions during the upstroke phase allows for full lung expansion during inspiration.*

5. Rescuer #2 palpates the pulse with each chest compression during the first full minute. *Palpating the pulse with each chest compression during the first full minute assures that adequate stroke volume is being delivered with each compression.*

6. Rescuer #2 is responsible for calling for a change when fatigued following this protocol. Two rescuers are needed, because one person cannot maintain CPR indefinitely. *When a rescuer becomes fatigued, chest compressions can become ineffective, decreasing the volume of oxygenated blood circulated to key organs and tissue.*

7. Rescuer #1 calls for a change and completes the five chest compressions. *So either rescuer does not tire prematurely.*

8. Rescuer #2 administers 2 breaths and then moves to a position parallel to the sternum and assumes the proper hand position. *So compressions can be delivered as needed.*

9. Rescuer #1 moves to the rescue breathing position and checks the pulse for 5 seconds. If the arrest persists, rescuer #1 says, "continue CPR" and delivers one breath. Rescuer #2 resumes cardiac compressions immediately after the breath. *So CPR continues without interruption.*

V. Neonate or premature infant

A. Follow the infant guidelines with the following changes for chest compression. *Improper hand placement can cause internal organ damage or other medical complications in premature infants or newborns.*

1. Encircle the chest with both hands. *Chest small enough to accommodate hands.*

2. Position the thumbs over the midsternum. *To prevent injury to ribs.*

3. Compress the midsternum with both thumbs. *Heel of hand is too large for neonate/premature CPR.*

4. Compress ⅓–1⅖ cm (¼–½ inch) at a rate of 100–120 times/minute. *Provides enough compression to circulate blood; provides sufficient rate to circulate blood.*

Refer to Table XV-1 for an overview of the various cardiopulmonary standards.

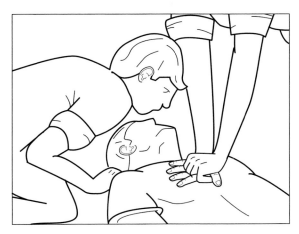

FIGURE XV-19 Two-rescuer positioning. One person kneels on each side of the client.

DOCUMENTATION

1. Time and date.
2. Condition of adolescent/child/infant when found.
3. Interventions implemented.
4. Personnel involved in CPR.

Table XV-1   Cardiopulmonary standards

Client	Hand Position	Chest Compression Depth (cm)	Chest Compression Depth (Inches)	Chest Compression Rate (Min⁻¹)	Chest Compression-to-Ventilation Ratio
Adult, adolescent, and larger child	Two hands on top of each other, heel on sternum, two finger widths above xiphoid	3.8–5.0	1½–2	80–100	15:2 (one rescuer), 5:1 (two rescuers)
Child (~1–7 years)	One hand, heel on sternum, two finger widths above xiphoid	2.4–3.8	1–1½	80–100	5:1 (one rescuer), 3:1 (two rescuers)
Infant (1–12 months)	Two fingers (index and middle) midsternum 1 cm below nipples	1.3–2.5	½–1	100	5:1 (one rescuer), 3:1 (two rescuers)
Neonate, premature infant	Encircle chest with hands, thumb over midsternum	1.3–1.8	½–¾	100–120	5:1 (one rescuer), 3:1 (two rescuers)

5. Orders received by physician or qualified health care provider during CPR.
6. Any medications administered.
7. Vital signs.
8. Status of adolescent/child/infant afterward.
9. Other information needed for code record.

- CPR is successful and there is a return of spontaneous respiration and circulation.
- Advanced life support measures are implemented (in the acute care setting) or the child is transferred to a facility that provides advanced life support.

- A rescuer is alone and unable to continue CPR due to fatigue.
- A physician or other qualified health care provider declares the child dead and discontinues CPR.

⧖ **Estimated time to complete procedure:** *This skill must be initiated as soon as possible and continued indefinitely until one of the following occurs:*

Community and Camp Nursing Procedures

Community and Camp Nursing Procedures

OVERVIEW

Many children receive insect bites, develop dermatitis when they come in contact with chemically irritating natural substances (poison ivy), or receive small wooden splinters when hiking or playing. It is important that all of these situations are treated efficiently and effectively so complications do not develop later.

PROCEDURE 105

REMOVING A TICK

OVERVIEW

Most tick bites are from the Ixodidae family of ticks, which attach and feed for several days if not removed. Although any tick may be a vector for one of more diseases, each species is a potential transmitter of only a subset of tick-borne disease agents. Tick bites often occur during the night when the victim does not know what caused the bite. Other tick bites occur when the child is in heavy underbrush or heavily wooded areas (forests, wood piles, tall grasses, bushes). Tick bites produce a firm, discrete, intensely pruritic nodules at the site of attachment and may cause urticaria or persistent edema that is localized to the site of the bite.

Ticks should be removed as soon as possible to reduce the likelihood of disease transmission if the tick was infected and to reduce the amount of cutaneous immune response. Irritants or petroleum jelly should never be applied to the tick. Rather, the best chance of removing the tick and all of the mouth parts from the skin is by using a curved-tip forceps.

To avoid ticks, long pants tucked into the socks and a long-sleeved shirt should be worn when walking or playing in wooded areas.

EQUIPMENT

Curved forceps
Nonsterile gloves
Liquid antiseptic
Antihistamine lotion/cream
Sterile needle

PROCEDURE

1. Prepare child. *Enhances cooperation and participation; reduces anxiety and fear.*
2. Assemble equipment. *Promotes organization and efficiency.*
3. Wash hands and put on gloves. *Reduces transmission of microorganisms.*
4. Obtain a short history relative to where child has been, when he/she might have been exposed to ticks, what type of clothing child may have been wearing, and where tick bite may be. *Assists in determining whether or not child was exposed to a tick.*
5. Examine child's skin (especially head) for tick. *Ticks are visible to the eye.*
6. When the tick is isolated, place the curved forceps parallel to the skin to grasp the tick firmly as close to the skin as possible. Avoid puncturing the child's skin and the tick's body. *Curved-tip forceps are best because the outer curve can be laid against the skin while the handle remains far enough from the skin to grasp easily.*
7. Pull the forceps slowly and steadily directly away from the skin without twisting. *Prevents tick body from breaking.*
8. Examine skin for any remaining body parts. *Sometimes the tick's body will come apart during removal.*
9. If any remaining body parts are seen, carefully remove them with the forceps or a sterile needle. *Important to remove all body parts.*
10. Apply an antiseptic to the area. *Cleanses area of broken skin.*
11. If local swelling and discoloration of the skin are apparent, apply an antihistamine. *Decreases swelling.*
12. Send tick to laboratory for analysis. *To detect etiologic agents of tick-borne diseases in geographic area where child received tick bite.*

DOCUMENTATION

1. Time and date.
2. Site of tick bite.
3. Appearance of skin and where tick bite was found.
4. Appearance of tick.
5. Whether or not entire tick was removed.
6. Child's condition after removal.

Estimated time to complete procedure: *5–8 minutes.*

PROCEDURE 106

TREATING CONTACT DERMATITIS CAUSED BY POISON IVY OR POISON OAK

OVERVIEW

Contact dermatitis is an inflammatory response of the skin due to contact with a chemical substance that is either naturally occurring or synthetic. A hypersensivity reaction occurs, itching is common, and early on there is a sharp delineation between the normal and inflamed skin.

Any part of the poison ivy, oak, or sumac plants can cause localized dermatitis as soon as contact is made. The chemical urushiol causes the reaction, which is manifested by redness, swelling, and itching at the site of contact. The rash can be evident 2 days after contact, and blisters oozing serum from damaged cells will appear several days later. By 10–14 days, the lesions will dry and heal spontaneously, and itching will stop.

Burow's solution compresses, calamine lotion, and/or Aveeno baths will relieve discomfort; topical corticosteroid ointment, if applied before blisters form, will prevent or relieve the inflammation. Benedryl or oral corticosteroids may also be useful. The best treatment is to avoid contact with the plants; teach children what the plants look like. The initial treatment is described below.

EQUIPMENT

Cold running water
Mild soap
Washcloth
Fresh change of clothes
Nonsterile gloves
Calamine lotion

PROCEDURE

1. Prepare child. *Enhances cooperation and participation; reduces anxiety and fear.*

2. Assemble equipment. *Promotes organization and efficiency.*
3. Wash hands and put on gloves. *Reduces transmission of microorganisms.*
4. Using cold running water, immediately flush skin that has had direct contact with the plant. *To neutralize the urushiol not yet bonded to the skin.*
5. Wash area with mild soap (if possible); avoid scrubbing. *Helps remove the urushiol; scrubbing may damage the skin.*
6. Remove all clothing that has had contact with the plants and launder in hot water and detergent. *Clothing may contain the urushiol and can spread it to other areas of the skin that did not come in direct contact with the plant.*
7. Help child put on a fresh change of clothes. *Prevents exposure from clothing that may have had contact with plant.*
8. Apply calamine lotion to skin where exposed to plant. *Helps prevent itching.*
9. Remove gloves; wash hands. *Reduces transmission of chemical.*

DOCUMENTATION

1. Time, place, and date of exposure.
2. History of exposure.
3. Procedure followed to rinse skin.
4. Appearance of any skin rash or blisters.
5. Lotions or medications administered.
6. Child's condition after skin rinsed.
7. Change of clothing.

 Estimated time to complete procedure: *5–10 minutes.*

PROCEDURE 107

REMOVING A SPLINTER

OVERVIEW

Often, children receive small wooden splinters when playing or hiking. Most of the time, parents are able to remove the foreign body and can be taught the following information. Camp nurses may also need to know how to remove splinters correctly.

EQUIPMENT

Sterile needle
Sterile tweezer
Nonsterile gloves
Soap and water
Antiseptic ointment or cream
Small bandage (if needed)

PROCEDURE

1. Prepare child. *Enhances cooperation and participation; reduces anxiety and fear.*
2. Assemble equipment. *Promotes organization and efficiency.*
3. Wash hands and put on gloves. *Reduces transmission of microorganisms.*

4. Wash area where splinter is embedded in the skin. *Reduces transmission of microorganisms into the splinter area.*
5. Use the needle to expose the splinter. *Allows better visibility for removal.*
6. Grasp the splinter with the tweezers and pull the splinter out with a horizontal motion, pulling it in the direction the splinter entered the skin. *Prevents the splinter from breaking.*
7. Apply small amount of antiseptic cream or ointment; cover with small bandage if needed. *Decreases chance of infection at site where splinter was embedded in the skin; protects area.*
8. Remove gloves; wash hands. *Reduces transmission of microorganisms.*

DOCUMENTATION

1. Time and date.
2. Site of splinter.
3. Procedure used to remove splinter.
4. Whether or not entire splinter was removed.

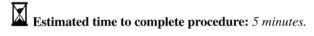 **Estimated time to complete procedure:** *5 minutes.*

UNIT XVII

Hygiene Skills

Hair Care

OVERVIEW

Children's hair should be brushed and combed daily unless contraindicated by the hair style. The child's hair should not be cut without parental permission unless it is necessary to access a scalp vein for intravenous access. Hair should be shampooed as part of the bath when needed (adolescents may need their hair washed more frequently than infants or small children) and styled according to the child's and parent's wishes.

For African-American children, combs with widely spaced teeth are preferred. Special hair dressing or pomade may be requested and can be brought in from home. Plaiting or braiding should be done loosely when the hair is damp.

PROCEDURE 108

ASSISTING WITH ORAL HYGIENE

OVERVIEW

The oral cavity functions in mastication, and may secrete mucus to moisten and lubricate the food before it enters the digestive system. Common problems occurring in the oral cavity of children include bad breath, dental caries, plaque, inflammation of the gums, or inflammation of the oral cavity. Daily oral care is essential to maintain the integrity of the mucous membranes, teeth, gums, and lips and includes flossing and brushing. Daily care may also include either rinsing with fluoride or taking fluoride tablets.

Fluoride prevents dental caries, is a common component of many toothpastes, and has been added to the water supply of many cities. However, if the local drinking water exceeds .3 ppm concentration of fluoride, the child does not need fluoride supplements. Infants as young as 2 weeks of age can be given fluoride drops, which are available without a prescription. If the water supply does not exceed .3 ppm, children should receive fluoride tablets. Flossing should be performed daily in conjunction with brushing. Flossing prevents the formation of plaque and removes plaque and food debris from between the teeth. Teeth should be brushed after each meal with toothpaste that contains fluoride. Brushing removes plaque and food debris as well as promoting blood circulation of the gums.

Young children are unable to brush all areas of the mouth, so parents will need to assume some responsibility for effective teeth cleaning. Young children (toddlers, preschoolers) may use only water, disliking the taste and foam of toothpaste. There is some danger if fluoridated toothpaste is swallowed, so parents should be cautioned to use toothpaste sparingly (about the size of a pea). Small toothbrushes that are soft with short, rounded bristles are appropriate for young children, and flossing is recommended after cleansing the teeth.

In addition to routine dental care, children should also see a dentist. The child's first visit should be soon after the first teeth erupt, at about 1 year of age. An important aspect of the visit is assessment of oral health, education of parents regarding correct methods of dental hygiene, and counseling on strategies to prevent caries.

EQUIPMENT

Toothbrush
Toothpaste with fluoride
Emesis basin (if needed)
Cup of water
Nonsterile gloves
Towel
Dental floss
Mirror

PROCEDURE

1. Prepare child. *Enhances cooperation and participation; reduces anxiety and fear.*
2. Assemble equipment. *Promotes organization and efficiency.*
3. Ask child to sit up, or have child stand at sink. *Decreases chance of aspiration.*
4. Wash hands and put on gloves. *Reduces transmission of microorganisms.*
5. Put toothpaste on toothbrush. Be sure amount is appropriate for child. *Promotes organization and efficiency.*
6. Assist child with brushing, being sure toothbrush moves up and down the front and back of teeth. *Permits cleaning back and sides of teeth and decreases microorganism growth in mouth.*
7. Help child floss teeth by moving floss up and down the sides of each tooth, using mirror if needed. *Removes plaque and food debris; prevents gum disease and dental caries.*
8. Help child rinse mouth with water and spit into emesis basin or sink. *Removes toothpaste.*
9. Help child dry mouth with towel. *Removes toothpaste and water from mouth area.*
10. Remove gloves, wash hands, and document care. *Reduces transmission of microorganisms and exposure to body fluids; documents care provided.*

DOCUMENTATION

1. Time and date.
2. Any unusual findings.
3. How well child was able to brush teeth independently.

⧖ **Estimated time to complete procedure:** *5 minutes.*

PROCEDURE 109

BATHING A CHILD

OVERVIEW

The type of bath provided depends on the purpose of the bath and the child's ability to participate. The therapeutic bath was discussed in an earlier skill related to fever management. Most children are able to take a tub bath or shower unless they are bedridden, when a bed bath may be needed.

SAFETY

1. If the child is to be bathed in a tub, place a towel on the bottom of the tub or basin to prevent the child from slipping and falling.
2. Ensure that the room temperature is warm so the child does not become chilled.
3. Do not leave a child under age 7 years alone in a tub.
4. Supervise children over the age of 7 who may be able to bathe independently.
5. Check the water temperature before bathing the child.
6. Hold on to an infant who is unable to sit alone in the tub.

EQUIPMENT

Washbasin or bathtub
Water should feel warm to touch
Washcloths
Dry towels and/or bath blanket
Plastic sheet to protect bed (optional)
Soap
Clean gown or pajamas
Nonsterile gloves

PROCEDURE

1. Gather equipment. *Promotes organization and efficiency.*
2. Explain procedure to child and family. *Enhances cooperation and participation; reduces anxiety and fear.*
3. Wash hands and put on gloves. *Reduces transmission of microorganisms.*
4. Undress child and place in tub. *Facilitates bathing.*
5. Shampoo hair; try to avoid getting shampoo in child's eyes. *Promotes hair cleanliness; avoids shampoo burning eyes.*
6. Bathe child; start with face and work down to legs and perineal area. Do not allow child to become chilled. *Reduces transmission of microorganisms.*
7. Dry child with a towel. *Reduces chilling.*
8. Dress child in clean gown or pajamas. *Promotes comfort.*
9. Remove gloves and wash hands. *Reduces transmission of microorganisms.*

DOCUMENTATION

1. Time and date.
2. How child tolerated bath.
3. How much child participated.
4. Any observations regarding child's abnormal behavior or physical condition.

 Estimated time to complete procedure: *5–10 minutes.*

UNIT XVIII

Special Skills

Special Skills

OVERVIEW

Two skills are important for nurses to know when caring for newborns. One skill relates to umbilical care. The other relates to male circumcision.

PROCEDURE 110

PERFORMING UMBILICAL CORD CARE OF THE NEWBORN
OVERVIEW

The newborn's umbilical cord is clamped in the delivery room and begins to necrose almost immediately because its blood supply is interrupted. However, until it falls off, the cord needs to be kept clean and dry because of organisms that may invade the cord stump and surrounding area. Cord care is done to control bleeding, prevent infection, and promote healing. Cord care should be provided after the cord falls off and continue until the skin appears normal. It is important to never pull the cord or attempt to loosen it. Since the cord falls off 7–10 days after birth, parents need to be taught cord care when their newborn is discharged.

EQUIPMENT

70% isopropyl alcohol or hydrogen peroxide
Cotton balls
Nonsterile gloves
Culture applicator and tube (if needed)

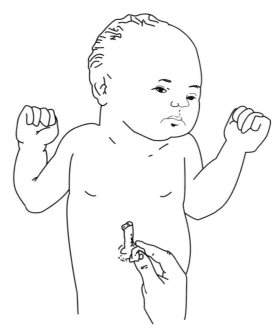

FIGURE XVIII-1   Cleaning the umbilical cord.

PROCEDURE

1. Prepare family. *Enhances cooperation and participation; reduces anxiety and fear.*
2. Assemble equipment. *Promotes organization and efficiency.*
3. Wash hands and put on gloves, *Reduces transmission of microorganisms.*
4. Inspect area around cord; obtain a culture of drainage if present. *Allows for evaluation of effectiveness of treatment.*
5. Clean base of cord with cotton balls soaked with alcohol or hydrogen peroxide with each diaper change (Figure XVIII-1). A*ssists in wound healing and drying of cord.*
6. Reapply diaper, being sure to fold the diaper down so the cord is not covered by the diaper (Figure XVIII-2). *Facilitates drying of cord.*
7. Discard gloves; wash hands. *Reduces transmission of microorganisms.*

DOCUMENTATION

1. Time and date.
2. Appearance of umbilical cord and surrounding area.
3. Cord care given.
4. Whether or not umbilical cord has fallen off.

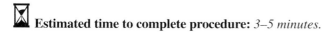 **Estimated time to complete procedure:** *3–5 minutes.*

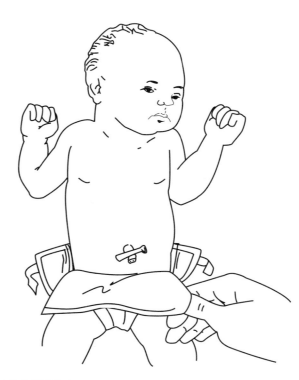

FIGURE XVIII-2   Turning diapers off of the umbilical cord.

PROCEDURE 111

PERFORMING CIRCUMCISION CARE

OVERVIEW

Circumcision is the surgical removal of the foreskin—the skin that covers the glans, or head, of the penis. It may be performed at any age and is a choice of many parents living in the United States and a ritual requirement of Islam and Judaism as well as many primitive tribes. Although there may be no medical indication for the circumcision, there is a decreased incidence of urinary tract infections in male infants and a decreased incidence of sexually transmitted diseases in those who have been circumcised.

The decision to have the newborn male circumcised is left up to the parents. Factors that may affect their decision include cleanliness, tradition, possible prevention of cancer, and personal preference. As with any surgery, there are risks involved when a circumcision is performed. Although rare, they may include hemorrhage; infection; injury to the penis, urethra, or scrotum; deformity; and scarring. Newborns who are premature, ill, or distressed at birth or have hemophilia or any genitourinary abnormality may have the circumcision delayed or not performed at all.

Care of the circumcised newborn, typically performed during the newborn's bath and at each diaper change, is dependent on the procedure performed. Parents should know how to care for the circumcision area when their son is discharged from the hospital.

If the Ring Was Not Used

EQUIPMENT

Nonsterile gloves
4 × 4 gauze
Sterile water
Petroleum gauze (if applicable)

PROCEDURE

1. Prepare family. *Enhances cooperation and participation; reduces anxiety and fear.*
2. Assemble equipment. *Promotes organization and efficiency.*
3. Wash hands and put on gloves. *Reduces transmission of microorganisms.*
4. Remove diaper. *Allows visualization of circumcision area.*

5. Inspect the circumcision site; assess penis for bleeding. *Allows for evaluation of effectiveness of treatment.*
6. Gently clean around the glans with a 4 × 4 sterile gauze moistened with sterile water (Figure XVIII-3). *Removes any exudates; assists in wound healing.*

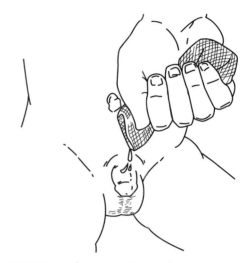

FIGURE XVIII-3   Cleaning the penis.

7. If the petroleum gauze is soiled with stool, replace it with new petroleum gauze. *Reduces transmission of microorganisms.*
8. Loosely reapply diaper. *A tight diaper may interfere with healing.*
9. Discard gloves; wash hands. *Reduces transmission of microorganisms.*

DOCUMENTATION

1. Time and date.
2. Appearance of circumcision site.
3. Condition of petroleum gauze.
4. Whether or not petroleum gauze was replaced.

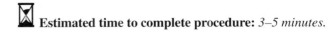 **Estimated time to complete procedure:** *3–5 minutes.*

If the Plastic Ring Was Used

NOTE: *The ring will fall off in 7–10 days when the circumcision has healed. Do NOT pull it off.*

EQUIPMENT

Nonsterile gloves
Cotton balls
Sterile water

PROCEDURE

1. Prepare family. *Enhances cooperation and participation; reduces anxiety and fear.*
2. Assemble equipment. *Promotes organization and efficiency.*
3. Wash hands and put on gloves. *Reduces transmission of microorganisms.*
4. Remove diaper. *Allows visualization of circumcision area.*
5. Inspect the circumcision site; assess penis for bleeding. *Allows for evaluation of effectiveness of treatment.*

6. Gently lift the ring and squeeze warm water from a cotton ball onto the tip of it.
7. Loosely reapply diaper. *A tight diaper may interfere with healing.*
8. Discard gloves; wash hands. *Reduces transmission of microorganisms.*

DOCUMENTATION

1. Time and date.
2. Appearance of circumcision site.
3. Presence/absence of bell.

 Estimated time to complete procedure: *3–5 minutes.*

REFERENCES AND BIBLIOGRAPHY

Adkins, L. (1997). Cast changes: Synthetic versus plaster. *Pediatric Nursing, 23*(4), 422, 425–427.

Altman, G. B. (2004). *Delmar's fundamental and advanced nursing skills.* (2nd ed.) Clifton Park, NY: Thomson Delmar Learning.

American Academy of Pediatrics Committee on Pediatric Emergency Medicine (2004). The use of physical restraint interventions for children and adolescents in the acute care setting. *Pediatrics, 99*(3), 497–498.

American Heart Association (2000). 2000 guidelines for cardiopulmonary resuscitation and emergency cardiac care. *Circulation, 102* (Special Supplement), 1–384.

American Heart Association (2004). The science behind the BLS guidelines. Retrieved November 4, 2004 from http://www.americanheart.org/downloadable/heart/1054743769661bls_2001Science_Guides.ppt

Arrowsmith, H. (1996). Nursing management of patients receiving gastrostomy feeding. *British Journal of Nursing, 5*(5), 268–273.

Axton, S. E., Smith, L. F., Bertrand, S., Dy, E., & Liehr, P. (1995). Comparison of brachial and calf blood pressures in infants. *Pediatric Nursing, 21*(4), 323–326.

Barton, S. J., Gaffney, R., Chase, T., Rayens, M. K., & Piyabanditkul, L. (2003). Pediatric temperature measurement and child/parent/nurse preference using three temperature measurement instruments. *Journal of Pediatric Nursing, 18*(5), 314–320.

Beckstrand, J., Ellett, M., Welch, J., Dye, J., Games, C., Henrie, S., & Barlow, R. S. (1990). The distance to the stomach for feeding tube placement in children predicted from regression on height. *Research in Nursing and Health, 13*(6), 411–420.

Beyer, J., Denyes, M., & Villarruel, A. (1992). The creation, validation and continuing development of the Oucher: A measure of pain intensity in children. *Journal of Pediatric Nursing, 7*(5), 335–346.

Bieri, D., Teeve, R., Champion, G., Addicoat, L., & Ziegler, J. (1990). The Faces pain scale for self-assessment of the severity of pain experienced by children: Initial validation, and preliminary investigation for ratio scale properties. *Pain, 41,* 139–150.

Broscious, S. K. (1995). Preventing complications of PEG tubes. *Dimensions of Critical Care Nursing, 14*(1), 37–34.

Buglass, E. (1999). Tracheostomy care: Tracheal suctioning and humdification. *British Journal of Nursing, 8*(8), 500–504.

Calagiovanni, L. (1999). Nutrition. Taking the tube . . . nasogastric tube-feeding . . . methods to test tube position. *Nursing Times, 95*(21), 63–64, 67, 71.

Carroll, P. (1997). Pulse oximetry at your fingertips. *RN, 60*(2), 22–26.

Chen, C. A., Paxton, P., & Williams-Burgess, C. (1996). Feeding tube placement verification using gastric pH measurement. *The Online Journal of Knowledge Synthesis for Nursing, 3.* Doc. No. 10, 1–9.

Clemence, M. A., Walker, D., & Farr, B. M. (1995). Central venous catheter practices: Results of a survey. *American Journal of Infection Control, 23*(1), 5–12.

Cummings, R. (1992). Understanding external ventricular drainage. *The Journal of Neuroscience Nursing, 24*(2), 84–87.

Danek, G. D., & Noris, E. M. (1992). Pediatric IV catheters: Efficacy of saline flush. *Pediatric Nursing, 18*(2), 111–113.

Dickinson, L. (1997). Central venous catheter site care: Chlorhexidine vs. povidone-iodine. *ANNA Journal, 24*(3), 349, 358.

Eland, J., & Anderson, J. (1997). The experience of pain in children. In A. Jacos (Ed.), *Pain: A sourcebook for nurses and other health professionals* (pp. 453–473). Boston: Little, Brown & Co.

Ellett, M. L. & Beckstrand, J. (2001). Predicting the distance for Nasojejunal tube insertion in children. *Journal of the Society of Pediatric Nurses, 6*(3), 123–132.

Ellett, M. L. C. (1997). What is the prevalence of feeding tube placement errors and what are the associated risk factors? *The Online Journal of Knowledge Synthesis for Nursing, 4.* Doc. No. 5.

Ellett, M. L. C., & Beckstrand, J. (1999). Examination of gavage tube placement in children. *Journal of the Society of Pediatric Nurses, 4*(2), 51–60.

Epps, C. K. (1996). The delicate business of ostomy care. *RN, 59*(11), 32–37, 53.

Erhardt, A. S., & Graham, H. (1990). Pulse oximetry. *Nursing90, 20*(3), 50–54.

Erickson, R., & Woo, T. M. (1994). Accuracy of infrared ear thermometry and traditional temperature methods in children. *Heart & Lung, 23*(3), 181–195.

Estes, M. E. (2002). *Health Assessment and Physical Examination, 2nd edition.* Clifton Park, NY: Delmar Thompson Learning.

Fitchie, C. (1992). Central venous catheter-related infection and dressing type. *Intensive and Critical Care Nursing, 8*(4), 199–202.

Fowler, S., Knapp-Spooner, C., & Donohue, D. (1995). The ABC's of tracheostomy care. *The Journal of Practical Nursing, 45*(1), 44–48.

Frankenburg, W. K. (1994). Preventing developmental delays: Is developmental screening sufficient? *Pediatrics, 93(4),* 586–593.

Freiberger, D. (1994). The use of Hibiclens™ in pediatric central venous line skin care. *Journal of Pediatric Nursing, 9*(2), 126–127.

Frey, A. M. & Schears, G. (2001). Dislodgment rates and impact of securement methods for peripherally inserted central catheters (PICCs) in children. *Pediatric Nursing, 27*(2), 185–189.

Gharib, A. M., Stern, E. J., Sherbin, V. L., & Rohrmann, C. A. (1996). Nasogastric and feeding tubes. The importance of proper placement. *Postgraduate Medicine, 99*(5), 165–168, 174, 176, passim.

Gibson, I. (1995). Making sense of . . . external ventricular drainage. *Nursing Times, 91*(23), 34–35.

Goodfellow, L. T., & Jones, M. (2002). Bronchial hygiene therapy. *American Journal of Nursing, 102*(1), 37–43.

Grady, N. P., et al. (2002). Guidelines for the prevention of intravascular catheter-related infections. *Pediatrics, 110*(5), 51–75.

Gray, M. (1996). Atraumatic urethral catheterization of children. *Pediatric Nursing, 22*(4), 306–310.

Griggs, A. (1999). Tracheostomy: Suctioning and humidification. *Emergency Nurse, 6*(9), 33–40.

Guide to medical devices. Getting an accurate temperature with an ear thermometer. (1996). *Nursing96, 26*(8), 24n.

Haddock, B. J., Merrow, D. L., & Swanson, M. S. (1996). The falling grace of axillary temperatures. *Pediatric Nursing, 22*(2), 121–125.

Hanna, D. (1995). Guidelines for pulse oximetry use in pediatrics. *Journal of Pediatric Nursing, 10*(2), 124–126.

Harken, H. (1998). Tracheostomy management. *Nursing Times, 94*(21), 56–58.

Hester, N. O., & Barcus, C. S. (1986). Assessment and management of children in pain. *Pediatrics: Nursing Update, 1,* 2–8.

Hilton, B. A. (1994). How do you flush your peripheral and central venous lines? Is it the most effective way? Let research guide your practice! *Canadian Oncology Nursing Journal, 4*(2), 64–65.

Holder, C., & Alexander, J. (1990). A new and improved guide to IV therapy. *American Journal of Nursing, 90*(2), 43–47.

Holder, C., Sexton, E., & Paul, D. (1996). Enteral nutrition. *Pediatric Nursing, 8*(5), 28–35.

Holmes, S. (1996). Percutaneous endoscopic gastrostomy: A review. *Nursing Times, 92*(17), 34–35.

Hooper, M. (1996). Nursing care of the patient with a tracheostomy. *Nursing Standard, 10*(34), 40–43.

Houlder, L. C. (2000). The accuracy and reliability of tympanic thermometry compared to rectal and axillary sites in young children. *Pediatric Nursing, 26*(3), 311–314.

Huddleston, K. C., & Ferraro, A. R. (1991). Preparing families of children with gastrostomies. *Pediatric Nursing, 17*(2), 153–158.

Huff, K. (2000). Seizures and epilepsy. In C. Berkowitz (Ed.), *Pediatrics: A primary care approach* (2nd edition, pp. 559–565). Philadelphia: Saunders.

Jansson, J. M. (1991). Dermatologic complications of ostomy care. *Dimensions of Oncology Nursing, 5*(3), 10–13.

Jordan-Marsh, M., et al. (2004). The social ecology of changing pain management: Do I have to cry? *Journal of Pediatric Nursing, 3*(19), 133–139.

Kandt, K. A. (1991). An implantable venous access device for children. *The American Journal of Maternal Child Nursing, 16*(2), 88–91.

Kankkunen, P., Pietila, A. M., & Vehvilainen-Julkunen, K. (2004). Families' and children's postoperative pain—literature review. *Journal of Pediatric Nursing, 2(19)*.

Kennedy, A. H., Shelley, S., & Mittrucker, C. (1994). Accuracy and reliability of temperature measurement by instrument and site. *Journal of Pediatric Nursing, 9*(2), 114–123.

Klein, T. (2001). PICCs and midlines—fine-tuning your care. *RN, 64*(8), 26–29.

Klien, N. C., & Cunha, B. A. (1996). Treatment of fever. *Infectious Disease Clinics of North America, 10*(1), 211–215.

Larsen, L. L., & Thurston, N. E. (1997). Research utilization: Development of a central venous catheter procedure. *Applied Nursing Research, 10*(1), 44–51.

Lindeke, L. L., Hauck, M. R., & Tanner, M. (2000). Practical issues in obtaining child assent for research. *Journal of Pediatric Nursing, 15*(2), 99–104.

Loan, T., Magnuson, B., & Williams, S. (1998). Debunking six myths about enteral feeding. *Nursing98, 28*(8), 43–48.

Lombardi, T. P., Gundersen, B., Zammett, L. O., Walters, J. K., & Morris, B. A. (1988). Efficacy of 0.9% sodium chloride injection with or without heparin sodium for maintaining patency of intravenous catheters in children. *Clinical Pharmacy, 7,* 832–836.

Mateo, M. A. (1994). Maintaining the patency of enteral feeding tubes. *The Online Journal of Knowledge Synthesis for Nursing, 1.* Doc. No. 9, 1–13.

McConnell, E. A. (1990). Clinical do's and don'ts: Administering a bolus gastrostomy feeding. *Nursing90, 20*(11), 102.

McConnell, E. A. (1997). Clinical do's and don'ts: Inserting a nasogastric tube. *Nursing97, 27*(1), 72.

McEleney, M. (1998). Update: Endotracheal suction. *Professional Nurse, 13*(6), 373–376.

Medem Medical Library (2004). Circumcision information for parents. Retrieved November 5, 2004 from http://www.medem.com/search/article_display.cfm?path=\\TANQUERAY/M_ContentItem&mstr=/M_ContentItem/ZZZJZMEMH4C.html&soc=Medem&srch_typ=NAV_SERCH

Metheny, N., Reed, L., Wiersema, L., McSweeney, M., Wehrle, M. A., & Clark, J. (1993). Effectiveness of pH measurements in predicting feeding tube placement: An update. *Nursing Research, 42*(6), 324–331.

Metheny, N. A., Stewart, B. J., Smith, L., Yan, H., Diebold, M., & Clouse, R. E. (1997). pH and concentration of pepsin and trypsin in feeding tube aspirates as predictors of tube placement. *Journal of Parenteral and Enteral Nutrition, 21*(5), 279–285.

Metheny, N. A., Stewart, B. J., Smith, L., Yan H., Diebold, M., & Clouse, R. E. (1999). pH and concentration of bilirubin in feeding tube aspirates as predictors of tube placement. *Nursing Research, 48*(4), 189–197.

Metheny, N. A., Wehrle, M. A., Wiersema, L., & Clark, J. (1998). pH, color, and feeding tubes. *RN, 61*(11), 25–27.

Munoz, C. (2005). *Transcultural Communication in Nursing, 2nd edition*. Clifton Park, NY: Delmar Thompson Learning.

O'Brien, B., Davis, S., & Erwin-Toth, P. (1999). G-tube site care: A practical guide. *RN, 62*(2), 52–56.

O'Brien. R. (1991). Starting intravenous lines in children. *Journal of Emergency Nursing, 17*(4), 225–231.

O'Connell, F. M., & Heard, S. O. (1998). Central venous catheter infections: Practical bedside measures to reduce risk. *The Journal of Critical Illness, 13*(9), 569–573, 576–578.

Ouwendyk, M., & Helferty, M. (1996). Central venous catheter management: How to prevent complications. *ANNA Journal, 23*(6), 572–579.

Padula, C., Kenny, A., Planchon, C., & Lamoureux, C. (2004, July). Enteral feedings: What the evidence says. *AJN, 104, 7*, 62–69.

Patient care services. *Protocol & procedure manual*. (2000) Salt Lake City, UT: Primary Children's Medical Center.

Perry, A. G., & Potter, P. A. (2004). *Clinical nursing skills & techniques* (5th ed.). St. Louis: Mosby.

Pontious, S., Kennedy, A. H., Skelley, S., & Mittrucker, C. (1994). Accuracy and reliability of temperature measurement by instrument and site. *Journal of Pediatric Nursing, 9*(2), 114–123.

Pontious, S. L., Kennedy, A., Chung, K. L., Burroughs, T. E., Libby, L. J., & Vogel, D. W. (1994). Accuracy and reliability of temperature measurement in the emergency department by instrument and site in children. *Pediatric Nursing, 20*(1), 58–63.

Prior, M. & Miles, S. (1999). Continuing professional development: Casting: part one. *Emergency Nurse, 7*, 33–42.

Rakel, B. A., Titler, M., Goode, C., Barry–Walker, J., Budreau, G., & Buckwalter, K. C. (1994). Nasogastric and nasointestinal feeding tube placement: An integrative review of research. *Clinical Issues in Critical Care Nursing, 5*(2), 194–206, 218.

Rowsey, P. J. (1997a). Pathophysiology of fever part 1: The role of cytokines. *Dimensions of Critical Care Nursing, 16*(4), 202–207.

Rowsey, P. J. (1997b). Pathophysiology of fever part 2: Relooking at cooling interventions. *Dimensions of Critical Care Nursing, 16*(5), 251–256.

Savedra, M., Tesler, M., Holzmer, W., & Ward, (1992). Adolescent pediatric pain tool: User manual. San Francisco: University of California.

Scheinblum, S. T., & Hammond, M. (1990). The treatment of children with shunt infections: External ventricular drainage system care. *Pediatric Nursing, 16*(2), 139–143.

Selekman, J., & Snyder, B. (1996). Uses of and alternatives to restraints in pediatric settings. *Clinical Issues in Critical Care Nursing, 7*(4), 603–610.

Selekman, J., & Snyder, B. (1997). Institutional policies on the use of physical restraints on children. *Pediatric Nursing, 23*, 531–537.

Sharber, J. (1997). The efficacy of tepid sponge bathing to reduce fever in young children. *The American Journal of Emergency Medicine, 15*(2), 188–192.

Smith, R. D., Fallentine, J. K., & Kessel, S. (1995). Underwater chest drainage. *Nursing95, 25*(2), 60–63.

Smith, S. F., Duell, D. J., & Martin, B. C. (2000). *Clinical nursing skills: Basic to advanced skills*. Upper Saddle River, NJ: Prentice Hall Health.

Snydman, D. R., Donnelly-Reidy, M., Perry, L. K., & Martin, W. J. (1987). Intravenous tubing containing burrettes can be safely changed at 72 hour intervals. *Infection Control, 8*(3), 113–116.

Swiech, K., Lancaster, D. R., & Sheehan, R. (1994). Use of a pressure gauge to differentiate gastric from pulmonary placement of nasoenteral feeding tubes. *Applied Nursing Research, 7*(4), 183–189.

Taylor, D., Meyers, S. T., Monarch, K., Leon, C., Hall, J., & Sibley, Y. (1996). Use of occlusive dressings on central line venous catheter sites in hospitalized children. *Journal of Pediatric Nursing, 11*(3), 169–174.

Teasdale, G., Knill-Jones, R., & Jennett, W. (1974). Assessing and recording "consciousness level". *Journal of Neurosurgical Psychiatry, 37*, 1286.

Terry, D., & Nisbet, K. (1991). Nursing care of the child with external ventricular drainage. *The Journal of Neuroscience Nursing, 23*(6), 347–355.

Thomas, D. O. (1995). Fever in children. Friend or foe? *RN, 58*(4), 42–48.

Thomas, V., Riegel, B., Andrea, J., Murray, P., Gerhart, A., & Gocka, I. (1994). National survey of pediatric fever management in practices among emergency department nurses. *Journal of Emergency Nursing, 20*(6), 505–510.

Thomas-Masoorli, S. (1996). Combating infection. Questions and answers about CVCs. *Nursing, 26*(11), 28–29.

Togger, D. A., & Brenner, P. S. (2001). Metered dose inhalers. *American Journal of Nursing, 101*(10), 26–32.

Treston-Aurand, J., Olmsted, R. N., Allen-Bridson, K., & Craig, C. P. (1997). Impact of materials on central venous catheter infection rates. *Journal of Intravenous Nursing, 20*(4), 201–206.

Trombly, J. (1996). Listen up: Don't trust tympanic thermometers. *Nursing96, 26*(2), 58–59.

Valencia, I. C., Falabella, A. F., & Schachner, L. A. (2001). New developments in wound care for infants and children. *Pediatric Annals, 30*, 211–218.

Wong, D., & Baker, C. (2001). Smiling faces as an anchor for pain intensity scales. *Pain, 89*, 294–300.

INDEX